THE KEY TO

PROSTATE

CANCER

30 EXPERTS EXPLAIN 15 STAGES
OF PROSTATE CANCER

MARK SCHOLZ, MD

THE KEY TO PROSTATE CANCER

Library of Congress Cataloging-In-Publication Data: 2017908411

Publisher's Cataloging-In-Publication Data
(Prepared by The Donohue Group, Inc.)

Names: Scholz, Mark.
Title: The key to prostate cancer : 30 experts explain
15 stages of prostate cancer / Mark Scholz, MD.
Description: Marina del Rey, CA : Mark Scholz, [2017] |
Includes bibliographical references and index.
Identifiers: ISBN 978-0-9990652-0-4 (hardcover) |
ISBN 978-0-9990652-1-1 (paperback) | ISBN 978-0-9990652-2-8 (ebook)
Subjects: LCSH: Prostate—Cancer. | Prostate—Cancer—Treatment.
Classification: LCC RC280.P7 S36 2017 (print) |
LCC RC280.P7 (ebook) | DDC 616.99463—dc23

ISBN: 978-0-9990652-1-1 (print)
978-0-9990652-2-8 (ebook)

DISCLAIMER

The content of this book is intended as a compilation of current methods and means of treating prostate cancer. This book is not to be used as medical advice for any particular patient. Rather, it is intended to provide information to patients enabling them to discuss their disease and treatment options with their physicians.

The authors have made every effort to provide accurate telephone numbers and Internet addresses at the time of publication, but neither the publisher nor the authors assume any responsibility for errors, or for changes that occur after publication of this book. Moreover, the publisher does not have any control over and does not assume any responsibility for author or third-party websites or their content.

To Ralph Blum

TABLE OF CONTENTS

PREFACE:
A PATH TO SELF-EDUCATION

Mark Scholz, MD

PATIENTS FACE A REAL DILEMMA when selecting among so many treatments with potentially irreversible consequences. Why can't we let the doctors decide? The conclusion of my last book, *Invasion of the Prostate Snatchers,* was that the urologists, the doctors who manage prostate cancer, lack objectivity. Although sincere, intelligent, and skilled, they are biased in favor of their chosen specialty—surgery. And there is no counterbalancing resource for a second-opinion. Nonsurgical doctors specializing in prostate cancer hardly exist.

The goal of *Invasion* was to calm people down by introducing various proven and developing nonsurgical alternatives and to demystify prostate cancer, enabling patients to think more clearly and make better decisions. However, *Invasion* was written primarily for men with *newly-diagnosed* disease. Many readers requested a more in-depth guide for treating all stages of prostate cancer. This new book, by 30 experts*, is a tool for helping patients and doctors work together on a level playing field to intelligently discuss the latest options.

---

* See Appendix IV for author biographies.

The term "prostate cancer" is an umbrella term that covers five major stages and 15 subtypes. It is not a singular disease. There are many distinct varieties. This book enables men to accurately identify their stage. Since fear disrupts clearheaded thinking, we have boldly altered the traditionally disturbing terminology by creating the "Five Stages of Blue." For example, the scary term *"High-Risk* prostate cancer" is renamed *Azure.*

The Five Stages are based on the most popular staging system used by doctors. The first three Stages, *Sky, Teal,* and *Azure,* represent the categories created by Dr. Anthony D'Amico, which divides newly diagnosed men into *Low-, Intermediate-* and *High-Risk.* The last two Stages, *Indigo* and *Royal,* represent the categories of *relapsed disease* and *metastatic disease,* respectively. To help recall this new terminology, the first letter of each Stage makes the acronym STAIR.

The method for assigning everyone's Stage is described in Chapter 1. Each of these five stages is a different breed of prostate cancer that requires a different type of treatment. A man's treatment *intensity* should be matched to his disease's severity, sufficient to control the cancer without overdoing it. Overtreatment causes unnecessary side effects without improving the survival rate.

THIS BOOK IS MUCH SHORTER THAN IT LOOKS

The book is divided into seven sections. Five of the sections cover each of the Five Stages of Blue. The average reader, therefore, will only need three sections: Section I, which covers PSA, Gleason score and body scans; Section VII, which covers lifestyle, diet, exercise and supplements; and *one* of the remaining five sections, the one that is related to that patient's stage. The other sections, the ones provided for the other four stages, can be skipped over.

FOREWORD:
THE PARADOX OF CHOICE

Peter Scholz

*It is our choices, Harry, that show what we
truly are, far more than our abilities.*
J.K. ROWLING

WHEN INITIALLY DIAGNOSED with prostate cancer, the first step is to seek information. Thankfully, there is a vast amount available. But the sheer volume becomes an unexpected burden, creating something called the "Paradox of Choice." Outside of a proper context, massive amounts of information *hinder* the decision-making process. Without a framework, people despair and default to a simplistic solution: "Cut it out." Others, are simply overwhelmed. They face mental paralysis, unable to figure out where to begin. The Paradox of Choice can be diminished by categorizing the cancer accurately.

The pathway leading out of this confusion is to know your Stage of Blue. This creates a distinct advantage: the ability to focus on the options appropriate for that Stage.

The advantages are fourfold: 1) It locates you on the map of prostate cancer information using "coordinates" from your medical records; 2) it protects you from getting sidetracked by irrelevant information related to other Stages; 3) it points you to the optimal choices for your stage of prostate cancer; and 4) it helps you understand the staging process used by doctors. When you appreciate how your doctor thinks about prostate cancer, you can participate in *shared* decision-making.

Achieving these goals will require a commitment of time to learn about your Stage of Blue and to reflect on your lifestyle priorities. If you gain understanding of your situation in advance of your physician visit, you can present your preferences concisely to your doctor. Then, together, you can develop an effective and personalized treatment plan.

INTRODUCTION:
SYNOPSIS OF TREATMENTS

Mark Scholz, MD

Everything should be made as simple as possible, but not simpler.
ALBERT EINSTEIN

MY ENTIRE PROFESSIONAL LIFE has been about a single disease—prostate cancer. As a result, besides seeing patients four
days a week, I write, speak, conduct research, arrange conferences, make
videos, teach classes, image prostates (with color Doppler ultrasound),
and, yes, even do digital rectal exams. Many people would consider
what I do overwhelming. Personally, I enjoy it (well, at least most of it).
There are times, however, when I do wonder … *Am I in over my head?*
I understand that many newly diagnosed patients have similar self-
doubts. The amount of prostate cancer information on the Internet, for
example, is overwhelming.

How can the information about one disease be so vast? As we've
said, it really isn't one disease. Prostate cancer comes in hundreds of
varieties: it can be slow- or fast- growing, responsive or unresponsive to
treatment, metastatic or nonmetastatic. In fact, if prostate cancer were

restricted to these black-and-white examples alone, the situation would be semimanageable. Most cases do not lie at the extremes. They are somewhere in the middle, making predictions about future outcome even more difficult. If the name hadn't already been taken, we could have titled our book *Fifty Shades of Grey*.

I. Staging Prostate Cancer

People often mistakenly assume that the different ways prostate cancer behaves—life threatening vs. benign—are due to seeing the *same* illness at *different* time points. In reality, distinct *varieties* of prostate cancer exist. *It's not all the same disease.* The *clinical stage* and the *pathologic stage* are important, but it's not the whole picture. Patients frequently ask, "Am I stage A, B, C, or D?" without realizing that the old lettering system was merely created to describe the size of a nodule (if one is present) when the surgeon feels the prostate during a digital rectal exam. Relying on a digital exam (the *clinical* stage alone) is a totally outdated approach! These days the staging process integrates multiple factors in addition to the clinical stage: PSA level, Gleason score, pathologic stage, scan results, and the results of previous treatments. Chapter 1 explains how these factors are obtained from your medical chart and combined to assign your Stage of Blue. Readers at this point who want a broader overview of the Five Stages of Blue can jump ahead to Chapter 50 and to Appendix I and then return here. However, I don't necessarily recommend doing this, since one of the main goals in this book is to *limit exposure* to unessential information and focus mainly on your Stage.

II. The Treatments

The goal of this book is to align men with a treatment that best fits their cancer profile. When you really get down to the basics, we only need to introduce four broad categories of treatment: observation, local treatments, systemic treatments and combination therapy.

OBSERVATION

Also known as "active surveillance," observation is the process of monitoring the cancer without any immediate medical intervention. It is now clear that over the last 20 years, several million men have undergone treatment for a type of prostate cancer that was essentially harmless. Now, with a better understanding of how *Low-Risk (Sky)* prostate cancer behaves, active surveillance is becoming increasingly popular.

LOCAL TREATMENTS

Treatment strategies focused on the prostate gland are called "local treatments." Examples are surgery (radical prostatectomy), radioactive seed implantation, varieties of external beam radiation therapy (IMRT, Proton, CyberKnife), and cryosurgery. In addition, "focal" options have been developed in which only a subsection of the gland is treated, namely, the area where the cancer is located. Local and focal options, when administered by accomplished experts, eliminate the cancer in the gland with a reasonably high degree of consistency.

SYSTEMIC THERAPIES

The main danger from prostate cancer is the possibility of spread outside the prostate. In its earlier stages, metastatic disease is *microscopic*. After a period, once the metastases increase in size, they become detectable on a scan. Men with either microscopic or visible metastases require *systemic* treatment that circulates through the blood and treats cancer throughout the whole body. Examples of systemic treatments are hormonal therapies, chemotherapy, immunotherapy, and, most recently, a new type of radiation therapy that circulates in the blood, called Xofigo.

COMBINATION THERAPIES

When a local therapy is combined with a systemic therapy, or if multiple systemic therapies are used at the same time, it is called "combination therapy." Improved survival rates have been documented when combination therapy is administered to men with higher grade or more advanced prostate cancer. When combination therapy is being considered with the goal of improving survival, the survival advantages need to be balanced against the potential for greater side effects.

III. The Challenge

The prostate world is a multibillion-dollar industry, with many powerful financial and professional incentives that can work against a patient's best interests. The treatment-selection process can be complex. Nevertheless, difficult problems can be broken down into manageable pieces. There are too few full-time prostate cancer experts to handle the 160,000 new cases that occur in the US every year. It's crucial, therefore, for patients and their families to educate themselves and take control of their treatment planning. As Francis Bacon said, "Knowledge itself is power."

SECTION I
STAGING AND PROGNOSIS

Chapter 1

QUIZ TO ASSIGN
A STAGE OF BLUE

Peter Scholz

*Patient empowerment is not about becoming a medical expert;
it is about learning how to become an expert patient.*
Peter Scholz

THE *RAISON D'ÊTRE* OF STAGING is patient empowerment, which
comes through learning. Empowerment grows a patient's confidence,
providing the strength to confront industry biases and respectfully stand
up to doctors who may be less-than-fully informed. Many treatments
have *irreversible* consequences, so it is worth getting it right the first
time. Long-term survival is improved by receiving optimal treatment
up front. The first shot is the best chance to eradicate the cancer. The
initial step in the selection process is to determine your Stage of Blue,
the specifics of which are addressed at the end of this chapter. But first,
let's review one more time why empowerment through education is so
critically important.

INDUSTRY BIAS

Empowerment helps you understand industry bias, which is prevalent in the prostate cancer world. Financial incentives often overshadow patient needs. Many studies show that doctors are much more likely to recommend a treatment related to their specialty. If there is a preset agenda is to push one form of treatment, you won't be hearing all the alternatives in a fair and balanced light. Your knowledge of the other treatments that are available, as well as knowing the risks and benefits of each, will help you reset the doctor's agenda to one more aimed at determining what is optimal for you.

UNINFORMED DOCTORS

Due to rapidly growing knowledge, many doctors are unable to stay current for complex diseases like prostate cancer. This is compounded because so few doctors specialize in prostate cancer. Most of the time, these deficiencies have nothing to do with their competency and everything to do with managing high demands on their time. Doctors are not intentionally giving suboptimal treatment. However, suboptimal treatment is the net outcome when there is a lack of current knowledge about the disease and its treatment.

NURTURE THE RELATIONSHIP WITH YOUR DOCTOR

It is a risk, once you get a taste of patient empowerment, to take it too far and trivialize the opinion of your doctor. It is not beneficial to look down on your doctor, even if you know about certain advancements that he is unaware of. This mentality is detrimental to your goal to obtain the best possible care. No matter how much research you do, you are not a medical expert. You need a good doctor and a good relationship with your doctor. You cannot prescribe a treatment for yourself; and you are unqualified to determine what is truly safe or beneficial.

The goal is to create a doctor-patient relationship based on mutual trust. Only you know the type of risks you are willing to take. Sharing your personal information—and the new prostate cancer developments you learn—should prompt your doctor to learn more about the disease and to think about how to integrate this information into an individualized plan.

THE MEDICAL CHART

The first step to empowerment is obtaining a copy of your medical records. You have every right to your records. Some offices may charge a nominal fee to provide them, which is reasonable. There is no universal format for charts, and some offices keep more complete records than others. It may even be necessary to request the information from more than one office to compile all the necessary information.

You don't need a complete understanding of everything contained in the chart. However, there are certain specific items you need to look for:

1. **Prostate Specific Antigen (PSA) Chronology:** You need to construct a chronological history of every PSA measurement that has ever been taken and the date that it was performed. The PSA results are found in the *Lab Reports* section of your chart. The testosterone level is also in this section of the chart. If you do not find a testosterone level, ask your doctor to request one the next time you have your blood tested.

2. **Clinical Stage:** The results from the *finger exam* of the prostate, called the digital rectal examination (DRE) is called the *clinical* stage or the *T* stage. The clinical stage will usually be found in the *Progress Notes* section of the chart. The notes will indicate the doctor's assessment of whether a nodule can be felt by the doctor's finger. The T stage, which describes the results of the DRE, are recorded in the *Physical Examination* section of the chart as in the table on the following page.

3. **Radiology Reports (Imaging Studies):** will be found in the *Radiology* section of the chart. These reports may be written by the urologist (in the case of an ultrasound) or by a specialist devoted to reading scans called a radiologist. Look

for the section in the report that summarizes the findings of the scan titled: "Impression." Ultrasound reports or MRI reports list the *size* of the prostate measured in grams or cubic centimeters (cc); this is the essential information for calculating the ratio of the PSA to the gland's size, which is called the PSA density (Chapter 2). Men's prostate glands vary in size, ranging from the size of a ping pong ball to the size of a small orange. Larger glands lead to a higher PSA, which impacts how PSA is interpreted.

4. **Biopsy Report:** The biopsy report will be in the *Pathology* section of the chart. For each biopsy core that contains cancer, the Gleason score and the percentage of the core involved with cancer (as opposed to normal prostate gland tissue) should be noted. Gleason is reported as 3+3=6, 5+4=9, etc. The total number is the "score." If several scores are present in the chart, the highest score on this report is used to describe your status (Chapter 3).

Table: Clinical Stage

Stage	Description
T1:	Tumor that cannot be felt by digital rectal examination
T2:	Tumor confined within the prostate
	T2a: Tumor that can be felt by DRE but involves 50 percent or less of one lobe
	T2b: Tumor felt by DRE involving more than 50 percent of one lobe but not both lobes
	T2c: Tumor felt in both lobes
T3:	Tumor felt by DRE that extends through the prostate capsule
	T3a: Extracapsular extension
	T3b: Tumor felt by DRE that invades seminal vesicle(s)
T4:	Tumor felt by DRE that invades the rectum or bladder

THE QUIZ: FINDING YOUR STAGE OF BLUE

The above four segments of information, which are obtained from the medical chart, provide the information necessary for assigning a Stage of Blue. Once you know your stage (upon completion of Quiz A or Quiz B) you should jump ahead to Chapter 2 and resume reading. All patients should start with Quiz A. Some patients will be able to determine their stage with Quiz A alone. Others, after starting Quiz A will be directed to complete Quiz B.

QUIZ A:

QUESTION 1: Have you had surgery, radiation or cryotherapy for prostate cancer *and* now have persistent cancer or a rising PSA? If no, continue to question 2; if yes, skip to **Quiz B** (see below).

QUESTION 2: Do you have a pathology report or a Bone, PET, CT or MRI scan that shows *any* bone metastases or metastases in lymph nodes that are located *outside* the pelvis area of the body? If yes, skip to **Quiz B.** If no, or if the metastases are located exclusively in the lymph nodes in the pelvis area, continue to question 3.

QUESTION 3: #_____ What was your PSA at the time of your diagnosis?

a.	Less than 10	(write #1)
b.	Between 10 and 20	(write #2)
c.	More than 20	(write #5)

QUESTION 4: #_____ What was the highest Gleason score on your biopsy?

a.	6 or less	(write #1)
b.	7	(write #2)
c.	8 or more	(write #5)

QUESTION 5: #____ What "T Stage" does your digital rectal exam (DRE) show? (See the table on the previous page titled "Clinical Stage").

    a. Small or no nodule (T1c, T2a)   (write #1)

    b. Larger nodule (T2b)   (write #2)

    c. Bilateral nodule or extracapsular
       extension (T2c, T3, T4)   (write #5)

QUESTION 6: #____ Do you have an MRI, color Doppler, or PET/CT scan showing cancer outside the prostate?

    a. No extracapsular extension   (write #0)

    b. Overt extracapsular extension   (write #3)

    c. Seminal vesicle invasion   (write #4)

    d. Abnormal pelvic nodes   (write #4)

Write the total of questions 3 through 6 _____. Your Stage of Blue is indicated by the sum:

3 = *Sky*   4–6 = *Teal*   7+ = *Azure*

    Now that you know your Stage of Blue, you can jump ahead to Chapter 2 and finish reading the remainder of Section I. The remaining chapters in this section provide a "behind-the-curtains" view of the basic components of prostate cancer—PSA, Gleason score, prostate scans and body scans. Although the Stages of Blue can serve you perfectly well without all these background fundamentals, the goal of this book is to introduce basic vocabulary and thought processes that are utilized throughout the prostate cancer world, enabling you to better communicate with your doctor. At the end of Section I you will be directed to read *another* section of the book specifically related to your Stage of Blue.

QUIZ B:

Use the following three questions to determine your Stage of Blue (if you were directed to complete Quiz B).

QUESTION 1: #_____ Is your current PSA?

   a. Less than 100   (write #0)

   b. More than 100   (write #1)

QUESTION 2: #_____ Do you have a rising PSA *and* a low testosterone under 50?

     a. No   (write #0)

     b. Yes   (write #1)

QUESTION 3: #_____ Does an MRI, PET/CT, bone scan or surgery show:

     a. Metastases not detected or are
            limited only to the pelvic nodes   (write #0)

     b. Metastases detected outside
            the pelvic lymph nodes   (write #1)

Write the sum of these three questions here: #_____ Your Stage of Blue is indicated by the sum:

$$0 = \textit{Indigo} \qquad 1+ = \textit{Royal}$$

Now that you know your Stage, you can continue to Chapter 2 and complete reading the remainder of Section I. The remaining chapters in this section provide a "behind-the-curtains" view of the basic components of prostate cancer—PSA, Gleason score, prostate scans and body scans.

Although the Stages of Blue can serve you perfectly well without all these background fundamentals, the goal of this book is to introduce basic vocabulary and thought processes that are utilized throughout the prostate cancer world, enabling better communication with your doctor. At the end of Section I you will be directed to *another* section of the book specifically related to your Stage.

Chapter 2
THE PSA BLOOD TEST

Stanley Brosman, MD

Any fool can know. The point is to understand.
ALBERT EINSTEIN

ONE CANNOT REALLY TALK intelligently about prostate cancer without a working knowledge of the prostate specific antigen (PSA) blood test. Prostate cancer is totally silent until it metastasizes, after which it is usually too late for a cure. Prior to the FDA's approval of PSA testing in 1987 (along with random prostate needle biopsy that same year), the behavior of early-stage prostate cancer was shrouded in mystery. Since then doctors have been detecting and quantifying early-stage prostate cancer with ever-increasing accuracy. All this new information has opened the door to the possibility of more personalized treatment. Unfortunately, powerful tools can also be misused.

THE VARIED ROLES OF PSA

PSA plays a variety of different roles. The most familiar is screening to detect prostate cancer at an early stage. This is weighty, considering that 160,000 cases are detected in the United States annually. However, PSA has other uses. One example is how PSA helps to define the Stages of Blue. For example, a PSA under 10 is representative of *Sky*. PSA levels over 20 are characteristic of *Azure*. Another role of PSA is to detect cancer relapse after surgery or radiation. Lastly, in advanced prostate cancer, rises or declines in PSA after hormone therapy or chemotherapy help determine whether the treatment is working.

PSA FOR PROSTATE CANCER SCREENING

PSA screening greatly improves the chance of detecting prostate cancer at an early stage while it is still curable. Delayed diagnosis increases the chance of cancer spreading and limits treatment options, mandating more aggressive treatment. How, then, can anyone be opposed to PSA screening? Can an early diagnosis of cancer be bad? Surprisingly, the answer is yes. PSA screening often leads to the detection of small "un-cancers" that are totally innocuous. Even without treatment these harmless cancers will never spread outside the prostate.

Ideally, all these un-cancers would be monitored rather than treated. However, doctors and patients alike struggle with the concept of a "harmless cancer." People naturally overreact, rushing into unnecessary radical treatment, risking irreversible impotence and incontinence. Overtreatment of un-cancers is such a big problem that in 2011 a government-sponsored team of experts, the US Preventive Services Task Force, issued a dire warning recommending against PSA screening. Many primary care physicians have taken this to heart and have decided to forgo routine annual PSA screening, since they believe it leads to unnecessary treatment.

MULTIPARAMETRIC MRI SCANS: THE SALVATION OF PSA SCREENING

PSA elevations, however, are not really the problem. A high PSA only *suggests* the possibility of cancer. Only a needle biopsy diagnoses cancer.

The real problem, therefore, is that doctors routinely recommend doing a 12-core *random* biopsy whenever PSA is slightly elevated. Over a million men are biopsied every year. Thankfully, this terrible problem does not have to continue. We now have a better alternative. Studies clearly show that multiparametric MRI imaging is more accurate than biopsy.[1] When an MRI scan detects an abnormality, it can be further investigated with a *targeted* biopsy. *Men with clear scans can avoid biopsy altogether.* Adopting an imaging policy that substitutes MRI for random biopsy solves the problem of over-diagnosis in men with high PSA (Chapter 4).

SCANS ALSO MEASURE THE SIZE OF THE PROSTATE

Imaging also improves the interpretation of PSA. Many men run high PSA levels from Benign Prostatic Hyperplasia (BPH), an enlarged gland, a condition that is totally unrelated to cancer. PSA rises as the gland increases in size. PSA, therefore, needs to be interpreted in the *context* of the prostate volume. Imaging the gland and finding that it is enlarged can be good news, providing a *benign* explanation for why the PSA is high.

The method used to determine when the PSA is elevated, higher than what would be expected for a *specific-sized* prostate, works by dividing the prostate size (in cubic centimeters) by 10. For example, a normal *30cc* prostate should have a PSA around 3.0; for a normal 50cc prostate the PSA should be around 5.0. A 100cc prostate will be approximately 10. PSA is only *abnormal* (the official term is a "high PSA density") when it's 50 percent higher than would be expected, based on the prostate's size. For example, a man's PSA is abnormal if he has a 30cc prostate and his PSA is above 4.5. An abnormal PSA for a 50cc prostate is above 7.5. For a 100cc gland, PSA would need to be above 15 to be suspicious.

PSA DENSITY

Doctors use a less intuitive way to calculate when the PSA is higher than what can be attributed to an enlarged prostate. The net effect, however, is the same. Instead of dividing PSA into the gland volume, they do the opposite. They divide the gland volume into the PSA. Using this inverted formula, an abnormal PSA relative to a specific-sized prostate is anything above 0.15. Men above 0.15, using this formula, are said to have a "high PSA density."

A SUGGESTED PSA SCREENING PROTOCOL

It's reasonable to start checking PSA yearly in men over the age of 45. Men with a family history of prostate cancer or who are African American should start annual testing at age 40. Men over age 75 who are in good health should continue screening.

So, at what level of PSA should one consider performing an MRI scan? Younger men who generally have small prostate glands (as estimated on digital rectal examination by a physician) might want to consider doing a scan when the PSA is over 2.5. If a man is older, or if the estimated size of the prostate gland determined via the digital rectal (DRE) is big, a PSA over 4.0 should trigger further investigation with imaging. Anytime an abnormality is felt on DRE, further investigation with a scan is warranted.

USING PSA TO *STAGE* PROSTATE CANCER

Despite the controversies that surround the use of PSA for screening, there are no controversies about using PSA for staging, once a diagnosis is established. Men with a higher PSA at the time of diagnosis, above 10 or 20, for example, are more likely to have cancer that has spread outside the gland. The exact methodology for determining a man's Stage of Blue, using PSA in combination with other factors, is explained in Chapter 1.

MONITORING FOR CANCER RELAPSE AFTER SURGERY OR RADIATION

A rising PSA is an accurate way to detect relapse after previous treatment. Normally, after surgery, the PSA should drop to undetectable levels. Even a small rise in PSA is significant. After radiation, the PSA should generally remain under 1.0. However, there are exceptions. First, PSA may decline slowly after radiation, sometimes taking several years to reach its lowest point. Second, a noncancerous PSA increase, termed "PSA bounce," can develop one to four years after radiation. The bounce is thought to be from a delayed immune reaction in the prostate. The bounce is further described in Chapters 14 and 36.

A true cancer recurrence is always signaled by a rising PSA. The *rate of PSA doubling* is a very important indicator of the tumor's aggressiveness. For example, recurrences associated with sequentially rising PSA levels requiring over 12 months to double, are low-grade. On the other hand, PSA that doubles in less than three months signals aggressive disease. The whole process of interpreting, diagnosing and treating a PSA relapse after therapy is fully elaborated in Section V of the book on *Indigo*.

DETERMINING THE RESPONSE TO HORMONE THERAPY OR CHEMOTHERAPY

PSA is very important for monitoring the effectiveness of anticancer therapy. For example, a PSA decline of more than 30 percent within a couple of months of starting chemotherapy provides a strong indication that the treatment is working.[2] However, not every treatment, even when it is effective, makes an impact on PSA. Two new therapies for *Royal*—Xofigo and Provenge—clearly prolong life but may show little or no impact on PSA. Accurately determining disease response requires more than simply checking PSA. Multiple blood indicators—such as alkaline phosphatase (ALP), lactate dehydrogenase (LDH), prostatic acid phosphatase (PAP), and circulating tumor cells (CTC), as well as the bone scan and other scans—are all necessary to track a treatment's effectiveness (Chapter 37).

PSA IS AN AMAZING TOOL

The wide-ranging clinical impact of PSA far surpasses the wildest dreams of the doctors who discovered it. Like any powerful tool, however, misuse can lead to harm. PSA results must be interpreted in the context of each patient's overall circumstances by an expert with experience managing prostate cancer. Unexpected PSA results should always be retested. Laboratory errors can certainly occur. Variations also occur between labs. Special care should always be taken when interpreting PSA results.

Wrong conclusions can lead to precipitous and ill-advised treatment decisions, potentially causing more harm than good.

References

1. HU Ahmed and others. The PROMIS study: A paired-cohort, blinded confirmatory study evaluating the accuracy of multiparametric MRI and TRUS biopsy in men with an elevated PSA. *Journal of Clinical Oncology* 34 suppl: abstr 5000, 2016.

2. DP Petrylak and others. Evaluation of prostate-specific antigen declines for surrogacy in patients treated on SWOG 99-16. *Journal of the National Cancer Institute* 98.8: 516, 2006.

Chapter 3

INTERPRETING THE PATHOLOGY REPORT

Jonathan Epstein, MD

*Education is the most powerful weapon which
you can use to change the world.*

NELSON MANDELA

PATIENTS SHOULD PERSONALLY REVIEW their pathology report. The report is an expert description of the information obtained from the needle biopsy. Typically, a copy of the report can be provided by the treating physician. Although a urologist will typically be the person who presents the results of the biopsy to the patient, the official pathology report is generated by a pathologist such as myself, a specialized physician with many years of training in the study and diagnosis of specimens removed by surgery or by needle biopsy.

The two major components communicated in the pathology report from a random 12-core biopsy are the *Gleason score,* which is a measure of how aggressive the tumor appears under the microscope, and the *quantity* of cancer in the 12-core specimen. The quantity is judged by the percentage of cancer replacing normal gland tissue within each single core of tissue removed from the prostate by the biopsy needle. The amount of cancer in each core can vary between 1 percent to 100 percent. Also, the *number* of biopsy cores that contain cancer can range from one to 12 (assuming, as is usually the case, that the biopsy was performed using standard random techniques). For example, if only two of 12 cores contain small amounts of cancer, the *quantity* of cancer (the presumed size of the tumor) would be small. At the other end of the spectrum, if the pathologist reports that 10 of the 12 cores contain cancer and each core is more than 50 percent replaced with cancer, the presumed amount of the tumor within the prostate would be large. So, the quantity of the cancer within the prostate, as judged by the needle biopsy, is based both on how many cores contain cancer as well as the percentage of cancer replacement seen in each core.

The field of prostate pathology is vast. Because of this, it is practically impossible to compress it into a single chapter. To convey the basic elements of prostate pathology, however, the most efficient and concise approach is to address 15 common questions that I frequently encounter:

1. What is the "Gleason grade" or "Gleason score"? What do the numbers in the Gleason score mean (for example, 3+4=7 or 3+3=6)?

The Gleason grading system assigns a "pattern" to the cancer cells, depending upon their appearance under the microscope. The patterns are graded from 1 to 5. However, it is important to realize that nowadays, patterns 1 and 2 are only very rarely assigned, since these patterns are so low grade they are hardly even considered to be cancer. Therefore, on a needle biopsy the pathologist almost always reports the grade as 3, 4 or 5. A higher number is assigned by the pathologist when the appearance of the cancer cells deviates more from the visual appearance of normal prostate gland tissue.

For example:

- If the cancerous tissue looks very similar to normal prostate tissue, it is pattern 1.

- If the cancer cells and their growth patterns look very abnormal, it is pattern 5.

- Patterns 2 through 4 have features in between these extremes.

Since prostate cancers in a single patient often have areas with different grades, the first pattern, when assigning a "score," is the most common pattern seen after a review of all the biopsy specimens, i.e., the pattern that applies to most of the cancer seen in the biopsy. The second pattern that is assigned is the one showing the next most common pattern. These two different grades are then added together to yield the Gleason score (also called the Gleason grade). For example, if the Gleason score is written as "3+4=7", it means that most of the tumor is primarily pattern 3 and, to a lesser amount, pattern 4. These two numbers are then added together to create a Gleason score of 7. If the tumor has only one pattern throughout the whole tumor, the same pattern is counted twice in order to keep the grade in scale. For example, a biopsy core that is involved by only Gleason pattern 4 would have a Gleason score of 4+4=8.

2. What does it mean to have a Gleason score of 3+3=6?

Tumors with Gleason scores of 2 through 5 are very rare because they cannot be identified accurately on needle biopsy. So, even though it is technically correct to say that the Gleason score can range from 2 to 10 (suggesting that 6 would be "in the middle"), *in actual practice*, the Gleason score ranges only between 6 and 10. Therefore, a Gleason 6 actually represents the lowest, most favorable grade possible. Assigning the number 6 can lead to potential misinterpretation by patients. For example, Gleason score 6 cancer is almost always cured (see Table 1). On the other hand, most men with higher-grade tumors will be recommended to undergo some type of treatment. Gleason score 6 cancers behave so benignly that most men with these tumors are candidates for active surveillance (Chapter 9). I have proposed a modification of the way we report the Gleason score that more accurately transmits the favorable message about Gleason 6. Question #5, below, expounds further on this proposal, the full details of which were published in *European Urology* in September 2015.

Table: Risk of PSA Relapse in the First Five Years After Surgery
Based on Various Biopsy Gleason Scores

		Relapse Rate
Group I	Gleason Score 3+3=6	5%
Group II	Gleason Score 3+4=7	17%
Group III	Gleason Score 4+3=7	35%
Group IV	Gleason Score 4+4=8	37%
Group V	Gleason Score 4+5, 5+4 or 5+5	76%

3. What does it mean to have a Gleason score of 7?

A Gleason score of 7 can mean 3+4=7 or 4+3=7, depending on whether grade 3 pattern or grade 4 pattern is predominant. There is a big difference between these two grades. The table shows the substantial difference in five-year cure rates. The biggest therapeutic difference between these grades is that more aggressive radiation therapy protocols are often recommended for Gleason scores of 4+3=7 and above.

4. What does it mean to have Gleason scores of 8 to 10?

Gleason score 8 cancers are aggressive, and Gleason score 9 or 10 tumors are more so. However, some patients with Gleason scores 9 or 10 can still be cured. The actual outlook for a specific patient is also dependent on additional factors, such as PSA, clinical stage (Chapter 1) and the extent of cancer on biopsy.

5. What is the best way to simplify the Gleason scores?

The best and simplest way to get a sense of what Gleason scores predict regarding the future behavior of the biopsy-detected tumor is by grouping them from I to V, with Group I having the best outlook and V having the worst. For example, the table shows how these Gleason groupings predict cure rates with surgery. As can be seen, cure rates decline as the group number increases.

6. What does it mean when there are different biopsy cores with different Gleason scores?

Different biopsy cores may sample different areas of the same tumor, or the cores may sample different *tumors* in the prostate. (It is fairly common for men to have more than one tumor). Because the grade may vary within the same tumor or between different tumors, different cores taken from the prostate may have different Gleason scores. The *highest* Gleason score observed in a particular patient is the one selected for predicting prognosis and deciding therapy.

7. Can the Gleason score from a random biopsy really tell what the cancer grade is in the entire prostate?

The Gleason score on biopsy *usually* reflects the cancer's true grade. However, in about 20 percent of cases the biopsy underestimates the true grade, resulting in *undergrading*. This can occur because randomly directed biopsy needles occasionally miss a higher-grade (more aggressive) area of the cancer. Undergrading is statistically more likely to occur in men with: 1) larger tumors; 2) higher PSA levels; or 3) smaller prostates.

Somewhat less commonly, *overgrading* occurs. This occurs when the true grade of the tumor is *lower* than that which is seen on the biopsy. For example, studies show that 16 percent of cases with a Gleason score of 3+4=7 on biopsy will change to a Gleason score of 6 when the surgically removed prostate is examined by the pathologist. Discrepancies between the biopsy Gleason and the final Gleason after surgery may be caused by inaccurate overgrading of the biopsy specimen by an inexperienced pathologist, or because the actual quantity of pattern 4 originally detected in the biopsy core turns out to be so small that it cannot be found by the pathologist who examines the surgically removed prostate.

8. What does it mean if the biopsy report mentions special studies, such as high molecular weight cytokeratin (HMWCK), ck903, ck5/6, p63, AMACR (racemase), 34BE12, or PIN4 cocktail?

These are special tests that the pathologist sometimes uses to help make the diagnosis of prostate cancer. Not all cases need these tests. Whether or not the report mentions these tests, they have no effect on the accuracy of the diagnosis.

9. What does it mean if the biopsy mentions that there is "perineural invasion"?

"Perineural invasion" means that cancer cells were seen surrounding or tracking along a nerve fiber *within the prostate*. When this is found on a biopsy, it means that there is a slightly higher chance that the cancer has spread along the nerves alongside the prostate. Still, perineural invasion doesn't necessarily mean that the cancer has spread outside the gland. Actually, other factors, such as the Gleason score and the quantity of cancer in the cores, are better indicators of cancer spread outside the gland. And even when some of the tumor has microscopically spread beyond the edge of the prostate, most men are still cured with either radiation therapy or radical prostatectomy.

10. What does it mean if, in addition to cancer, the biopsy report also says "high-grade prostatic intraepithelial neoplasia" or "high-grade PIN"?

"High-grade prostatic intraepithelial neoplasia" (also called "high-grade PIN") is a *precancer* of the prostate. PIN means abnormal, but not cancerous, cell-growth and really has no importance whatsoever to someone who already has cancer. The word "high-grade" refers to the PIN and not the cancer, so it has nothing to do with the Gleason score or how aggressive the cancer is. However, in someone *without* cancer the presence of PIN suggests that this individual is at higher risk for being diagnosed with cancer in the future.

11. What does it mean if the biopsy report also says "atrophy" or "adenosis" or "atypical adenomatous hyperplasia" or "seminal vesicle"?
All of these terms are things that the pathologist sees under the microscope that are benign (*not* cancer). They are mentioned merely for completeness in the report, because sometimes, to a physician with a less experienced eye, they might be *misinterpreted* as cancer. They are of no concern to the patient.

12. What does it mean if, in addition to cancer, the biopsy report also says "atypical glands" or "atypical small acinar proliferation (ASAP)" or "glandular atypia" or "atypical glandular proliferation"?
All these terms mean that the pathologist saw something under the microscope that *suggests* cancer *may* be present. However, the actual evidence for cancer is insufficient for a conclusive diagnosis. If cancer has already been diagnosed in another part of the biopsy, ASAP is of no relevance to the overall outlook. However, men with ASAP who have not been diagnosed with cancer are at greater risk for being diagnosed with cancer in the future.

13. How do pathologists measure the amount of cancer in the core?
There are multiple techniques of quantifying the amount of cancer found on needle biopsy. The most common are: 1) number of positive cores; 2) total millimeters of cancer among all cores; 3) percentage of each core occupied by cancer; and 4) total percent of cancer in the entire specimen. All of these different methods of measuring cancer volume on needle biopsy give similarly reliable results, and it is difficult to demonstrate the superiority of one technique of measuring over the other. In general, a report that has the number of positive cores along with one of the other measurements is sufficient.

14. How can a patient be sure that the Gleason grade in the report is accurate?

Assigning the correct Gleason score is a skill that, like any other, is developed through experience and practice. It is often prudent to submit the biopsy material for a second opinion to a center managing a large number of patients with prostate cancer, to confirm the accuracy of the initial Gleason score. In certain cases, a targeted biopsy may be necessary to ensure that the needle biopsy is sampling the most aggressive area of the tumor (Chapters 4 and 5).

15. Does genetic testing with Prolaris and Oncotype DX provide additional useful information?

In a minority of patients, preliminary studies seem to indicate that these tests can provide additional information about a cancer's future behavior. In addition, these tests may also have some value in "cross-checking" the accuracy of the Gleason score that has been assigned, though testing for this purpose has yet to be evaluated in a clinical trial.

CONCLUDING THOUGHTS

A few years ago, there was a news story about a polar bear attacking a man in Canada. Shockingly, the report said that the bystanders did nothing to help the poor man. However, upon further review it turned out that the reporter had neglected to report that the "bear" was only a cub, whose reach was lower than the man's knees.

When facing a monstrous behemoth like "cancer," the most important question to ask is "What *kind* of cancer am I dealing with?" With currently available medical knowledge and technology, there can be no excuse for not knowing the cancer's exact grade to make an informed treatment (or nontreatment) decision. Men facing a new diagnosis of prostate cancer should scrutinize the pathology report and reflect carefully on its implications before rushing to make, or allowing themselves to be pressured into making, hasty treatment decisions.

Chapter 4

MULTIPARAMETRIC MRI AND TARGETED BIOPSY

Daniel Margolis, MD

*If you want to make a substantial contribution to medicine
for this decade and maybe for the century, address yourself to
the problem of imaging cancer within the prostate gland.*
PATRICK WALSH

MULTIPARAMETRIC MRI (MP-MRI) PROVIDES a three-dimensional image of the prostate, giving important information about the cancer's location, size, and how "aggressive" it appears. For example, its likelihood of having a Gleason score above 6 if a targeted biopsy is performed. As such, MP-MRI is an excellent way to stage men with newly diagnosed disease. When used as a guide for targeted biopsy, the accuracy of the Gleason score is greatly improved compared with the older, hit-and-miss, random biopsy technique. MP-MRI also greatly increases the confidence that higher-grade cancers are not being overlooked in men embarking on active surveillance.

STAGING NEWLY DIAGNOSED DISEASE

For the purposes described above, MP-MRI is usually performed *without* an endorectal coil. However, men who are considering a radical prosta-tectomy should have an endorectal coil. It provides the best view of the capsule of the prostate. Imaging is the most accurate way to determine capsular status for surgical planning, to determine whether it is safe to spare one or both of the nerve bundles that control erections.

EVALUATING UNDIAGNOSED MEN WITH HIGH PSA LEVELS

Using MP-MRI to evaluate men with an elevated PSA (but no confirmed cancer) is still controversial. However, there are notable advantages of MP-MRI over the random 12-core biopsy. First, it is less likely to diagnose *clinically harmless* cancers, sparing patients from unnecessary anxiety, overtreatment, and damage to their quality of life. Second, well-performed MP-MRI only misses significant cancer about 10 percent of the time, and these missed cancers tend to be small and unlikely to spread. Periodic follow-up with regular annual screening should detect most of them before they have a chance to spread. To put this informa-tion in perspective, a well-performed 12-core random biopsy misses high-grade cancer 25 percent of the time.[1]

A consensus policy about undergoing an MP-MRI *prior* to a random biopsy, and whether random biopsies should be performed in addition to a targeted biopsy, is still being debated. While the "MRI-first" approach is still uncommon in the United States, in Great Britain it is becoming routine to use MP-MRI to evaluate men with elevated PSA, rather than starting with doing a random biopsy.

MRI FOR ACTIVE SURVEILLANCE

Until recently, men on active surveillance have been monitored with periodic random 12-core biopsies. MP-MRI provides three advantages over random biopsy. First, imaging is noninvasive. Second, imaging can find suspicious areas that might have been missed by previous random biopsies. Third, imaging provides a baseline measurement of the cancer's size that can be used for follow-up monitoring to detect enlargement.

As logical as imaging sounds, active surveillance strategies currently performed in most academic centers do not yet routinely use MP-MRI to detect cancer progression. Nevertheless, this concept of substituting imaging for periodic follow-up biopsies is gaining traction, and new data suggests that this approach may be workable.

"MULTIPARAMETRIC" MEANS FOUR SCANS IN ONE

There are four different imaging components to MP-MRI. The first is "T2-weighted," which creates the clearest images and gives the most capsular detail. The second and third parameters are called diffusion-weighted imaging (DWI) and the apparent-diffusion coefficient (ADC). These provide information about the *aggressiveness* of the tumor. The fourth parameter, called dynamic-contrast enhancement (DCE), maps the blood flow of the tumor.

THE STANDARD REPORTING FORMAT—"PI-RADS"

PI-RADS (prostate imaging reporting and data systems) scores the T2, DWI/ADC, and DCE parameters on a 1-to-5 scale. Lesions with a score of 4 or 5 are more likely to represent clinically significant prostate cancer (Gleason 4+3=7 or higher). PI-RADS 3 lesions are much less than 50 percent likely to have clinically significant cancer. PI-RADS 1 and 2 are generally not even reported, since they are no more likely to show cancer than a random biopsy.

THREE WAYS TO PERFORM A TARGETED BIOPSY

Once MP-MRI detects a suspicious lesion, a targeted biopsy can be performed in one of three ways. The simplest is called "cognitive fusion." Cognitive fusion means that the doctor reviews the MRI images to get a mental picture of where the cancer is located. The same area of the gland is then targeted using an ultrasound.[2] The second way is called "image-fusion." Software and hardware "fuse" the MRI image with an ultrasound image. A third approach is called "in-bore" biopsy. This is performed in the MRI itself. A robotic device guides the biopsy needle to the exact place seen by the MRI scan.

The best technique for performing a targeted biopsy will vary, based on the clinical scenario. For a large tumor in the posterior prostate (near the rectum), any of the techniques would likely work quite well. For a *small* tumor in the *anterior* part of an enlarged prostate, the in-bore technique probably holds the greatest likelihood of accurately sampling the tumor.

THE FUTURE OF PROSTATE MRI

The same imaging techniques for identifying prostate cancer for targeted biopsy can also be used to direct treatment, so-called "focal therapy." Focal therapy spares much of the surrounding normal prostate tissue from unnecessary damage. It is probably just a matter of time before focal treatment becomes a new treatment method of choice. Given the increasing reliance on accurate imaging for state-of-the-art care, the importance of finding centers of excellence with skilled and experienced physicians will assume progressively greater importance.

References

1. HU Ahmed and others. The PROMIS study: A paired-cohort, blinded confirmatory study evaluating the accuracy of multiparametric MRI and TRUS biopsy in men with an elevated PSA. *Journal of Clinical Oncology* 34 suppl: Abstract 5000, 2016.

2. S Vourganti and others. Multiparametric magnetic resonance imaging and ultrasound fusion biopsy detect prostate cancer in patients with prior negative transrectal ultrasound biopsies. *Journal of Urology* 188.8: 2152, 2012.

Chapter 5

COLOR DOPPLER ULTRASOUND AND TARGETED BIOPSY

Duke Bahn, MD

*The most pathetic person in the world is
someone who has sight but no vision.*
HELEN KELLER

NEWLY DIAGNOSED CANCER PATIENTS face the enormous task
of understanding the disease and choosing the most appropriate
treatment. Cancer characteristics and staging information that is based on
undirected random biopsy are often no more than *"guestimations"* of the
cancer's extent. Today's more informed patients, those who seek answers
through patient advocacy groups and the Internet, often discover that
the "specialist," to his consternation, actually knows less about the latest
technology than he does. These patients are often left with the feeling
that the ball is in their court and that they alone must make the elusive
three-point shot. State-of-the-art imaging can help compensate for all
this uncertainty. Sound clinical decisions are based on obtaining the

most accurate staging information. In most cases, that requires accurate imaging of the prostate.

Since the advent of PSA and random needle biopsy in the late '80s, the number of men diagnosed with prostate cancer has doubled. Ironically, even though some men's lives are saved by early diagnosis, many more are diagnosed with *insignificant tumors that do not need treatment.* Random biopsy in every man with a slightly elevated PSA is causing a terribly high incidence of overdiagnosis and overtreatment.[1-3] This problem is so out of control that the US Preventive Task Force recommended that PSA testing only be offered after a careful discussion of the risks and benefits.[4]

Evaluation of high PSA levels with high-resolution imaging rather than a random biopsy circumvents the problem of overdiagnosis and overtreatment. In Chapter 4, MP-MRI technology combined with a targeted biopsy was discussed. This chapter will discuss an alternative type of imaging, called color Doppler ultrasound (CDU). Unfortunately, CDU followed by targeted biopsy is available in only a few centers around the United States. Even so, this chapter will expound the many advantages of CDU for the diagnosis and staging of prostate cancer.

PSA, GLAND VOLUME, AND DIAGNOSIS

Using an arbitrary PSA level as a trigger for random biopsy casts such a broad net that overdiagnosis becomes inevitable. Men's prostates vary greatly in size—so the amount of PSA they produce varies greatly. My policy is to use a relatively low PSA threshold of 2.5 as an initial trigger to recommend a CDU evaluation in a younger man whose prostate size is small, as determined by digital rectal examination. However, in men with risk factors such as family history or African American descent, I use an even more conservative cut point of 2.0 to recommend a CDU. In older men with larger prostate glands, a threshold of 4.0 is reasonable.

The first step should be to measure the *size* of the prostate. If a patient's PSA is higher than that expected for the individual's prostate size, it increases the likelihood that an underlying high-grade prostate cancer may be present (Chapter 2 explains how to calculate a normal PSA level in light of a man's prostate size). Men whose PSA levels are in the normal range for their prostate size should not be subjected to invasive diagnostic procedures unless other suspicious findings are uncovered during the performance of the CDU.

IMAGING WITH COLOR DOPPLER

Imaging with CDU utilizes two components; grayscale imaging and color Doppler evaluation of vascularity. Cancer tissue has a different appearance on grayscale compared with normal prostate tissue, due to a loss of normal glandular pattern and more compact tissue density. Cancerous lesions appear hypoechoic, (e.g., as a dark spot). In addition, cancer can show increased blood vessel density or "hypervascularity." A specific lesion detected by CDU is more likely to be cancerous if it is both hypoechoic and hypervascular.

High-resolution CDU readily identifies tumors over 5 mm in diameter. Cancers that are visible on CDU are more likely to be clinically significant (Gleason 4+3=7 or above). Hypervascularity tends to indicate tumors with a higher grade.[5] Studies comparing the use of CDU to detect suspicious lesions that are subsequently targeted by biopsy show that CDU-directed biopsy uses fewer biopsy cores than random biopsy, while also reducing the chance of detecting clinically insignificant tumors (those that are grade 6 or less). However, accurate color Doppler imaging requires skill, experience, training, and good equipment.

TARGETED BIOPSY TECHNIQUE

The biopsy protocol should include one sample from the center of the suspicious lesion. Additional biopsy samples may also be obtained from just outside the prostate capsule near the suspicious lesion to detect the presence of early microscopic spread outside the capsule, should it be present. One study shows that 26 percent of patients[7] previously diagnosed with random biopsy were diagnosed with higher-grade disease after undergoing a CDU-targeted biopsy. The detection of a previously unsuspected extracapsular extension alters the prognosis and choice of treatment.

QUESTIONS THAT COLOR DOPPLER AND TARGETED BIOPSY CAN ANSWER

- Where is the tumor located within the gland?

- Does the tumor remain confined within the prostate?

- Is the tumor close to the neurovascular bundle or seminal vesicle, areas of more easy spread of the tumor outside the gland?

- What is the tumor's diameter in millimeters? Does the size of the lesion detected by imaging coincide with the length of cancer reported in the needle biopsy by the pathologist?

- What is the true Gleason score?[6,7]

- Is tumor size or vascularity on sequential scanning increasing over time for men who are on active surveillance?[8]

FINAL THOUGHTS ON PROSTATE IMAGING

Prostate imaging with MP-MRI, CDU, or both dramatically reduces the need for random biopsy which relies on sampling with multiple needles. In addition, the information provided by imaging is of a higher quality, compared with what a random biopsy provides. Imaging should precede invasive needle biopsy. When a biopsy is indicated, it should be targeted rather than random.

References

1. FH Schroder and others. Screening and prostate cancer mortality in a randomized European study. *New England Journal of Medicine* 360: 1320, 2009.

2. GL Andriole and others. Mortality results from a randomized prostate cancer screening trial. *New England Journal of Medicine* 360.13: 1310, 2009.

3. D Ilic and others. Screening for prostate cancer. The Cochrane Library, 2013.

4. K Lin and others. Benefits and harms of prostate-specific antigen screening for prostate cancer: An evidence update for the US Preventive Services Task Force. *Annals of Internal Medicine* 149.3: 192, 2008.

5. M Mitterberger and others. Comparison of contrast enhanced color Doppler targeted biopsy to conventional systematic biopsy: Impact on Gleason score. *Journal of Urology* 178.2: 464, 2007.

6. DK Bahn and others. The role of TRUS-guided biopsies for determination of internal and external spread of prostate cancer. *In Seminars in Urologic Oncology* 16.3: 129, 1998.

7. O Ukimura and others. Image visibility of cancer to enhance targeting precision and spatial mapping biopsy for focal therapy of prostate cancer. *British Journal of Urology International* 111.8: E354, 2013.

8. MM Eltemamy and others. Serial anatomical prostate ultrasound during prostate cancer active surveillance. *Journal of Urology* 196: 727, 2016.

Chapter 6

BODY SCANS AND OTHER PROGNOSTIC FACTORS

Fabio Almeida, MD

I look to the future because that's where I'm
going to spend the rest of my life.
GEORGE BURNS

PSA, BIOPSY AND SCAN RESULTS are the tools used to assign the Stage of Blue. The preceding chapters acquainted you with PSA, Gleason score and prostate imaging. In this chapter, we will talk about body scans and some additional factors related to staging and prognosis. The Stages of Blue themselves are *prognostic,* (i.e., they give insight into the future behavior of the cancer). Developing an accurate prognosis, predicting how the cancer is going to behave, is the critically important first step in the prostate cancer treatment-selection process. Higher-grade cancers need aggressive treatment. Low-grade cancers require little or no treatment, or at least treatment can be postponed.

People naturally have reservations about anyone who claims to fore-tell the future. However, prostate cancer forecasting is pretty accurate. Inaccuracy usually results from a lack of thoroughness in gathering infor-mation. One way to optimize accuracy is by cross-checking the results between different tests. For example, something is probably amiss if the prostate MRI scan shows a large tumor, but the pathology report from a random biopsy shows only minimal amounts of disease. In a scenario like this, one can surmise that the needles from the random biopsy *missed* the main cancer. Gathering further data by doing a *targeted* biopsy may be necessary. Bottom line: If test results don't agree with each other, further investigation is needed. Once all the information is properly compiled, the overall picture should hang together and make sense.

The process of selecting the best treatment—avoiding overtreatment or undertreatment—is much more challenging with prostate cancer than it is with other types of cancer. This is because the *longevity* after diagnosis with prostate cancer is drastically extended—decades, rather than months or years, as is the case with other cancers. Long survival is a good thing. However, it means there is a potential for extended suf-fering if treatment is botched. Bluntly stated, elderly men want to savor the last decade or two of their lives need to be careful. A quality of life blunder can be just as disheartening as a mistake that diminishes sur-vival. Quality of life questions are front and center with prostate cancer because of the gland's precarious location near the bladder, rectum and nerves that control erections. The risk of urinary and sexual problems is very high, even with the best surgeons.

There are varieties of prostate cancer *even within the confines of each Stage of Blue*. Treatment, therefore, will certainly vary from patient to patient. As we draw near to the end of the first section of this book, which has introduced basic concepts related to staging, scanning and prognosis, it is appropriate to review two additional prognostic indicators that refine the D'Amico system upon which the Stages of Blue system is partially based: The first is the tumor's size in which regard the D'Amico system is imprecise because it measures tumor size indirectly (see below). The second is whether any cancer is located outside the prostate in another area of the body. This is determined with body scans. Scan results contribute to determining all the Stages except *Sky*.

THE SIZE OF THE TUMOR

Tumor size (not to be confused with prostate gland size) is a universally important predictive factor for every type of cancer, including prostate cancer. Bigger tumors are more dangerous than smaller ones. The D'Amico system *estimates* tumor size by relying on *the degree of PSA elevation* and the size the nodule (felt by the doctor's finger during the DRE) if a nodule is present. However, DRE information is less precise than a scan or biopsy. While this book advocates targeted biopsies, most doctors still perform randomized biopsies. When a 12-core random biopsy is performed, *the total number of cores with cancer* indicates the tumor's size more accurately (Chapter 3). A greater number of cancerous cores signals a larger tumor. As will be seen in the following sections of the book, the Stages of *Sky*, *Teal* and *Azure* are subdivided using the extent of disease as indicated by the number of biopsy cores that contain cancer.

THE LOCATION OF THE TUMOR IN THE REST OF THE BODY

While multiparametric MRI and color Doppler ultrasound are excellent tools for staging and monitoring disease *inside* the prostate, scanning for cancer that may have spread to the lymph nodes or bones is also critical. Using a wartime analogy, imaging provides accurate reconnaissance about the exact location of the enemy. Knowing the cancer's location in the body opens the door to targeted therapies that can concentrate their firepower directly at the cancer. Traditionally, doctors have relied on CT scans and bone scans. However, their accuracy is quite disappointing. They frequently fail to detect cancer in its early stages of spread. *Undetected spread is the most common reason for cancer recurrence after the initial treatment.* Therefore, better methods of scanning are critically needed.

Positron emission tomography (PET) scanning technology is revolutionizing the way prostate cancer is treated. PET scans provide three-dimensional images of the whole body—evaluating the lymph nodes, the prostate gland region and other organs such as the lungs and the bone.

There are several types of PET scans, which are discussed in greater detail on my Prostate Cancer Research Institute blog titled: *Overview of PET Scans*. The most recent and exciting development has been the momentous discovery that prostate cancer generally relies on *fat* as its primary energy source.[1-2] Since prostate tumors rapidly absorb fat that is injected into the bloodstream, if the fat is made radioactive by the insertion of radioactive carbon (C^{11}), the tumors "light up" on a scanner.[3-7] Lymph node metastases as small as 5–6 mm can be detected. Knowing the location of the cancer guides toward less-invasive treatment when cancer appears localized to the prostate, or more aggressive treatment when disease in the lymph nodes is detected.

BONE SCANS

Careful imaging of the bone is important because, after lymph nodes, bone is the next most common site of metastatic spread. The detection of a metastatic lesion almost always signals a marked change in the treatment plan. Standard bone scans (not PET) use a radiotracer called Technetium[99], which is fairly sensitive but, unfortunately, not very specific. The problem with Technetium[99] is that other changes in the bone, such as arthritis or benign lesions, can be mistaken for cancer metastasis.

More recently, another type of PET scan, called NaF^{18} (radioactive sodium fluoride), has been shown to have superior sensitivity since it can detect smaller lesions. It also provides superior specificity (metastases can be distinguished from arthritic and benign changes to the bone more easily) when compared with Technetium[99]. Bone lesions as small as 2 to 3 mm can be seen. NaF^{18} PET imaging used in combination with C^{11} acetate PET imaging in the same patient offers the most comprehensive method currently available for detecting cancer metastases.

FUTURE DIRECTIONS

C^{11} acetate PET scanning for prostate cancer is a giant leap forward over older scanning techniques, but C^{11} has practical and economical limitations. The scan center must be located immediately adjacent to a cyclotron facility. Other new types of scans are therefore being explored such as

Ga^{68} PSMA. Since Ga^{68} PSMA can be produced without a cyclotron, it has the potential to be available at many sites. Another promising new agent is FACBC (Axumin), which detects increased amino acid metabolism similar to how C^{11} exploits increased lipid metabolism. FACBC is now FDA approved and has recently become commercially available for men with prostate cancer.

References

1. F Almeida and others. C^{11}-Acetate PET/CT compared to F-18 FDG PET for Men with Early Recurrent Prostate Adenocarcinoma. *Radiologic Society of North America Annual Meeting* 2012.

2. E Fricke and others. Positron emission tomography with ^{11}C-acetate and ^{18}F-FDG in prostate cancer patients. *European Journal of Nuclear Medicine and Molecular Imaging* 30.4: 607, 2003.

3. H Hautzel and others. The (11C) acetate positron emission tomography in prostatic carcinoma. New prospects in metabolic imaging. *Urologe A* 41.6: 569, 2002.

4. J Kotzerke and others. Carbon-11 acetate positron emission tomography can detect local recurrence of prostate cancer. *European Journal of Nuclear Medicine and Molecular Imaging* 29.10: 1380, 2002.

5. R Bar-Shalom and others. Clinical performance of PET/CT in evaluation of cancer: Additional value for diagnostic imaging and patient management. *Journal of Nuclear Medicine* 44.8: 1200, 2003.

6. G Sandblom and others. Positron emission tomography with C11-acetate for tumor detection and localization in patients with prostate-specific antigen relapse after radical prostatectomy. *Urology* 67.5: 996, 2006.

7. H Vees and others. 18F-choline and/or 11C-acetate positron emission tomography: Detection of residual or progressive subclinical disease at very low prostate-specific antigen values (< 1 ng/mL) after radical prostatectomy. *British Journal of Urology International* 99.6: 1415, 2007.

Chapter 7
PICKING THE RIGHT DOCTOR

Ralph Blum

A patient who is mortally sick may yet recover from
his belief in the goodness of his physician.

HIPPOCRATES

WAS ORIGINALLY DIAGNOSED WITH prostate cancer in 1990 at the age of 58. I describe the details of my long relationship with prostate cancer in "Invasion of the Prostate Snatchers", the book I cowrote with Dr. Mark Scholz. Basically, without any real physician supervision, I placed myself on a type of "active surveillance" of my own design for 12 years before I embarked on any treatment at all. My method was to check my PSA levels and fly to San Francisco (from Hawaii) to get periodic MRI scans of my prostate. In 2002, my PSA was up to 13, and for the first time my MRI scan showed tumor growth. I decided to consult with Dr. Mark, and we mutually decided to start hormonal therapy. I was treated for 12 months. Over the subsequent 11 years, my PSA slowly rose back to 13. During that time, I was monitored by Dr.

Duke Bahn with periodic color Doppler ultrasound scans as described in Chapter 5. In 2013, Dr. Bahn indicated that the tumor was growing again. So finally, at the age of 81, I decided to undergo IMRT, which fortunately did not cause any notable side effects.

Throughout the 23 years of living with prostate cancer before I underwent radiation treatment, I lived with the premise that even if the prostate cancer is not low-risk, it is still likely to grow slowly. Moreover, I was really turned off by the standard treatments that have very unpleasant side effects and complications that seem to be worse than the disease. I decided to withhold treatment until I was convinced that the cancer was growing or spreading. Little did I know the type of steely conviction that would be required to fend off the many impassioned "experts," all of whom kept recommending surgery. Over the years, I learned that doctors vary greatly in the way they present treatment options to their patients. Far too many doctors advocate radical treatment because it's what they know and what they do. It goes against the grain for doctors *not* to treat cancer.

Your decision about who will manage your prostate cancer is one of the most critically important decisions you will ever make. So how do you go about choosing a good doctor? Depending on where you live and your type of health insurance, you and your primary care doctor will need to decide who is the best specialist for you. Usually you will be referred to a local urologist for a diagnosis, but before you take this step, you need to be aware of the five medical specialties that can participate in prostate cancer management: urology, radiation oncology, radiology (reading scans), pathology (reading biopsy specimens under the microscope), and medical oncology. Each of these specialties is very different from the other. They all require four or five years of intensive training *after* finishing medical school.

Ideally, the process of deciding on the best treatment would begin with supervision from a doctor who specializes in *treatment selection*, rather than one who performs a *specific type* of treatment. However, this is very rarely the case. Prostate cancer patients are typically managed by urologists, who specialize in surgery. Since the early 1900s, urologists have dominated the prostate cancer realm. Throughout much of this long history, surgery has been the only effective cancer treatment available.

Therefore, up to the present, the urologists who diagnose the cancer by performing the initial biopsy *invariably take on the primary role of guiding the treatment-selection process.*

With just about any other type of cancer (breast, colon, lung, bone lymphoma, etc.) full-time cancer specialists—board-certified *medical oncologists*—assume the leadership role in creating a treatment plan. Oncologists are also board-certified in internal medicine and therefore trained in *treatment-selection* and how to administer different types of medications—both for cancer treatment and for overall health needs. Unfortunately, of the 10,000 medical oncologists in the United States outside of academia, *less than 20 doctors in the whole country* specialize exclusively in prostate cancer! So, the medical oversight of men with newly diagnosed prostate cancer remains largely on the shoulders of urologists, who, with occasional exceptions, are *generalists* in urologic care, *not* prostate cancer specialists.

If there were a universal consensus about how to select optimal treatment, the fact that urologists are generalists could be safely overlooked. Simple, straightforward problems usually can be solved without the aid of a specialist. The problem is that the definition of "optimal treatment" in the prostate realm is changing very rapidly. Until about 12 years ago, surgery was clearly better than radiation, achieving higher cure rates with fewer side effects. Thus, radiation oncologists had a much smaller role. Back then, surgery could justifiably be called the "Gold Standard." These days, however, we don't hear the Gold Standard argument very often. Even many urologists are beginning to concede that modern radiation is better than surgery.

However, there remains fierce competition between doctors who consciously or unconsciously try to sway patients toward the treatment in which they specialize. Urologists hold a very powerful advantage in this behind-the-scenes struggle because, in the prostate world, the urologist makes the cancer diagnosis (with a biopsy). He decides which radiation doctor to refer to, if any. Patients should be aware that some radiation doctors will agree to the premise that surgery is better for *younger* men, just to keep their referring urologist happy. They can still treat the older patients, the ones who everyone agrees are bad candidates for surgery.

If you end up with a urologist as your cancer doctor, as most men do, realize that they are not all created equal. The average urologist's medical practice mainly involves treating problems like impotence, infections, incontinence, kidney stones, bladder problems, and enlarged prostates. He sees between 20 and 40 patients a day, and has reports to write and meetings to attend. He may be a talented doctor, but he may not have the time to keep up with the evolving prostate cancer field. So ideally, you want a urologist who manages a higher volume of prostate cancer patients.

If you are considering surgery, bear in mind that, although it has the advantage of a possible cure, it also has a high risk of causing side effects such as impotence and incontinence (Chapters 12 and 13). Furthermore, sometimes the cancer will recur after surgery and additional therapy will be needed. But, if you plan to go ahead with surgery, the most vital information you need to know is that *the average local urologist performs fewer than five prostatectomies a year.* Given that, anatomically, the prostate is in absolutely the worst place for a simple surgical solution, five cases a year are nowhere near enough operations to be proficient. There is no doubt that men who are treated by specialists with the most experience have better surgical outcomes. Unless you are in a position to consult one of the top prostate cancer surgeons who performs hundreds of these complex and challenging surgeries each year, or unless you are able to travel to a major medical center, surgery is a really bad option.

Arguably, your most important task when choosing a doctor for your prostate cancer is to find a specialist with a good track record who is skilled at diagnosing and treating the disease. It is also important to choose a doctor with whom you feel comfortable, and who is caring and compassionate. He doesn't have to be your new best friend, but he should be someone you feel you can trust. Typically, you will want to have at least a one-time consultation with doctors from several specialties: a urologist, a radiation oncologist, and a medical oncologist. Each of these doctors will look at your case through the lens of his own training and experience.

A good doctor will give you a thorough explanation of the pathology report in patient-friendly language and will thoroughly discuss all viable treatment options for your type and stage of cancer in an even-handed manner. A significant part of any doctor's job is to create a relationship with his patient based on trust, confidence, and hope. In an essay titled, "Complications: Surgeon's Notes on an Imperfect Science," Atul Gawande, surgeon, writer, and professor at Harvard Medical School, wrote: "Just as there is an art to being a doctor, there is an art to being a patient. You must choose wisely when to submit and when to assert yourself."

As children, most of us were taught to believe in the infallibility of doctors, but in the highly commercialized prostate cancer world, a "Whatever you say, doc" passive attitude will not serve you well. You have the right, even the responsibility, to ask questions, but you need to know what questions to ask. Go on the Internet. Search PCRI.org. Call the PCRI Helpline at (800) 641-7274. Increase your knowledge so you are confident enough to say "No" if you feel the treatment your doctor recommends is not for you. And if your doctor tells you, "There's nothing more we can do" or "You have only a few months to live," don't believe it. Head for the door, and find another doctor.

You have reached the end of Section I of this book, which has introduced the basic tools used for staging and monitoring prostate cancer. Armed with this, along with information from Chapter 1 that enables you to determine your Stage of Blue, it is now possible for you to jump ahead to the Section of the book that addresses your Stage specifically:

Sky:	Section II	Chapter 8
Teal:	Section III	Chapter 16
Azure:	Section IV	Chapter 26
Indigo:	Section V	Chapter 31
Royal:	Section VI	Chapter 37

After you finish the Section related to your Stage of Blue, you can then jump to Section VII to complete the remainder of the book.

SECTION II
THE *SKY* STAGE OF BLUE

Chapter 8
OVERVIEW OF *SKY*

Mark Scholz, MD

Patience is bitter, but its fruit is sweet.
Jean-Jacques Rousseau

PROSTATE CANCER GROWS AT a snail's pace compared with other cancers. However, this fact is underappreciated by patients and doctors alike. When a celebrity dies from prostate cancer, it's trumpeted on the evening news. That's the media's job—to get the public's attention. The celebrity may have been fighting his prostate cancer for two decades; but that detail is never mentioned in the story. The reality is that 91.5 percent of men who have prostate cancer live to a normal life expectancy.[1] *The small minority who succumb live for an average of 13 years after their diagnosis.* That means that the men with the "deadly" type of prostate cancer who are diagnosed in 2017 are likely to benefit from future technology that will be invented in 2030.

BE CAREFUL OF WHAT YOU THINK YOU KNOW

The biggest challenge of educating people about prostate cancer is reversing preconceived notions, (i.e., *what they already think they know about cancer*). In this modern age of random biopsies, the majority of "prostate cancers" are so tiny that even if they grow while under observation, they will still be curable. If well-informed men have patience to forgo immediate treatment and actively watch for a while, to see if their cancer starts to enlarge, at least when they undergo treatment, they will proceed with conviction, knowing that treatment is truly required.

All of this is rather comforting, but how much confidence can I place in an expert who tells me that I have the harmless type of prostate cancer? What if my doctor makes a mistake and informs me that I have the harmless type when I really have the bad type? Are the predictions about prostate cancer accurate? This question has been studiously evaluated, and the answer turns out to be an absolute "yes." PSA, Gleason score, imaging studies, and new genetic tests enable us to accurately predict which prostate cancers are potentially dangerous.

As good as these predictors are, there is an additional layer of protection against being misinformed—active surveillance. Surveillance means *ongoing monitoring*. Low-grade cancers are expected to remain stable for years without growing. If, however, while being closely monitored, a small tumor starts to enlarge, curative treatment can still be initiated in a timely fashion. Ongoing surveillance is how we double check and confirm that the tumor is not misbehaving.

It is certainly necessary to exercise great care when selecting treatment for anything called cancer. And, if there is any doubt, it is sensible to err on the side of being careful. However, studies show that the good and bad types of prostate cancer can be accurately distinguished. The table provides a rough idea of how active surveillance candidates are selected:

Table

	Favorable	Ambiguous	Unfavorable
PSA	Under 8	9–14	15 and Over
Imaging	Organ-confined	Larger-sized tumor	Extracapsular extension
Highest Gleason Score	Grade 3+3=6	3+4=7	4+3=7 or higher

The application of active surveillance is not simply a good theory; it is a scientifically proven methodology. Ten years ago, surgery was called the "Gold Standard." Now you rarely hear the Gold Standard argument. What changed? In 2012, *The New England Journal of Medicine* published a study by Dr. Timothy Wilt comparing the long-term outcome of surgery versus observation.[2] Between 1994 and 2002, 731 men volunteered to undergo either observation or immediate surgery based on a coin flip. The average age for the whole group was 67. Their median PSA was 7.8. Ten years into the study, survival rates between both groups were the same! The only exception was in men whose PSA level was above 10. However, even in this higher-risk group, surgery only improved the 10-year survival rate by seven percent (94.5 percent 10-year survival for surgery vs. 87.2 percent 10-year survival for observation).

Studies of men volunteering for active surveillance show the same thing. At Johns Hopkins, 1,298 men were observed for up to 18 years. Only two died of prostate cancer.[3] In addition to these studies, simple common sense argues in favor of active surveillance: Autopsy studies of healthy men dying of unrelated causes show that prostate cancer is so prevalent that practically every man has prostate cancer toward the end of his life. So if prostate cancer is so common, it would be illogical to assume that every case is deadly.

Avoiding the side effects from surgery and radiation is what makes active surveillance appealing. However, there are some drawbacks to active surveillance. Withholding treatment for something that patients have been made to view as "cancer" can create an emotional burden. Periodic blood tests, prostate scans, and doctor visits are required. Plus, physicians continue to maintain the policy of doing repeated prostate biopsies, even though monitoring with multiparametric MRI is a feasible alternative (Chapter 4). Despite these inconveniences, treatment with surgery or radiation can have much worse side effects. Chapters 11 through 14 describe the notable risks faced by men who choose to undergo surgery or radiation.

Unfortunately, these side effects are routinely downplayed by doctors and patients alike. Doctors underemphasize them because, after years of working in the field, they become desensitized; they grow accustomed to the daily occurrence of impotence and incontinence in their patients. And a minority of their patients do beat the odds, emerging relatively unscathed after surgery. These individuals sing the praises of their treatment. They took a radical step to have treatment and were fortunate enough to avoid the worst consequences. Regrettably, though, most men who undergo surgery have long-lasting side effects. These men usually remain silent, because they are too embarrassed to talk about wearing a diaper or being impotent. They downplay the negative effects, emphasizing their gratefulness because they are "free from cancer."

No one, not even the finest surgeons or radiation therapists, can promise that impotence and incontinence will be avoided. For a vivid, first-hand description of the potential complications from surgery—surgery performed by Patrick Walsh, the world's best prostate surgeon—read Michael Korda's excellent book, *Man to Man: Surviving Prostate Cancer.* Mr. Korda was the editor-in-chief at Simon & Schuster. In his book, he describes his tribulations undergoing a radical prostatectomy performed by Dr. Walsh.

Surgery and radiation cause *permanent* side effects with astounding frequency. In a study of 475 men, fewer than 20 percent of men described their sexual function as "returning to normal."[4] In another study of 785 men, fewer than 20 percent of men who had surgery and fewer than 50 percent of the men who had radioactive seed implants described their sexual function as returning to normal.[5]

In the study by Dr. Wilt cited earlier, as would be expected, the men undergoing surgery experienced dramatically more side effects than the men placed on observation. During the first 30 days after the operation, there were a number of very serious side effects, including one death. Two men developed blood clots in their legs, one suffered a stroke, two had blood clots in their lungs, three suffered heart attacks, one man had renal failure requiring dialysis, 10 required additional corrective surgery, six required additional blood transfusions, and six still wore urinary catheters more than 30 days after surgery.

Over the longer term, the disadvantages of surgery persisted. Forty-nine men (17 percent) who had surgery compared with 18 men (6 percent) who underwent observation "had a lot of problems with urinary dribbling," some losing larger amounts of urine than "dribbling but not all day," others having "no control over urine," and the remainder having "an indwelling catheter." Two-hundred-thirty-one men (81 percent) who had surgery, compared with 124 men (44 percent) who underwent observation, had erectile dysfunction, defined as the inability to attain an erection sufficient for vaginal penetration.

In view of these risks, active surveillance is the plausible alternative. Appropriately selected men can forgo immediate intervention, in most cases postponing destructive treatments indefinitely. The men who are on active surveillance have another advantage. If a nontoxic treatment is discovered in the future, they will be eligible. The rationale for choosing active surveillance, therefore, stands on two legs: the scientific validation of its safety, and the realization that sexual and urinary dysfunction from surgery or radiation are common.

In the next chapter, Laurence Klotz, the doctor who invented the term "active surveillance," explains the undergirding science and rationale for this approach. He shares his deep insight into prostate cancer biology, an understanding that helped him to foresee the need for active surveillance long before anyone else. He also presents his long-term experience providing active surveillance to over 1,000 men beginning back in the 1990s.

In chapter 10, Dr. Duke Bahn presents a treatment approach that uses *focal* freezing of a section of the prostate with liquid Argon. In chapters 12 through 14, world-class experts review the most common side effects caused by surgery and radiation. These chapters provide a clear picture of the potential risks associated with surgery and radiation and the most common approaches used to correct them.

References

1. SE Eggener and others. Predicting 15-year prostate cancer specific mortality after radical prostatectomy. *Journal of Urology* 185.3: 869, 2011.

2. TJ Wilt and others. Radical prostatectomy versus observation for localized prostate cancer. *New England Journal of Medicine* 367.3: 203, 2012.

3. JJ Tosoian and others. Intermediate and longer-term outcomes from a prospective active-surveillance program for favorable-risk prostate cancer. *Journal of Clinical Oncology* 33.30: 3379, 2015.

4. JL Gore and others. Survivorship beyond convalescence: 48-month quality-of-life outcomes after treatment for localized prostate cancer. *Journal of the National Cancer Institute* 101.12: 888, 2009.

5. JB Malcolm and others. Quality of life after open or robotic prostatectomy, cryoablation or brachytherapy for localized prostate cancer. *Journal of Urology* 183.5: 1822, 2010.

Chapter 9

THE SCIENCE BEHIND ACTIVE SURVEILLANCE

Laurence Klotz, MD

All truth passes through three stages.
First it is ridiculed. Second, it is violently opposed.
Third, it is accepted as being self-evident.

ARTHUR SCHOPENHAUER

N A RECENT SPECIAL PUBLICATION titled "200 Years of Surgery," Awul Gawande, MD, concluded that "If the past quarter century has brought minimally invasive procedures, the next may bring *the elimination of invasion*."[1] This observation is nowhere more apt than in the management of localized prostate cancer. The field of prostate cancer treatment is rapidly transitioning toward prostate-sparing treatments, including active surveillance and focal therapy. Progress in these areas will be reviewed in this chapter.

THE RATIONALE FOR SURVEILLANCE: THE NATURAL HISTORY OF *SKY*

It is now clear that prostate cancer is part of the normal male aging process. It develops in men of all races and regions. In Caucasians and African Americans, the chance of a normal man on the street harboring prostate cancer is approximately the same as his age: 30 percent of men in their 30s, 40 percent in their 40s, and so on.[2] Most of these "cancers" are less than a millimeter in diameter and low grade. The high prevalence of tiny prostate cancers has been confirmed in autopsy studies of Caucasians, Asians, and other racial groups. A recent autopsy study of Japanese and Russian men who died of causes not related to prostate cancer showed that 35 percent of both groups had prostate cancer. Surprisingly, 50 percent of the cancers in Japanese men over age 70 were Gleason score 7 or above, a supposedly more dangerous form of the disease.[3] Considering the extremely low mortality rates from prostate cancer in Japan, these findings suggest that, particularly in men over 70, small amounts of Gleason 3+4=7 might be just as harmless as 3+3=6.

GENETICS FORETELL A CANCER'S BEHAVIOR

A prostate *cancer* cell is merely a prostate *gland* cell that is genetically altered. Just as human genetic information remains stable and is faithfully transmitted from father to son in *healthy* gland cells, so prostate cancer cells of one type of lineage continue to produce offspring with the same *cancerous* genetic makeup. The behavior of malignant cells varies, depending on their specific genetic makeup.

Multiple genetic alterations must occur before a normal prostate gland cell starts behaving like a cancer. The genetic pathways responsible for these hallmarks of malignancy have been worked out with precision, and I have described the specifics in a blog titled *An Update on Active Surveillance* that is posted on the PCRI website. The hallmarks of cancer cells that behave more aggressively—i.e., ones that grow more quickly, disseminate throughout the body, and place a man's life at risk—have been described by Hanahan and Weinberg.[4,5] The aggressive cancer cell has:

1. The potential ability to replicate without limit

2. Sustained development of new blood vessels (angiogenesis)

3. The capacity for tissue invasion

4. Insensitivity to the signals from other cells that limit growth

5. The capacity to metastasize

6. The ability to hide from the immune system

GLEASON SCORING ACCURATELY PREDICTS GENETICS

It is amazing that a relatively simple scoring system that relies on a trained observer (a pathologist) looking at the visual appearance of the cells under a microscope (the Gleason scoring system) has an uncanny ability to segregate prostate cancer into genetically normal and abnormal cells. The Gleason scoring system has been proven over and over in numerous studies, to be amazingly accurate at predicting what types of prostate cancer are potentially dangerous and what types are not. (It is rumored that, over 40 years ago, Don Gleason, the pathologist who described the eponymous grading system, argued that Gleason pattern 3+3=6 *should not be called cancer* but was unsuccessful in convincing his colleagues).

A couple of large clinical studies illustrate the accuracy of the Gleason score: In one study, 12,000 men with *surgically confirmed* Gleason 6 cancer were followed for 20 years.[6] The mortality from prostate cancer was only 0.2 percent. In a subgroup of 4,000 men, only one single man died of prostate cancer, but a second review of his archived pathology specimen showed that his original tumor had been graded incorrectly: it was actually Gleason 4+3, not 3+3.[7] In another study involving 14,000 men with surgically confirmed Gleason 3+3=6, 22 of them (0.157 percent) had cancer spread into the lymph nodes. The initial implication is that Gleason 3+3=6 can indeed metastasize. However, once again, subsequent reviews of the archived pathologic specimens showed that every single one of these 22 men had occult (hidden, or hard-to-detect), higher-grade disease in the prostatectomy specimen that was missed on the original report.[8]

Other studies have modeled survival rates of active surveillance compared with surgery and radiation. One analysis compared 452 men on active surveillance with 6,485 men having surgery, 2,264 men treated with external beam radiation, and 1,680 treated with brachytherapy. *There was no difference in prostate cancer mortality,* and, amazingly, there was an *improved* overall survival in the surveillance group (due to an increase in other-cause mortality in the radiation patients).[9] Surveillance clearly offers the highest quality of life.[10]

Now that the medical profession has finally figured out that Gleason 3+3=6 has no metastatic ability, the terminology used to describe this condition to patients needs to be radically overhauled. Terms like "pseudo-cancer," "pseudo-disease," "part of the aging process," and "precancer" are accurate descriptive terms that should be used when describing Gleason 3+3=6 to men. Eliminating the poisonous word "cancer" is essential to reassure patients and derail their headlong rush into overaggressive treatment.

Being younger is definitely *not* a reason to avoid choosing surveillance. To no one's surprise, younger men are very eager to avoid the loss of erectile function that comes with surgery or radiation. Since we now know that low-grade cancer is present in 40 percent of men in their 40s,[11] it's illogical to conclude that it is universally dangerous. The diagnosis of Gleason 3+3=6 on random biopsy does not mean that the disease will necessarily progress.

WHEN IS THERE *TOO MUCH* GRADE 6 FOR ACTIVE SURVEILLANCE TO BE SAFE?

Men with *larger quantities of Gleason 6* are known to be at higher risk of harboring occult, higher-grade cancer that may have been missed on the random biopsy. The exact threshold of what constitutes a "large quantity" of grade 6, for example, is variable. A threshold effect of more than 8 mm of total cancer on random biopsy has recently been described as one potential starting point.[12] Another proposed upper limit of Gleason 6 is with a cancer volume of over 1.3cc.[13] Patients with higher-volume Gleason 6 need to be evaluated with multiparametric MRI (MP-MRI) and with genetic testing (see below) to exclude the presence of higher-grade cancer. If rigorous review using these methods fails to detect higher-grade disease, even patients with larger quantities of Gleason 6 become reasonable candidates for active surveillance.

Several new genetic tests have recently been approved by the FDA that predict the risk of cancer progression. These include the Prolaris assay[14] (Myriad Genetics), which looks for abnormal expression of cell cycle–related genes; the Oncotype DX assay (Genomic Health), which identifies a panel of genes linked to a more aggressive phenotype;[15] and the Mitomics assay, which identifies the presence of a functional mitochondrial DNA deletion associated with aggressive prostate cancer.[16] These tests even have the capacity to predict the presence of higher-grade cancer missed by a random biopsy. The tests are performed on the archived biopsy specimen from the initial biopsy, so there is no need to perform additional blood tests or biopsies to get the information. In the United States, the cost of performing these tests is covered by most insurance companies.

SELECTING ACTIVE SURVEILLANCE CANDIDATES

Who, then, is a candidate for active surveillance? *Sky* disease is defined by a biopsy that shows Gleason 6 with a PSA under 10 and with no palpable nodule on digital rectal examination. *Sky* includes *45 percent of all the newly diagnosed patients in the US and Canada, which amounts to approximately 150,000 men per year. Sky* has been further divided into *Very Low-Risk* and *Low-Risk* subcategories, which, using the Stages of Blue system, are called *Low-Sky* and *Basic-Sky.* These subcategories are assigned depending on the number of biopsy cores and the extent of core involvement (see below). In addition, the ratio of the PSA level to the size of the prostate gland measured in cc (the PSA density) should be under 0.15 (Chapter 2).

The definition of *Very Low-Risk* cancer (*Low-Sky*) was proposed by Dr. Jonathan Epstein, the author of Chapter 3. Dr. Epstein proposes very stringent threshold criteria for pursuing active surveillance:

- A maximum of two positive cores containing cancer (regardless of how many cores were taken)

- No core that is more than 50 percent replaced with cancer

- A PSA Density (the ratio of PSA to the size of the prostate gland in cubic centimeters) i.e., the PSA ÷ gland volume that is under 0.15

Some doctors require patients to be *Low-Sky* to embark on active surveillance. I contend that any man with a PSA less than 10, Gleason 6, and, at most, a small nodule is potentially an excellent candidate for surveillance. I base my conclusion on the benign genetic profile of Gleason 3+3=6 (detailed in blog on the PCRI website titled *An Update on Active Surveillance*), and on the large studies cited above that prove the safety of forgoing immediate treatment. In my view, "high volume" Gleason 6 is only an indication of the *possible* existence of occult, coexistent, higher-grade cancer. In patients who have been carefully screened with state-of-the-art MP-MRI to ensure the absence of higher-grade cancer, future metastatic spread of the cancer is exceedingly unlikely. These patients do not require treatment. They do require close scrutiny to preclude the possibility of missing higher-grade disease developing sometime down the line.

OCCULT CANCER PRESENT SINCE DIAGNOSIS, VERSUS A BRAND-NEW CANCER

Based on our knowledge of the slow growing nature of prostate cancer, even when the Gleason score is high, it is generally believed that most active surveillance patients who are subsequently diagnosed with high-grade disease have been harboring it since the time of initial diagnosis. The higher-grade cells were simply missed by the original random biopsy. Biological grade progression, that is, Gleason 3 cells *transforming* into

Gleason 4 or 5 progeny, is known to be quite uncommon. For example, at our institution in Toronto, the observed rate of grade progression was one percent per year.[17] Therefore, detecting higher-grade disease that was missed on the original biopsy is the main problem. Grade progression, or the development of a completely new, higher-grade cancer, is relatively unlikely because in most cases the Gleason grade remains stable.

THE ROLE OF RACE

African Americans on surveillance have higher-grade disease diagnosed more frequently when compared with Caucasian men.[18] African Americans also have a higher incidence of cancers in the less-accessible "front" part of the prostate (transition zone cancers).[19] However, many African American patients diagnosed with low-grade prostate cancer have little or no probability of a prostate cancer-related death. Active surveillance is still an appealing option for those who have been appropriately screened with careful imaging.

ACTIVE SURVEILLANCE TECHNIQUE

The clinical management of men on surveillance is evolving. Currently, most clinicians use the following approach or a variation of it: Following the initial diagnosis of Gleason 6, PSA is performed every three months for the first two years, and then every six months. Another random biopsy is recommended within three to 12 months after the initial diagnostic biopsy. The second biopsy should target areas in the gland that are typically *under*-sampled on the initial diagnostic biopsy. This includes the anterior prostate, and the prostatic apex and base. If it is either negative or confirms a relatively small amount of Gleason 3+3, subsequent biopsies are performed every three to five years until the patient reaches age 80 or has a life expectancy under five years because of other maladies or serious medical issues.

Multiparametric MRI should be performed on those patients whose PSA levels have changed over time in a way that suggests more aggressive disease (usually defined as a PSA-doubling time of less than three years); whose confirmatory biopsy shows substantial volume increase;

or who are upgraded to Gleason 3+4 and who still desire surveillance as a management option. Identification of a lesion by MP-MRI that is suspected to be high grade should lead to a *targeted* biopsy. As quality MP-MRI centers become more widely available, it is possible that imaging will replace random biopsy altogether (see Chapter 4).

Over time, in men who were initially diagnosed via random biopsy, one-third of patients will be reclassified as being at higher risk for progression and so offered treatment. The rate of reclassification will vary depending on the criteria used for selecting active surveillance in the first place. An approach that offers surveillance to all patients with Gleason 6 and PSA less than 15, for example, will include more patients with undetected high-grade disease than a policy restricted to the Epstein criteria (less than or equal to two positive cores, less than 50 percent involvement of any one core, and PSA density under 0.15). However, *Epstein's stringent eligibility requirements deny surveillance to many men with nonlife-threatening disease,* that is, cancer that grows slowly. Experience shows that in men who are later upgraded, the majority (85 percent) have Gleason 3+4. Many of these men who have low-volume grade 3+4=7 are still appropriate candidates to remain on active surveillance.[20]

Far and away, the most common cause of death in men on surveillance is cardiovascular disease. Death from prostate cancer is very uncommon. In the active surveillance study with the longest follow-up,[21] men with Gleason 3+3=6 or with low-volume Gleason 3+4=7 were *10 times* more likely to die of causes other than prostate cancer. To date, the published literature on surveillance includes 13 "prospective" studies, encompassing about 5,000 men.[21-34] (A prospective study is one that follows a group of patients into the future to see how their disease progresses, to study what might affect their disease progression, or to try to answer some other such question.) These studies evaluating men who were mostly Gleason 3+3=6 fail to identify any increased risk of prostate cancer mortality, though one drawback is that the duration of observation in many of the studies is still short. A complete list of these studies has been posted in my *An Update on Active Surveillance* blog on the PCRI website.

There is one study from Sweden that raises a cautionary note about the possibility of prostate cancer becoming more aggressive in the long term, say 15 years after diagnosis. This particular study, however, did not involve men on active surveillance. They were on "watchful waiting."[35] Men on watchful waiting forgo immediate treatment similar to active surveillance. However, men on watchful waiting undergo a much less intense monitoring process. Typically, they never undergo curative therapy at all; treatment is withheld unless the cancer spreads to the bones, after which hormone therapy is initiated. Watchful waiting is usually reserved for very elderly men. In the active surveillance series that I presently supervise, we have 70 patients who have been on surveillance for over 14 years. So far, we have not observed any tendency for disease acceleration in these patients. Our rate of late progression is only 1.5 percent.[21]

IMAGING TO MONITOR MEN ON ACTIVE SURVEILLANCE

Multiparametric MRI has a rapidly emerging role in the management of surveillance patients (Chapter 4). Patients who undergo initial and regular scanning with MP-MRI enjoy two potential benefits: reassurance that higher-risk disease is absent, and earlier detection of higher-grade disease, should it develop while on surveillance. With respect to the former benefit, the real question is the accuracy of MP-MRI. In a group of about 300 surveillance candidates at Memorial Sloan Kettering, *97 percent of men with a negative MP-MRI were confirmed to have no high-grade disease.* This highly favorable observation, which is much more accurate than random biopsy, will require further validation. But, if this degree of accuracy is confirmed, MP-MRI could potentially replace the random biopsy altogether. A limitation of MP-MRI is the high level of skill required for accurate interpretation. As yet, these skills are not widely prevalent. However, this situation is improving rapidly.

PSA MONITORING ON ACTIVE SURVEILLANCE

PSA monitoring is helpful for identifying patients at higher risk. However, changes in PSA cannot be relied upon to make final decisions about treatment. This represents a shift from earlier practice. Until MP-MRI became available, men on surveillance with rapidly rising PSA levels (with a doubling time under three years) were usually offered treatment. One multi-institutional surveillance registry reported that 20 percent of the men participating in the study were treated because their PSA doubling time was less than three years.[22] Another report describes the cases of five men dying of metastatic prostate cancer, all five of whom had a PSA doubling time under two years.[20]

The main limitation of using the rate of PSA elevation to guide therapy is the lack of specificity. Vickers, in an overview of all active surveillance studies of more than 200 patients, concluded that *changes in PSA had no independent predictive value*.[36] In another study looking at the rate of PSA elevation to monitor disease progression in a large surveillance cohort, false positive PSA triggers (doubling time less than three years, or PSA rising at a rate of more than two points per year) occurred in 50 percent of stable untreated patients, none of whom went on to develop progressive cancer, require treatment, or die of prostate cancer.[37] These studies show that great care needs to be exercised when interpreting the significance of a rise in PSA. Otherwise men with moderate changes may overreact and seek aggressive treatment.

Active surveillance, with close monitoring and selective delayed intervention based on risk reclassification over time, is an appealing approach for *Sky* patients, and a welcome antidote for the 150,000 men in North America diagnosed every year with Gleason 3+3=6, who historically have been encouraged to undergo surgery or radiation. Furthermore, ongoing improvements in diagnostic accuracy based on multiparametric MRI and genetic biomarkers should be able to reduce the need for systematic biopsies and improve the early identification of occult, higher-risk disease. If active surveillance were pursued by every available candidate in North America and Europe, close to 300,000 men could be spared from unnecessary surgery and radiation every year.

References

1. AA Gawande. Two hundred years of surgery. *New England Journal of Medicine* 366.18: 1716, 2012.

2. WA Sakr and others. High grade prostatic intraepithelial neoplasia (HGPIN) and prostatic adenocarcinoma between the ages of 20–69: An autopsy study of 249 cases. *In Vivo* 8.3: 439, 1993.

3. AR Zlotta and others. Prevalence of prostate cancer on autopsy: Cross-sectional study on unscreened Caucasian and Asian men. *Journal of the National Cancer Institute* 105.14: 1050, 2013.

4. D Hanahan and R Weinberg. The hallmarks of cancer. *Cell* 100.1: 57, 2000.

5. D Hanahan and R Weinberg. The hallmarks of cancer: The next generation. *Cell* 144.5: 646, 2011.

6. SE Eggener and others. Predicting 15-year prostate cancer specific mortality after radical prostatectomy. *Journal of Urology* 185.3: 869, 2011.

7. SE Eggener, personal communication, archived content.

8. HM Ross and others. Do adenocarcinomas of the prostate with Gleason Score (GS)≤6 have the potential to metastasize to lymph nodes? *American Journal of Surgical Pathology* 36.9: 1346, 2012.

9. A Stephenson and L Klotz. Comparative propensity analysis of active surveillance vs initial treatment. *American Urological Association*, 2013.

10. JH Hayes and others. Active surveillance compared with initial treatment for men with low-risk prostate cancer: A decision analysis. *Journal of the American Medical Association* 304.21: 2373, 2010.

11. HB Carter and others. Early detection of prostate cancer: AUA Guideline. *Journal of Urology* 190.2: 419, 2013.

12. O Bratt and others. Upper limit of cancer extent on biopsy defining very low-risk prostate cancer. *BJU International* 116.2: 213, 2015.

13. T Wolters and others. A critical analysis of the tumor volume threshold for clinically insignificant prostate cancer using a data set of a randomized screening trial. *Journal of Urology* 185.1: 121, 2011.

14. J Cuzick and others. Prognostic value of a cell cycle progression signature for prostate cancer death in conservatively managed needle biopsy cohort. *British Journal of Cancer* 106.6: 1095, 2012.

15. D Knezevic and others. Analytical validation of the Oncotype DX prostate cancer assay—a clinical RT-PCR assay optimized for prostate needle biopsies. *BMC Genomics* 14.1: 690, 2013.

16. K Robinson and others. Accurate prediction of repeat prostate biopsy outcomes by a mitochondrial DNA deletion assay. *Prostate Cancer and Prostatic Diseases* 13.2: 126, 2010.

17. A Loblaw and L Klotz. Gleason upgrading in a surveillance cohort is time dependent. *American Urological Association,* 2014.

18. D Sundi and others. African American men with very low-risk prostate cancer exhibit adverse oncologic outcomes after radical prostatectomy: Should active surveillance still be an option for them? *Journal of Clinical Oncology* 31.24: 2991, 2013.

19. SP Porten and others. Changes in prostate cancer grade on serial biopsy in men undergoing active surveillance. *Journal of Clinical Oncology* 29.20: 2795, 2011.

20. L Klotz and others. Clinical results of long-term follow-up of a large, active surveillance cohort with localized prostate cancer. *Journal of Clinical Oncology* 28.1: 126, 2009.

21. M Bul and others. Active surveillance for low-risk prostate cancer worldwide: The PRIAS study. *European Urology* 63.4: 597, 2013.

22. MA Dall'Era and others. Active surveillance for the management of prostate cancer in a contemporary cohort. *Cancer* 112.12: 2664, 2008.

23. Y Kakehi and others. Prospective evaluation of selection criteria for active surveillance in Japanese patients with stage T1cN0M0 prostate cancer. *Japanese Journal of Clinical Oncology* 38.2: 122, 2008.

24. JJ Tosoian and others. Active surveillance program for prostate cancer: An update of the Johns Hopkins experience. *Journal of Clinical Oncology* 29.16: 2185, 2011.

25. S Roemeling and others. Active surveillance for prostate cancers detected in three subsequent rounds of a screening trial: Characteristics, PSA doubling times, and outcome. *European Urology* 51.5: 1244, 2007.

26. MM Soloway and others. Careful selection and close monitoring of low-risk prostate cancer patients on active surveillance minimizes the need for treatment. *European Urology* 58.6: 831, 2010.

27. MI Patel and others. An analysis of men with clinically localized prostate cancer who deferred definitive therapy. *The Journal of Urology* 171.4: 1520, 2004.

28. GA Barayan and others. Factors influencing disease progression of prostate cancer under active surveillance: A McGill University Health Center cohort. *BJU International* 114.6b: E99, 2014.

29. J Rubio-Briones and others. Obligatory information that a patient diagnosed of prostate cancer and candidate for an active surveillance protocol must know. *Actas Urológicas Españolas* 38.9: 559, 2014.

30. RA Godtman and others. Outcome following active surveillance of men with screen-detected prostate cancer. Results from the Göteborg randomised population-based prostate cancer screening trial. *European Urology* 63.1: 101, 2013.

31. FB Thomsen and others. Active surveillance can reduce overtreatment in patients with low-risk prostate cancer. *Danish Medical Journal* 60.2: A4575, 2013.

32. ED Selvadurai and others. Medium-term outcomes of active surveillance for localised prostate cancer. *European Urology* 64.6: 981, 2013.

33. M Popiolek and others. Natural history of early, localized prostate cancer: A final report from three decades of follow-up. *European Urology* 63.3: 428, 2013.

34. HA Vargas and others. Magnetic resonance imaging for predicting prostate biopsy findings in patients considered for active surveillance of clinically low risk prostate cancer. *Journal of Urology* 188.5: 1732, 2012.

35. Y Krakowsky and others. Prostate cancer death of men treated with initial active surveillance: clinical and biochemical characteristics. *Journal of Urology* 184.1: 131, 2010.

36. AJ Vickers and others. Systematic review of pretreatment prostate-specific antigen velocity and doubling time as predictors for prostate cancer. *Journal of Clinical Oncology* 27.3: 398, 2009.

37. A Loblaw and others. Comparing prostate specific antigen triggers for intervention in men with stable prostate cancer on active surveillance. *Journal of Urology* 184.5: 1942, 2010.

Chapter 10

FOCAL CRYOSURGERY

Duke Bahn, MD

*Prostate cancer comes in two forms, slow
growing and extremely slow growing.*
RALPH BLUM

THE EXTREMELY SLOW RATE of disease progression of localized
prostate cancer makes it difficult to develop a national consensus
regarding optimal treatment. This conundrum is further complicated by
early-detection strategies that are diagnosing thousands of men with very
small-volume, low-grade cancers that may not adversely affect survival.

Current treatment options are either active surveillance or radical intervention, such as surgery, radiation, or brachytherapy. Radical
therapy maximizes cancer control but is associated with sexual and
urinary complications. Active surveillance does not impact a patient's
sexual and urinary function, but reliance on constant monitoring and
periodic biopsy is a burden.

TARGETED FOCAL CRYOABLATION

When newly diagnosed, many prostate cancers are at a very early stage and localized in one lobe of the prostate. It is estimated that as many as a third of newly diagnosed men have only one spot of cancer. These are the patients who may be candidates for *focal* treatment. Focal cryotherapy is defined as the ablation—destruction—of a *section* of the prostate gland with ice. The known tumor site is treated, but the other lobe and surrounding structures are spared. The goal is to offer *targeted* local cancer control that maintains the preservation of sexual potency and urinary continence.

Multiple large, single-institution case studies and prospective trials have been reported for *total* cryoablation of the prostate. The cure rates, as measured by PSA status or negative biopsy rates, are comparable to surgery and radiation. However, there is a high incidence of erectile dysfunction and a small risk of incontinence in men undergoing *total* cryoablation.

Focal cryoablation provides acceptable cancer control rates while dramatically improving the chances of preserving sexual potency and urinary continence. *Focal* cryoablation, therefore, fills a niche between active surveillance on the one hand and radical therapy (surgery, radiation, or brachytherapy) on the other.

DEFINITION OF FOCAL THERAPY

There is no widely agreed upon simple definition of "focal therapy." Some researchers treat only the areas of known cancer, while others treat up to half of the prostate. Some researchers have even proposed treating the entire gland, excluding the nerves controlling erections that are located on the opposite side of the prostate to the tumor. This approach is termed "subtotal therapy" instead of "focal therapy."

PATIENT SELECTION FOR FOCAL CRYOABLATION

To be considered for focal cryoablation, the patient must have unilateral prostate cancer, that is, cancer in only one lobe. At the Prostate Institute of America, we perform a staging color Doppler ultrasound (Chapter 5) along with a *staging* biopsy (in addition to the initial random 12-core biopsy that was, usually, already performed by the patient's urologist). A staging biopsy, in my practice, targets all suspicious lesions detected by color Doppler ultrasound. Some centers advocate a *saturation* biopsy with 20 to 40 cores to confirm the absence of any additional tumor in the other lobe. Whatever system is used, if an unexpected cancer is found in the other lobe, the patient is no longer considered a candidate for focal cryotherapy.

In general, men with *Sky* are the preferred candidates for focal treatment, but *Teal* and even *Azure* cancers can also be considered. *Unilaterality*—the cancer being confined in one lobe—is the defining issue, not the PSA level or Gleason grade. Men with extra-capsular extension (disease that has extended outside the prostate capsule) or seminal vesicle invasion are also candidates for focal therapy, as long as the cancer is proven to be unilateral. Focal cryotherapy may also be offered as a salvage therapy for *Indigo* (relapsed disease after any type of organ-preserving treatment, such as radiation, cryotherapy, HIFU, or photodynamic therapy), as long as the recurrent disease is unilateral.

METHODS

The cryoablation procedure uses an extremely cold temperature to destroy the cancer tissue by circulating subzero Argon gas through cryoprobes strategically placed in the prostate. An expanding ice ball forms at the end of the cryoprobe. Argon is circulated for cooling, helium for warming. With the patient under general anesthesia or spinal block, the cryoprobes are placed via ultrasound guidance. If seminal vesicle invasion is present, a probe is placed in the seminal vesicle. Usually two to four cryoprobes are used, depending on the size of the lesion and the size of the prostate. A single probe may also be placed in the contralateral (opposite) lobe close to the urethra and external sphincter for warming purposes (to protect these structures from damage). A warming device to protect the urethra is also used.

This combination of aggressive freezing at targeted locations within the prostate (while maintaining the integrity of the urethra, external sphincter, and contralateral lobe, including the neurovascular bundle), is the premise of focal cryoablation. Cryotherapy can be an outpatient procedure performed at a same-day surgery facility. However, it is often convenient for the patient to remain for overnight observation and discharged on the following day, with a Foley catheter in his bladder that is then usually removed after three to five days.

After treatment, a surveillance protocol is followed that is very similar to the protocol used for active surveillance. PSA levels should be performed every three months for one year and every six months thereafter. Scanning with color Doppler, multiparametric MRI, or both is performed once a year.

SCIENTIFIC STUDIES SUPPORTING FOCAL CRYOABLATION

The scientific studies published on focal cryoablation show encouraging results. At the Prostate Institute of America, we evaluated 73 men with unilateral *Sky* or unilateral *Teal* cancer who were followed for a median of 3.7 years after focal cryoablation. There were no deaths or metastatic disease. No patient developed urinary incontinence. Potency sufficient for intercourse was preserved in 86 percent of patients. Only four (5.7 percent) of 70 patients needed further treatment for cancer. Three patients underwent a second round of focal cryotherapy and one had radiation therapy.

In a study that compared our focally treated patients with men at another center who had surgery, 8.8 percent of the surgically treated patients needed salvage therapy, compared with only 5.7 percent of those focally treated. The outcome of focal cryotherapy was therefore equal to surgery, with a significantly lower incidence of side effects and complications. The results of focal cryotherapy performed at other centers, as well as at ours, is presented in the table:

	Bahn	Lambert	Ellis	*Ward
Number of Patients	73	25	60	1160
Median Age	64	68	69	68
Years Follow-up	3.7	2.3	1.3	1.8
Gleason 6	30	13	47	844
Gleason 7	43	12	12	240
Gleason >7			1	64
Stage T1c	41	25	55	
Stage T2a	31		5	1013
Stage T2b	1			147
Stable PSA (%)	85	85	80.4	75
Incontinence (%)	0	0	3.6	1.6
Potency (%)	86	71	71	58

Data from COLD [Cryo On-line Database] registry.

OTHER TYPES OF FOCAL TECHNOLOGY

There are many other technologies that may turn out to be equally effective for administering focal therapy, such as High Intensity Focused Ultrasound (HIFU), Radiofrequency Tumor Ablation (RFTA), Microwave Thermal Ablation (MTA), Photodynamic Therapy (PDT), Focal Brachytherapy, or Nanotech-Laser treatment. Focal therapy, accomplished by these other methodologies, however, is a very new area of prostate cancer therapy. They are new because these other methodologies rely on multiparametric MRI imaging to guide treatment. Only recently has multiparametric MRI technology advanced enough to accurately guide treatment for focal therapy. Therefore, there is relatively little long-term experience at other centers offering focal therapy. Our reliance at the Prostate Institute of America on color Doppler, an imaging technology that has existed for over 20 years, has enabled us to hone our cryotherapy skills and build up clinical experience for more than 10 years.

To review, there are three essential criteria for successful focal treatment:

1. "Imaging visibility" on scanning is necessary to achieve precise cancer mapping for successful focal therapy. Without clear identification of the tumor, focal therapy will end up being a blind approach, resulting in a suboptimal outcome.

2. Unilaterality of the tumor in the prostate. Careful staging is necessary to ensure that focal therapy is appropriate. The risk of incomplete eradication of cancer is likely to be small in carefully screened men.

3. A skillful practitioner. Since only a portion of the prostate is targeted, precision targeting of the cancer is paramount. Experience, clinical judgment, and proper training are essential for obtaining consistently good results.

Assuming all three of these criteria are met, focal treatment offers the potential for excellent cancer control with a relatively low risk of erectile dysfunction and practically no risk of urinary problems.

References

1. DK Bahn and others. Focal prostate cryoablation: Initial results show cancer control and potency preservation. *Journal of Endourology* 20.9: 688, 2006.

2. GM Onik and others. "Male lumpectomy": Focal therapy for prostate cancer using cryoablation. *Urology* 70.6: S16, 2007.

3. JS Jones and others. Focal or subtotal therapy for early stage prostate cancer. *Current Treatment Options in Oncology* 8.3: 165, 2007.

4. MD Gillett and others. Tissue ablation technologies for localized prostate cancer. *Mayo Clinic Proceedings* 79.12: 1547, 2004.

5. TJ Polascik and others. Focal therapy for prostate cancer. *Current Opinion in Urology* 18.3: 269, 2008.

6. EH Lambert and others. Focal cryosurgery: Encouraging health outcomes for unifocal prostate cancer. *Urology* 69.6: 1117, 2007.

7. DK Bahn and others. Focal cryoablation of prostate: A review. *Scientific World Journal* 8: 486, 2008.

8. HD Nguyen and others. Focal cryotherapy in the treatment of localized prostate cancer. *Cancer Control* 20.3: 177, 2013.

9. DK Bahn and others. Focal cryotherapy for clinically unilateral, low-intermediate risk prostate cancer in 73 men with a median follow-up of 3.7 years. *European Urology* 62.1: 55, 2012.

10. RJ Babaian and others. Best practice statement on cryosurgery for the treatment of localized prostate cancer. *Journal of Urology* 180.5: 1993, 2008.

11. A Luis De Castro Abreu and others. Salvage focal and salvage total cryoablation for locally recurrent prostate cancer after primary radiation therapy. *BJU International* 112.3: 298, 2013.

Chapter 11
INTRODUCTION TO
TREATMENT-RELATED SIDE EFFECTS

Mark Scholz, MD

Long-range goals keep you from being
frustrated by short-term failures.
JAMES CASH PENNY

S URGERY AND RADIATION ARE known to cause irreversible side
effects. Side effects may be an acceptable price to pay if mortality
is reduced. And, prostate cancer survival rates with these treatment
regimens are amazingly good according to the American Cancer Society:

Mortality rate within the first five years after diagnosis: 1%
Mortality rate within the first 10 years after diagnosis: 2%
Mortality rate within the first 15 years after diagnosis: 4%

You might tend to think that these numbers are for *Sky*. No, they
include all five Stages of Blue! The fantastic survival rates for prostate

cancer patients are often overlooked because they are so different from other cancers. For example, colon cancer patients who relapse after surgery live an average of *13 months*. Prostate cancer patients who relapse after surgery live an average of *13 years!*

Keeping in mind the characteristically sluggish behavior of prostate cancer, let's consider another defining characteristic—its precarious location in the lower pelvis, positioned within millimeters of the bladder, the rectum and the nerves that control erections. Damage to these sensitive structures from treatment is very common.

The next three chapters review the common side effects from treatment. *Managing side effects is a gigantic industry.* Since patients in *Sky* are frequently advised to have treatment, they must be informed about the potential side effects. Many of these side effects are irreversible. Men in *Sky* have a *choice* to do active surveillance, a privilege unavailable to men in the other Stages of Blue (except for *Low-Teal*).

Patients routinely *underestimate* the side effects of surgery or radiation. They assume, perhaps, that it's like an appendectomy or gallbladder surgery. The doctors who administer surgery or radiation are poor sources of information about the risks. They become desensitized to treatment-related problems because they encounter them frequently in their everyday practice. They are not trying to be deceptive. They are influenced by a medical culture functioning on a false premise for the last 30 years—that every prostate cancer is life-threatening. With that mentality, collateral damage to a man's quality of life is easily justified; side effects are simply considered a necessary evil, inescapable in the normal process of saving lives. Doctors and patients alike become willing accomplices in the mutual underestimation of treatment-related risks.

The goal for the following chapters, therefore, is to educate men about what it takes to recover from treatment-related damage, if recovery is even possible. In addition, the following chapters will convey a realistic understanding of the risks related to standard treatment. For men in *Sky*, shedding light on side effects is more important than talking about cure rates. Mortality from *Sky* is extremely rare. However, treatment-related side effects are the norm. With *Sky*, preserving *quality of life* deserves as much attention as protecting longevity.

In the rush to achieve a cure, it is common for concerned patients to assume that side effects won't happen. This type of irrational reasoning needs to be countered. Men need to *visualize* what it would be like to visit a doctor to deal with leaking urine, sexual dysfunction, burning pain in the rectum, or a crooked penis. The following chapters, by world-class experts who specialize in correcting these frustrating side effects, are written for this purpose, to describe the problems that occur so commonly after treatment. The mad rush to treatment is energized by an impatient desire to "get the problem out." Men need to slow down and "count the cost," *in advance*. Careful investigation of the potential problems associated with treatment is the only way to avoid being stuck with unnecessary and permanent negative consequences.

Chapter 12
SEXUAL DYSFUNCTION

Kelly Chiles, MD
and
John Mulhall, MD

Perspective is the cure for depression.
BONO

THIS CHAPTER WILL DISCUSS A VARIETY of sexual dysfunctions that may occur after the treatment of prostate cancer. In addition, we will provide the means by which physicians can help in the management of sexual dysfunction. We will also introduce the concept of "penile rehabilitation" as a way of improving sexual outcomes. This frank discussion about sexual changes is not meant to frighten or cause anxiety. However, only by gaining a full understanding of problems that may arise, can an informed decision be made about how to manage prostate cancer.

ERECTILE DYSFUNCTION

Erectile dysfunction, commonly referred to as "ED," is the inability to either achieve or maintain an erection that is hard enough to take part in satisfactory sexual relations. Inability to maintain an erection means that some men may be able to get hard enough for penetration but then lose their erections too quickly—often just before penetration or during intercourse. Other men who have difficulty achieving erections may not achieve sufficient hardness for penetration, even though they stay somewhat hard for longer periods of time, while other men with ED may suffer from both: difficulty achieving and maintaining erections.

In order to understand what erectile dysfunction is and how prostate cancer treatment can cause it, it is important to know how erections normally work. The penis is actually a hydraulic pump with inflow provided by the arteries and outflow by the veins, and a few bells and whistles such as nerves and blood vessels. The two "erectile bodies" known as the *corpora cavernosa* are the specific parts of the penis that get hard during erection by becoming engorged with blood. An erection occurs when the inflow of blood into the erectile bodies via arteries exceeds the outflow of blood via veins, causing the penis to get larger and harder. Once you understand the anatomy, it is easy to see why a problem with too little arterial inflow, called "arterial insufficiency," or too much blood leaking through the veins, called "venous leak," can cause problems with erections.

In addition, the nerves that "switch" erections on and off pass directly alongside the prostate on their way from the spinal cord to the penis. The nerves, known as the "neurovascular bundle" because they are often intertwined with blood vessels, are so fine and thinly distributed that a high degree of skill is required for surgeons to perform a "nerve-sparing" prostatectomy. (Think about removing the skin from an apple.) Damage to these nerves can cause problems with erections because the neurovascular bundle is responsible for flipping the "switch" that releases nitric oxide, the molecule that promotes blood flow into the *corpora cavernosa*.

It is important to understand that the nerves that cause erections and keep the penis tissue healthy are entirely separate from the nerves that give the penis its tactile sexual sensations. The sensation nerves are not at risk of damage from prostate cancer treatment, because they are located far from where the prostatectomy surgery is performed. Therefore, penile sensation will usually be unaffected by any treatment you choose; when we talk about nerve damage, we specifically mean the nerves next to the prostate that cause erections.

Importantly, radiation treatment also causes ED through the same mechanism as surgery—by damaging these same nerves and vessels in the neurovascular bundle and by causing erectile tissue damage. Radiation treatment can take several forms, and the regimens are constantly changing. When we use the term "radiation," we are describing either external radiation, which is a broad term used to describe several different ways of delivering radiation beams to the prostate, or radioactive pellets or seeds that are surgically implanted into the prostate, a technique known as brachytherapy. When considering multiple different treatment possibilities, the question that men need to ask is, "What is my individual risk of sexual dysfunction after treatment of prostate cancer?"

Erectile dysfunction is a risk in every type of treatment for prostate cancer, but the exact risk that each treatment poses is very specific to each patient. In general, the better a man's erections are before prostate cancer treatment, the better chance he has of preserving his erectile function, no matter what treatment he chooses. Men who already have difficulty getting hard or staying hard are at greatest risk for permanent ED, regardless of the type of treatment. In fact, we very clearly see that one of the biggest risk factors for ED after prostate cancer treatment is having any decrease in erection quality before treatment. Additional factors that will affect the development of erectile dysfunction include one's age and overall general health. We will later discuss the types of lifestyle changes that can improve sexual function outcomes.

It is important to understand that there is one clear difference between surgery and radiation, and that is when the ED will occur. After *surgery*, men have an immediate, almost complete loss of erections, unless they use erection aids like pills or injections. ED after surgery often, but not always, improves over time. This improvement can take up to two years or, in some cases, longer. After *radiation*, men do not encounter an immediate loss of function. However, ED can slowly develop over the ensuing two to five years or, in some cases, longer. When men receive hormone therapy along with their radiation, erectile function will definitely worsen.

So what is the rate of ED after surgery or radiation? Individual surgeons have different degrees of success. The literature that has been published to date shows that results are heavily dependent on the surgeon's ability. However, even in the hands of the finest surgeons *only about 15 percent of men will have the same erectile function two years after surgery as they had prior to surgery.* With the advent of many erection aids, which we will discuss later, a significant number of men will be able to have satisfying sexual relations after their prostate cancer treatment.

A third treatment option that is known to cause ED is hormone treatment, also known as "androgen deprivation therapy" or "testosterone inactivating pharmaceuticals" (TIP). Doctors can use TIP alone or in conjunction with either surgery or radiation. The duration of TIP treatment varies, depending on the reasons why your doctor has recommended it. The longer a man is treated with TIP, the greater the impact on the quality of his erections. Short-term hormone treatment (four months or less) is unlikely to cause a permanent change in penile tissues, even though erections will probably decrease in frequency and quality while under treatment, as will sex drive. Longer treatment with TIP will likely cause damage to one's erectile tissue. (Think of this as "atrophy," or wasting away of tissue, which leads to a leaky valve in the penis, the condition known as "venous leak"). Once these tissue changes occur, they will be permanent and cannot be reversed.

CHANGES IN EJACULATION AND ORGASM

Many men and their partners are surprised to learn that changes in ejaculation or orgasm can and frequently do occur after prostate cancer treatment. Orgasm is the "sensation" that occurs with climax, and, although it occurs at the same time, this is separate from ejaculation in men, which is the process of fluid ejection from the penis. Importantly, *orgasm can occur without an erection,* and ED does not prevent men from achieving orgasm. Ejaculation and orgasm must be considered separately, because different things happen each after treatment.

Men will no longer ejaculate after surgery, as the prostate and semi-nal vesicles, which are responsible for 95 percent of semen production, are removed. After radiation, the vast majority of men will, over time, also develop dry orgasms, (i.e., orgasms without ejaculation). Indeed, 70 percent of men three years after radiation therapy, and 90 percent of men at five years, will no longer ejaculate fluid when their orgasm occurs. In addition, hormone therapy will also decrease the volume of ejaculate, often to zero. Thus, ejaculation will be affected by any treatment of prostate cancer. The only difference is when the changes will appear.

Orgasm, however, is a very different story. The sensation of orgasm is produced in the brain but is accompanied by the rhythmic contrac-tions of muscles around the penis that cause a throbbing sensation. This muscular mechanism should be unaffected by surgery. Interestingly, 5 to 10 percent of men consider their orgasms "better" or "more intense" after prostatectomy, and 25 to 30 percent of men have no change in orgasm sensation. An additional 33 percent of men complain of decreased orgas-mic intensity. The reason for this is poorly understood, but some experts think this might be due to dry orgasms. However, up to 33 percent of men are unable to reach orgasm after surgery, a condition known as "anorgasmia." Our experience leads us to believe the reason that those men who could achieve orgasm prior to prostate surgery, but become anorgasmic after surgery, is largely psychological.

Orgasm changes also occur at about the same frequency with radiation or TIP as with surgery. In our experience, radiation treatment has the same potential to cause orgasm changes as surgery, albeit over a longer time. Furthermore, it is very common that men on TIP fail to accomplish orgasm. Unfortunately, there is very little research into the causes of orgasm changes after radiation or TIP.

The struggle to reach orgasm after treatment may have other causes. The most common ones (not specifically in men with prostate cancer) include the use of antidepressant medications, low testosterone level, loss of penile sensation, and psychological problems. Some men welcome the "increased staying power" associated with this delay. However, many men find it frustrating. In particular, if the physical exertion associated with trying to achieve an orgasm becomes too great, a man can become too tired to continue, and delayed orgasm can turn into anorgasmia. Regardless, men who suffer from anorgasmia or delayed orgasm are treatable.

Painful orgasm (known as "dysorgasmia") can also occur after prostate cancer treatment. Although typically mild and generally lasting less than a minute, this discomfort can be significant enough to discourage a man from pursuing sexual activity. This pain is believed to be due to muscle spasms in the bladder neck and may improve with medications in the "alpha-blockers" family, which function by relaxing the bladder neck. Dysorgasmia will usually resolve over time, even without treatment.

Another change some men experience after surgery is urinary incontinence during sex. There are some men who leak urine when they are being sexually stimulated (called "arousal incontinence") or when they reach orgasm (called "climacturia"). These two issues will be discussed in detail in the next chapter, but it is important to realize that urinary issues could overlap with sexual dysfunction after prostate cancer treatment.

PENILE SIZE AND SHAPE CHANGES

One of the most devastating consequences of prostate cancer treatment involves the change in penile size: penile shrinkage. This involves not only a reduction in length, but also a decrease in girth. It is estimated that about 70 percent of men will observe a change in the size of the penis after surgery. On average there is about a one cm (.394 inch) loss of length. It is important to appreciate that, while there are only a few studies that look at penis-size changes after surgery, there are no studies that look at penis-size changes over time after radiation treatment. Recent evidence suggests that the loss of penile length can be offset with regular use of Viagra or Cialis.

LIBIDO CHANGES

"Libido" is another way to describe the *desire* or drive to take part in sexual activity. Libido loss is generally attributed to one of three things: hormone changes, medication use and psychological issues. In some men, the diagnosis of cancer alone can cause ED and decreased libido. One of the reasons this happens is because depression and anxiety can often develop after the diagnosis of cancer. Stressors completely unrelated to concerns about sexual function can also negatively impact erectile function and libido.

For instance, men who are following their PSA levels on active surveillance can become so consumed with this issue that they lose interest in sex or actually develop erection problems because of their preoccupation. Another example of how prostate cancer might negatively affect libido is found in men who develop some form of sexual dysfunction after treatment. Some men feel inadequate if their erections are changed, or fear that they cannot satisfy their partners or that they are no longer "as good as they were before." These feelings manifest themselves as "avoidance behavior." Men who suffer from this problem may end up avoiding participation in sexual activities altogether.

It is imperative for men and their partners to understand that there is a good chance for a psychological component to any sexual dysfunction, regardless of whether this dysfunction occurs before or after treatment for cancer. Fortunately, once identified, psychological sources of problems with erections and libido can be treated with appropriate counseling.

Obviously, not all men will have a psychological reason for their decreased libido. One of the more common correctable causes of decreased libido is a low testosterone level. While prostate cancer by itself may not cause low testosterone, the men who develop prostate cancer tend to be elderly, at an age when men typically experience low testosterone levels naturally. A very simple way for your physician to determine if low testosterone is affecting your libido is to do a blood test. Ideally, blood should be drawn before 10 a.m. (a time when testosterone is at its peak). If levels are too low, discuss with your physician whether testosterone replacement therapy is appropriate.

TIP medications are common culprits for medication-induced libido loss. Almost all men who are on TIP for a year or less will see their testosterone levels increase back to normal again within about a year after they stop their hormone treatments, whereas men with low testosterone from aging may not. However, about 15 percent of TIP patients will have a permanent decrease in testosterone level even after they stop their medications. Further help maintaining libido may be needed. In addition to hormone therapy, some antidepressants reduce libido. If you are on any of these medications and feel that you are suffering from decreased libido, you should discuss with a doctor the pros and cons of continuing the medications or changing to another type of antidepressant.

MANAGING ERECTILE DYSFUNCTION

The first step to minimizing the risk of ED starts even before a decision is finalized regarding how the prostate cancer will be treated. The single most important factor that predicts good erectile function after treatment is the quality of erectile function BEFORE any treatment. The health of the penis is maintained in the very same way as that of the heart. In fact, anything that is good for cardiovascular health is also good for penile health; and if it's bad for the heart, it's worse for the penis. Behaviors that improve penile function are eating a heart- and penis-healthy diet, quitting smoking, and exercising, as well as properly managing any chronic medical conditions such as high blood pressure, high cholesterol, or diabetes. As stated above, regardless of which treatment you choose, improving baseline penis health serves well for years to come. Because we know that not all men will return to their baseline erectile function after prostate cancer treatment, it is strongly suggested that you ask your doctor about methods to restore sexual fulfillment.

There are multiple ways that men can increase their erections. First-line treatment for men who have a decrease in erectile function is oral medication. All of the pills available in the US right now, such as Viagra, Levitra, Cialis and Stendra, belong to the same family: phosphodiesterase-5 inhibitors (PDE5i). Earlier in this chapter we talked about the steps involved in getting an erection, and one of those steps involves the release of nitric oxide (NO) from nerves that are part of the neurovascular bundle. NO helps relax the muscles, so blood flow into the penis increases greatly. A PDE5i will help maintain NO blood levels for a longer period of time than normal, and therefore the NO is continuously available to help relax the muscles.

How well a PDE5i works depends largely on how badly the nerves that trigger the release of NO were damaged from treatment; the only way a man can test his nerve function is through trying out a PDE5i after treatment. We recommend that even men who do not initially respond to PDE5i try these pills every now and then over time (months to years), because we know that nerves can heal and recover; some men who, for example, did not respond well to PDE5i immediately after surgery will become responsive to pills over time. Conversely, men who responded well to PDE5i immediately after radiation treatment might find that these pills become less effective over time, because the radiation damage takes years to develop. Furthermore, as with any pill, there are side effects and contraindications to using PDE5i. You cannot, for example, use PDE5i if you are taking certain medications such as nitrates. Doing so might cause headaches, vision changes (a blue halo effect), indigestion, or muscle aches.

What about other options besides pills? One extremely effective approach is to use "intracavernosal injections" (ICI). This involves using a small needle (much smaller than anything you would have ever seen used for drawing blood, for example) to inject medicine directly into the erection chambers of the penis. While this may initially be anxiety-provoking, it has proven to be very effective.

There are many formulations of medications and countless dosing regimens, so it is essential that your physician have broad familiarity with all the options. You must also have a detailed discussion with your physician—and preferably have something written out to refer to if the need arises—about what you do if you ever develop a prolonged erection, known as "priapism." While uncommon, priapism is a urologic emergency, so you must understand what to do in case of this emergency and have a plan in place.

Another way to deliver erection medication is by inserting a small pill in the urethra—the "pee channel"—and letting the penis absorb the medication. This is known as an "intraurethral alprostadil" (IUA) suppository. The most common trade name is "Muse." In our experience, IUA is not the most reliable way to produce erections. For example, a man who experienced a satisfactory erection the first time he used IUA might not get any erection the second time, and for no apparent reason. More importantly, many men claim that they have significantly more discomfort with this medication than with any other treatment option—including the injection. Because it is a medication that is very "hit or miss," and because it may cause the most discomfort of any medication we can prescribe, we don't often recommend it. Having said that, there are men in our practice who use IUA without any problems, and it is important for all men and their partners to know that IUA is an option.

Another option for increasing erectile rigidity and longevity is a vacuum erection device (VED). This involves inserting the penis into a plastic tube, which uses negative pressure to draw blood into the penis, and then slipping a ring around the base of the penis to keep the blood from draining out. As with any other erection aid, there are benefits and risks to this option, which include discomfort caused by the ring pinching the penis, and the risk that the penis could turn "cold and blue." However, it is a relatively inexpensive option compared with many medications, and it does not involve using needles or tolerating the side effects of PDE5i. For these reasons, many men feel that the VED is right for them.

The final treatment for ED is surgical. The inflatable penile prosthesis (IPP) can be used in men who do not achieve satisfactory erections through any of the previously described treatments. The IPP involves surgically inserting inflatable "balloons" into the penis. These balloons are connected by a small tube to a fluid-filled reservoir and pump, located in the abdomen and scrotum, respectively. The pump draws fluid out of the reservoir and into these balloons to produce an erection. When sex is over, a separate "deflate" button causes the pump to drain the balloons and let the fluid go back into the reservoir. Obviously, because this is the most invasive treatment for ED, it should be considered last. There are risks inherent in any surgery, including infection. Mechanical failure of the pump, with the need for further surgery, is also a risk.

This section was merely an overview, to give you an idea about how we help men manage ED and, for this reason, it was not all-inclusive. The most important thing to understand is that there are many pathways to the recovery of satisfying sexual relations. A doctor who is experienced with ALL the erectile aid options can help a man choose the best path to follow.

PENILE REHABILITATION

The concept behind penile rehabilitation involves the acknowledgement that the penis, like any muscle that needs to be exercised, is meant to have frequent erections. Otherwise, the ability to achieve an erection will be lost. Healthy men have up to six nocturnal erections a night. At our institution, we believe that the purpose of nocturnal erections is to keep the penile tissue (all the nerves, blood vessels, and muscle) in good working order, whether or not a man is sexually active.

Immediately after surgery, most men (regardless of whether or not the surgeon was successful at saving the critical nerves that enable erections) stop having nocturnal erections. This can persist for months. In our opinion, anything we can do to replicate nature's intent (that men should have nocturnal erections) is good for the penis. This proactive approach to the treatment of sexual dysfunction is called "penile rehabilitation" (PR). This means that not only do we recommend and encourage PR after surgery, we also want men undergoing radiation treatment to be proactive about their penis health.

So, what exactly is PR? PR entails taking a small dose of a PDE5i every day (usually a quarter of the maximal dose—one pill split up into four parts) and taking a maximum dose of PDE5i (one full pill) once a week. The daily small dose is based on the theory that PDE5i does multiple things in addition to increasing NO for erections—PDE5i also protects the penile tissue from atrophy and scarring. The full-dose pill is taken to ensure that a hard erection occurs at least once a week (just as nocturnal erections help keep the penis healthy).

One of the most important ways to keep the penis healthy is to regain erectile function as soon as possible after prostate cancer treatment. If the maximum dose of a PDE5i is ineffective, we switch the regimen to maintaining the same small *daily* dose of PDE5i, but instead of a maximum-dose PDE5i pill, we advocate using injections to achieve erections. In our experience, men who stick to the PR regimen are more satisfied with their sexual function than men who do not participate in PR.

So why doesn't every doctor put their prostate cancer patients on a PR regimen? It's important to realize that our opinions regarding the usefulness of PR are just "expert opinion," but that, as yet, there is no conclusive research published to support our claims. While we think that the preliminary research published to date strongly suggests that PR works, there are weaknesses in the studies that some doctors take as evidence that PR is not worth the time or the money. In our expert opinion, however, everything a man can do to keep his penis healthy is worth doing, because we know that many of the changes resulting from disuse are irreversible.

CONCLUSION

Sexual dysfunction after a man is diagnosed with prostate cancer takes many forms. Although we know that the vast majority of men will see some decline relative to their baseline erectile function, we have ways to treat this. The most important goal is to find a healthcare provider who appreciates how critically important sexual side effects are and has the knowledge about preventive care and the skills to manage all forms of dysfunction. Choose an experienced surgeon or radiologist with a proven track record of successful treatment.

References

1. JP Mulhall. *Saving Your Sex Life: A Guide for Men with Prostate Cancer.* 1st ed. Munster: Hilton Publishing, 2008.

2. BA Sherer and LA Levine. Current management of erectile dysfunction in prostate cancer survivors. *Current Opinion in Urology* 24.4: 401, 2014.

3. E Chung and G Brock. Sexual rehabilitation and cancer survivorship: A state of art review of current literature and management strategies in male sexual dysfunction among prostate cancer survivors. *Journal of Sexual Medicine* 10.S1: 102, 2013.

4. CR Mazzola and JP Mulhall. Impact of androgen deprivation therapy on sexual function. *Asian Journal of Andrology* 14.2: 198, 2012.

5. Prediction Tools–A Tool for Doctors and Patients. nomograms.org

Chapter 13

SURGICAL SIDE EFFECTS AFFECTING URINATION

Gary Leach, MD

Start by doing what's necessary; then do what's possible;
and suddenly you are doing the impossible.
FRANCIS OF ASSISI

INCONTINENCE

Loss of bladder control (urinary incontinence) after prostate surgery can be a devastating complication that can have a very negative impact on quality of life. The good news is that, with appropriate evaluation and treatment, incontinence is usually treatable.

PERCENTAGE OF MEN WITH BLADDER CONTROL PROBLEMS AFTER TREATMENT

Bladder control problems for the first few months following radical prostatectomy are to be expected. A biofeedback program (explained later) may be helpful during this period to help restore bladder control.

When urinary incontinence persists for more than three to six months, appropriate bladder testing, called "urodynamics," is critical to evaluate the function of the bladder and sphincter (valve) muscle to determine the exact cause. Urodynamic testing is performed in the doctor's office and takes about 20 minutes. It involves filling the bladder through a special catheter inserted into the penis while measuring pressures in the bladder. During the test, various maneuvers are performed to evaluate the muscular function of the bladder wall and to evaluate the ability of the urinary sphincter to control the flow. Basically, the goal is to define the cause of the urine loss.

Normally, as the bladder fills to capacity, there is very little change in bladder pressure and the sphincter remains closed, allowing a man to stay dry. When incontinence occurs following prostatectomy, this normal balance of bladder pressure and sphincter strength is disturbed.

Our own internal research has defined three main causes of incontinence based upon urodynamic findings, listed below. (Note that these percentages are not necessarily applicable to all prostate cancer patients but represent the patients who came to us for help with incontinence).

1. High bladder pressure with muscular "spasms" of the bladder that develop as the bladder fills occurs in **50 percent of men.** It is possible that these bladder spasms are related to nerve damage from prostatectomy. Bladder spasms may cause urge incontinence (the need to rush to get to the bathroom), frequent urination, and, sometimes, loss of urine at night. This type of "high-pressure" bladder dysfunction can also occur following pelvic radiation therapy.

2. Damage to the sphincter muscle occurs in **35 percent of men** after surgery. This results in stress incontinence with loss of urine during change in position, coughing, straining, or vigorous physical activity.

3. A *combination* of bladder spasms and sphincter damage occurs **10 percent of the time.** Men with this combined problem usually experience "mixed incontinence" symptoms, with a combination of both urge and stress incontinence.

BIOFEEDBACK

Biofeedback is also known as "Pelvic Floor Training." It may be the preferred treatment choice in men who desire immediate treatment for urine loss right after surgery. Biofeedback is also useful for long-standing incontinence of lesser severity. The treatment program involves weekly one-hour visits with a trained therapist. A special sensor is inserted into the rectum and attached to a biofeedback computer. During the treatment session, the patient is taught to contract and strengthen the pelvic muscles. His muscular contraction is displayed on a computer screen. Also, an electrical signal can be sent to his pelvic muscles to further strengthen them. Each week, the goal is to make the muscles progressively stronger through repetition. Many men experience significant improvement in bladder control with this biofeedback program.

When the main reason for incontinence is high bladder pressure, medications such as Enablex, Vesicare, Ditropan XL, Detrol LA, the Oxytrol patch, oxybutynin 3% gel and imipramine can relax the muscle in the bladder wall. Common side effects are dry mouth, constipation, and blurry vision. These drugs can't be used in patients with glaucoma or in men who do not empty their bladder well. A new medication, Myrbetriq, does not cause dry mouth or constipation. However, 10 percent of the men who take Myrbetriq will have an increase in blood pressure.

Another option for controlling high bladder pressures, when oral medications are not successful, is Botox injections into the bladder delivered through a scope inserted in the penis. The success rate is approximately 50 percent and the effects usually last for three to six months. There is, however, a five percent risk of urinary retention, necessitating self-catheterization three to four times per day until the effect wears off.

INTERSTIM BLADDER PACEMAKER

When the treatments to decrease high bladder pressures such as those described earlier are unsuccessful, the Interstim "bladder pacemaker" may be an excellent alternative. To determine if Interstim is likely to be effective, an initial one-week test with an external battery pack delivers an electrical signal that "tells" the bladder to relax. If the initial test is successful, about 70 percent of men will benefit by surgical placement of an internal Interstim device.

The permanent Interstim device requires placement of a stimulation electrode in the lower back, next to the main nerve that controls the bladder. Separately, an internal "pacemaker" generator that is attached to the stimulation electrode is implanted. The generator is similar to a heart pacemaker, with a battery that usually lasts eight to 10 years. This "bladder pacemaker" only helps patients who have bladder dysfunction from an overactive, spasmodic bladder wall.

MEN WHO HAVE SPHINCTER DAMAGE

Options for the treatment of sphincter damage include biofeedback, surgical placement of an artificial urinary sphincter, and a surgical procedure called the "male sling." Men with "mixed" bladder and sphincter malfunction usually undergo initial treatment with anticholinergic drugs or Botox to improve their bladder function and lower their bladder pressures. If that is successful, subsequent treatment to address the weak sphincter may be considered. The urodynamic studies described above are repeated periodically to evaluate the response to each stage of therapy.

THE ARTIFICIAL URINARY SPHINCTER (AUS)

The artificial urinary sphincter is used to correct incontinence in men with sphincter damage. The AUS has three components: a cuff that surrounds and helps close the urethra, a pump placed inside the scrotum, and a pressure-regulating balloon that is placed in the lower abdomen (See Figure). When a man wants to urinate, he squeezes the pump in the scrotum, which opens the cuff around the urethra.

After three to five minutes, the fluid returns into the cuff, causing it to close automatically.

Figure: Artificial Urinary Sphincter in place.

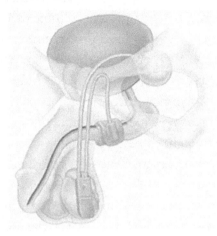

With the current model of the AUS, the mechanical malfunction rate is 15 percent at 10 years. However, despite these favorable results, some men are attracted to a less-extensive surgical procedure. For these men, as well as for those with more minor degrees of incontinence, the male sling is a promising alternative.

MALE SLING PROCEDURE

The best candidates for the male sling are men with more minor degrees of stress incontinence (using only one pad per day) and men with no previous history of pelvic radiation therapy. The sling *compresses* the urethra to reduce the risk of urine loss with coughing, sneezing, or vigorous activity. Surgical implantation takes about one hour and is placed via an incision between the scrotum and rectum. A catheter is usually left in place for 24 hours, with most men being able to urinate with good control immediately after the catheter is removed. Approximately 30 percent of men are completely dry, 40 percent are significantly improved, and 30 percent show no improvement. Should the male sling prove ineffective, an artificial urinary sphincter is often considered as a backup alternative.

CLIMACTURIA: EJACULATION OF URINE

"Climacturia" is defined as ejaculating urine at the moment of orgasm. Although the exact number of cases of climacturia after surgery for prostate cancer is unknown, different studies have estimated the incidence to be between 20 percent and 95 percent! Climacturia is thought to be more common in men who also have posttreatment erectile dysfunction and those who complain of penile shortening. Although the exact mechanism of climacturia has not been well studied, men who have climacturia usually have urinary incontinence as well. Thus, the pooling of urine in the urethra, along with relaxation of the sphincter mechanism during orgasm, are thought to be predisposing factors for climacturia. As a result of this problem, many men suffer from decreased libido and decreased sexual satisfaction.

Treatment suggestions for climacturia have included behavior modification (urinating before sexual activity), the use of condoms, and the use of a constriction ring at the base of the penis during intercourse. Although the results of these various treatments have not been well studied, patients should be informed regarding the possibility of this rather common posttreatment complication of radical prostatectomy, which can have a very significant impact on quality of life. Though there is very limited data, complaints of climacturia after radiation or focal therapy have been very uncommon.

STRICTURE

"Urethral stricture," scarring and constriction of the urethra, may occur after any invasive treatment of prostate cancer. Recent literature suggests that robotic prostatectomy is associated with much lower rates of urethral stricture than older surgical techniques, occurring in about two percent of men. Most strictures develop within three to six months of treatment. Stricture is also frequently associated with urinary incontinence (which commonly becomes even worse after stricture treatment).

Stricture treatment options include dilation of the stricture, incision of the stricture area, repeated self-catheterization and, in rare cases, major urethral reconstruction. The treatment of incontinence with any of the invasive options listed above should be postponed for at least three to six months to ensure that "stability" has been achieved, confirming that further stricture recurrence has been avoided.

SUMMARY

Recent advances in the evaluation and treatment of men with incontinence following prostate surgery offer hope for men to regain their urinary control and improve their quality of life. Men with significant incontinence following treatment for prostate cancer should have an appropriate evaluation (including urodynamic testing) to determine the exact cause of their incontinence. Appropriate treatment based upon the results of this testing usually results in significant restoration of bladder control and improvement in quality of life. Both climacturia and urethral stricture are potential complications following prostate surgery, with a major negative impact on quality of life.

References

1. GE Leach and others. Post-prostatectomy incontinence: Urodynamic findings and treatment outcomes. *Journal of Urology* 155.4: 1256, 1996.

2. F Haab and others. Quality of life and continence assessment of the artificial urinary sphincter in men with minimum 3.5 years of followup. *Journal of Urology* 158.2: 435, 1997.

3. E Chung and G Brock. Sexual rehabilitation and cancer survivorship: A state of art review of current literature and management strategies in male sexual dysfunction among prostate cancer survivors. *Journal of Sexual Medicine* 10.S1: 102, 2013.

4. R Wang and others. Risk factors and quality of life for post-prostatectomy vesicourethral anastomotic stenoses. *Urology* 79.2: 449, 2012.

Chapter 14

SIDE EFFECTS FROM RADIATION THERAPY

Henry Yampolsky, MD

"Side effects have been documented," he admits. "In a very small percentage of cases. Less than two percent."

"What kind of side effects?" Suddenly I'm feeling nauseous. Feels like the ants are crawling around inside me now, which is exactly as disturbing as it sounds.

"Memory loss. Synesthesia. And occasionally … vestigial growths."

"So I could forget my own name, start smelling purple everywhere and have an extra nipple sprout from my forehead?"

D.D. Barant

R ADIATION THERAPY FOR PROSTATE CANCER may cause short-term or long-term side effects. Radiation kills cancer by damaging the DNA of cancer cells. Even though the cancer cells are targeted, normal body tissues near the tumor can be affected. Fortunately, the normal body tissues are much better at repairing radiation damage than cancer cells (the poor radiation repair mechanisms of cancer cells may be a prerequisite for their capacity to sustain unrestrained growth).

Most radiation side effects are due to its effects on the adjacent organs. The organs located near the prostate or near the lymph nodes in the pelvis are most at risk. Specifically, we are talking about the rectum, small bowel, bladder, urethra, bone marrow, skin, and sexual organs. If these normal organs repair incompletely, the radiation effects may devolve into scar tissue, which can lead to long-term problems. Fortunately, most short-term side effects usually resolve within one to two months after completion of treatment. Long-term side effects, which are more rare than short-term side effects, can start right after radiation and last for years.

FATIGUE

There is one "global" radiation-related side effect—fatigue. Radiation-related fatigue is thought to be due to the release of inflammatory cyto-kines that circulate throughout the body via the bloodstream. Hormonal therapy, which is often used along with radiation, can also cause fatigue. The time course of fatigue from radiation is as follows: Once radiation to the prostate is initiated, fatigue may begin to be noticeable after two weeks or so. The maximum level of fatigue usually occurs after about four weeks of treatment and persists until the end of treatment. After the radiation is complete, normal energy levels typically recover in four to eight weeks. Evidence from a randomized trial performed in England[1] suggests that moderate-intensity exercise—walking 30 minutes at least three days each week—substantially reduced fatigue. Therefore, moderate-intensity aerobic exercise (walking, swimming, cycling) should be encouraged for all men who undergo prostate radiation.

GASTROINTESTINAL SYSTEM

Radiation can injure the bowel by delaying cell repopulation on the inner ("mucosal") wall of the intestine, resulting in inflammation and swelling of the bowel lining. These effects, if they occur, tend to begin

10 to 14 days after radiotherapy is started. Fortunately, after completion of the radiation, the body usually repairs the damage. However, in some cases, scar tissue leads to aberrant blood vessel formation and chronic inflammation of the intestinal lining that can persist for years after radiation treatment. Chronic symptoms from bowel damage are similar to those that occur in people with "irritable bowel syndrome" or IBS, mainly intermittent stomach bloating and discomfort. They also may have alternating problems with loose stools and constipation. These potential side effects can affect the large intestine, the small intestine, and the rectum. Symptomatic management with antispasmodic medication is the mainstay of therapy.

RECTUM

The frequency of rectal complications due to prostate radiotherapy has declined significantly in the 21st century with the use of intensity-modulated radiation therapy (IMRT) and image-guided radiation therapy (IGRT). These technologies allow much more accurate targeting, thus reducing the amount of rectal tissue exposed to radiation. Short-term rectal side effects are usually mild in intensity and may include increased bowel movement frequency, painful defecation, and blood in the stool. These effects occur in 5 to 10 percent of patients and usually appear during the third or fourth week of treatment, reaching maximum intensity toward the end of treatment, and dissipating four to eight weeks following completion of treatment.[2] Most patients are able to complete a standard course of radiation without any specific treatment, although in some cases dietary modifications and anti-inflammatory rectal steroid suppositories are required. Long-term rectal side effects are uncommon but may include chronic bowel frequency, rectal bleeding, and pain. In a study by Memorial Sloan Kettering Cancer Center using modern radiation therapy, gastrointestinal complications requiring *noninvasive* intervention occurred in 1.5 percent of patients treated with IMRT and in approximately five percent of patients treated with radioactive seed implants (brachytherapy), while complications requiring *invasive* interventions were reported in fewer than one percent of patients treated with either technique.[3] Steroid suppositories can ease symptoms, and in cases of significant rectal bleeding, a formaldehyde enema has been shown to be effective.[4] Severe long-term rectal complications, such as loss of anal sphincter control or "fistula" (a passageway connecting the rectum and another organ such as the bladder), are rare and occur in less than one in 1,000 treated patients.[5] It should be emphasized that these statistics are from a high-volume center of excellence utilizing state-of-the-art equipment and highly trained personnel. The risk of serious side effects is probably greater in radiation centers that do a smaller volume of business.

A new treatment called SpaceOAR can prevent rectal damage from radiation. SpaceOAR is a gel injected between the prostate and the rectal wall to create a separation large enough that rectal wall exposure to radiation is greatly reduced. SpaceOAR makes sense, and the clinical trials leading up to FDA approval have demonstrated a low incidence of rectal problems with SpaceOAR. SpaceOAR is new, so insurance coverage may be lacking. Even so, reducing the risk of rectal toxicity may be worth the out-of-pocket costs to patients who can afford them.

SMALL INTESTINE

By virtue of its anatomic location in the peritoneal cavity above the prostate, the small intestine is not usually affected when the prostate alone is being irradiated. However, when pelvic lymph nodes and seminal vesicles are also targeted, there is a risk of short- and long-term radiation effects on the small intestine. The lining of the small intestine normally undergoes continuous cell turnover by shedding and replenishing the cells. Radiation prevents normal growth of the cells lining the inner surface of the intestine, resulting in decreased absorption of nutrients. Short-term radiation effects, called "enteritis," can present as bloating, loss of appetite, nausea, colicky abdominal pain, or diarrhea. Enteritis can start after the second week of radiation and reach maximum intensity in the fourth week of treatment. Approximately 15 percent of patients with enteritis require medications or other interventions to control these symptoms.[6] Treatment of acute radiation enteritis is aimed at reducing the symptoms with antinausea medicines and antidiarrheal medications, as well as temporary diet modification to reduce fat and lactose content. These symptoms typically resolve within three months after the completion of treatment, and most patients do not require further intervention. Late small-bowel side effects from radiation may develop several months to many years after radiotherapy. The incidence of long-term complications requiring intervention is expected to be less than five percent in patients who have pelvic radiotherapy using modern techniques. The mechanism of late intestinal damage is likely due to an adverse effect on small blood vessels that supply the intestine, resulting in mucosal atrophy and ulceration that can occasionally lead to perforation, bleeding and obstruction. Patients with a prior history of abdominal/pelvic surgical procedures are at higher risk for small-intestine complications. Treatment of chronic radiation enteritis includes antinausea medications (Compazine or Ondansetron) and antidiarrheal medications (Lomotil or Imodium). Cholestyramine, which binds bile acids, can help reduce enteritis symptoms as well. Consultation with a dietitian experienced with radiation enteritis may be helpful. Treatment with hyperbaric oxygen may be beneficial, though the outcome of studies testing its effectiveness have been conflicting. Surgical evaluation and possible surgery to repair the damage may be necessary for rare patients who develop intestinal obstruction or perforation.

GENITOURINARY SYSTEM (GU)

Improvements in radiation technology have reduced the frequency of GU side effects. However, due to the close anatomic relationship between the prostate, the bladder, and the urinary passage (called the urethra), portions of the GU system receive high doses of radiation. Therefore, mild to moderate GU side effects during radiation are common. Severe short-term GU side effects are rare. Long-term complications are also rare.

Gentiourinary side effects during radiation therapy for prostate cancer are mostly caused by inflammation of the GU mucosa in response to radiation. Approximately three to four weeks after the start of radiation, symptoms including increased nighttime urination, bladder spasms, and urinary urgency may occur. These symptoms occur in 30 to 40 percent of patients and typically resolve within one to two months. Rarely, patients report blood in the urine ("hematuria") and painful urination ("dysuria") during treatment. Such symptoms are often alleviated by nonsteroidal anti-inflammatory drugs (NSAIDS) such as Ibuprofen or Naprosyn. Alpha-blockers such as tamsulosin (Flomax) also may be helpful. In the MSKCC study, late urinary complications requiring nonsurgical intervention were reported in approximately four percent of the IMRT patients and in about 16 percent of the brachytherapy patients. Complications requiring surgical intervention were noted in one percent of IMRT patients and two percent of brachytherapy patients.[3] Urinary incontinence during or after radiation therapy is extremely rare. Long-term scar formation leading to narrowing of the urethra (stricture) can occur in fewer than two percent of the patients. Patients with a prior history of transurethral resection of the prostate (TURP) have a higher risk of urinary stricture and urinary incontinence, especially after brachytherapy. Urinary strictures can be treated with variable success by urinary dilatation. Surgical intervention is required in a very small minority of cases. Some recent studies suggest that smokers may have an increased risk of GU complications after radiation therapy.[7]

SEXUAL FUNCTION

The function of the prostate is to produce seminal fluid. During the radiotherapy process, men have inflammation in the prostate. If they are sexually active, ejaculation may be painful. After radiation is completed, the inflammation dies down and over time, atrophy of the prostate glands and scar formation usually occur. As a result, the volume of seminal fluid becomes significantly reduced, causing some patients to experience reduction of volume or even absence of the ejaculate (dry orgasm).

The mechanism of erectile dysfunction (ED) occurring from radiation therapy is not well understood. Experts theorize that it is related to an alteration in the function of the blood vessels leading to the penis that are responsible for erections. A number of factors need to be considered when estimating the risk of ED, including age, blood pressure, smoking habits, and diabetes.

Across the board, considering all age groups, up to 50 percent of patients have reported a decline in erectile function following radiation therapy. This decline is seen as a gradual decrease in the ability to reach erections sufficient for sexual intercourse during the first two years after treatment. Recent studies suggest that prophylactic daily doses of sildenafil (Viagra), taken during and after radiotherapy, can improve erectile function.[8] Other studies suggest that limiting radiation exposure to the base of the penis by using careful targeting techniques decreases the risk of developing ED. A minority of men retain fertility after radiation. However, those desiring fertility preservation should consider sperm banking prior to treatment. Medical treatment for ED after radiation is essentially the same as the treatment of ED after surgery and is described in detail in Chapter 12.

PSA BOUNCE

A temporary increase in PSA can be noted long after radiation therapy has been completed. This benign increase of PSA, termed the PSA "bounce," occurs in about a third of patients undergoing brachytherapy. However, PSA bounce can also occur after external beam radiation. The timeframe for the occurrence of bounce tends to be between one and three years after treatment. Any increase of PSA greater than 0.2 from the lowest PSA level after therapy, and which subsequently declines without further treatment, is defined as PSA bounce. The magnitude of a bounce is usually around 1, but in rare patients, dramatic increases of PSA of more than 10 have been reported. A delayed inflammatory effect of radiation on benign prostate tissue is thought to be responsible for the PSA bounce. This temporary increase in PSA is *not* indicative of cancer progression or recurrence and does not warrant a prostate biopsy.

CANCER RECURRENCE VERSUS BOUNCE

The American Society for Radiation Oncology (ASTRO) defines cancer recurrence after radiotherapy as a persistent rise in PSA that is greater than 2 above the lowest PSA value. Using a "two-point" threshold is fairly effective at discriminating between a recurrence and a bounce, although, as noted above, in some patients the bounce is greater than 2. Careful follow-up and multiple PSA readings may ultimately be required to distinguish between the PSA bounce and treatment failure. Chapter 36 provides further information on how to distinguish a bounce from a recurrence.

CONCLUSION

Many of the historical problems related to radiation have been solved with modern targeting techniques. Reduction in sexual potency remains is the most frequent problem, and intervention for recovery has a varied record of success. Urinary issues, with increased frequency or painful urination, are the second most common problem. A variety of medications to reduce these symptoms was reviewed earlier in this chapter. GI problems are the least likely to occur. However, a small minority of men who undergo radiation therapy still encounter truly serious long-term GU and GI side effects that are difficult to manage. While treatment by knowledgeable experts can correct some treatment-related side effects, it's certainly important to minimize the risk of side effects by carefully selecting skilled and experienced radiation experts to perform the treatment.

References

1. PM Windsor and others. A randomized, controlled trial of aerobic exercise for treatment-related fatigue in men receiving radical external beam radiotherapy for localized prostate carcinoma. *Cancer* 101.3: 550, 2004.

2. MJ Zelefsky and others. High-dose intensity modulated radiation therapy for prostate cancer: Early toxicity and biochemical outcome in 772 patients. *International Journal of Radiation, Oncology, Biology, Physics* 53.5: 1111, 2002.

3. MJ Zelefsky and others. Comparison of tumor control and toxicity outcomes of high-dose intensity-modulated radiotherapy and brachytherapy for patients with favorable risk of prostate cancer. *Urology* 77.4: 986, 2011.

4. S Parikh and others. Treatment of hemorrhagic radiation *proctitis* with 4 percent formalin. *Diseases of the Colon and Rectum* 46.5: 596, 2003.

5. AK Lee and A Pollack. "The Prostate." *Radiation Oncology*, 9th. Edited by James D. Cox and Kie Kian Ang. St. Louis, MO: Mosby, 2009.

6. R Stacey and JT Green. Radiation-induced small bowel disease: Latest developments and clinical guidance. *Therapeutic Advances in Chronic Disease* 5.1: 15, 2014.

7. E Steinberger and others. Cigarette smoking during external beam radiation therapy for prostate cancer is associated with an increased risk of prostate cancer-specific mortality and treatment-related toxicity. *BJU International* 116.4: 596, 2015.

8. MJ Zelefsky and others. Prophylactic sildenafil citrate improves select aspects of sexual function in men treated with radiotherapy for prostate cancer. *Journal of Urology* 192.3: 868, 2014.

Chapter 15
SUMMARY OF *SKY*

Mark Scholz, MD

You are what you do, not what you say you'll do.

Carl Jung

IN 2012, A SURVEY FROM THE Mayo Clinic and Harvard was sent to 1,439 physicians. They were queried about their attitudes regarding active surveillance for men with *Very Low-Risk* prostate cancer (no more than two biopsy cores positive with Gleason 6). *Two-thirds* of the doctors were comfortable recommending active surveillance. For men who were merely *Low-Risk* (any number of biopsy cores positive with Gleason 6, and a PSA under 10), many of the doctors recommended surgery (47 percent) or radiation therapy (32 percent). *But only 21 percent of the doctors endorsed active surveillance.*

As has been shown in previous studies, radiation oncologists were 11 times more likely to recommend radiation, while urologists were 4.7 times more likely to recommend surgery, even for men who were *Very Low-Risk*. The conclusion of the doctors performing the study was that even though active surveillance is widely viewed as effective by both radiation oncologists and urologists, most urologists continue to recommend surgery, while most radiation oncologists recommend radiation therapy.

Decision-making, especially about such a critical issue, always has a strong emotional component. Sometimes, on the surface, it is unclear why people do what they do. Let's address the two most common questions that arise when discussing the possibility of pursuing active surveillance:

Why are Many Doctors Lukewarm About Monitoring?

1. Historically, cancer has always been treated, usually with surgery. Until recently, experts thought that all prostate cancer should be treated. It takes time for the industry to change.

2. Delaying treatment risks and being sued for medical malpractice if the cancer spreads. So far, no one has been successfully sued for recommending treatment.

3. The doctors who manage men with prostate cancer are surgeons (urologists), and they obviously tend to favor surgery. The old saying bears repeating, "If you are a hammer, everything looks like a nail."

4. Prostate cancer experts who specialize only in prostate cancer are extremely rare. Considering the complexity and rapidly changing nature of this vast field of medicine, it's hardly surprising that doctors struggle to stay abreast of the latest research.

5. Teaching frightened patients (and their frightened family members) about active surveillance takes time. It's hard for busy doctors to explain something complicated that may not come up very frequently in their day-to-day practice. In many cases, the doctors themselves only have a partial understanding of the active surveillance protocol.

6. Most doctors have not studied the issue thoroughly enough to become completely convinced that active surveillance is really safe. Their ambivalence is transmitted to the patients through their tone of voice and body language.

7. If all things are equal, doctors prefer to give patients what they want. Whenever "cancer" is in the discussion, patients are naturally biased toward treatment. Statistics, even though they are favorable, are cold and removed. When sitting across the table from a frightened patient, the doctor wants to satisfy the patient's urge for a cure.

8. Doctors are humans and are influenced by financial incentives. Treatment pays far better than observation.

Why are Many Patients Biased Toward Treatment?

1. In their frightened state, they don't fully understand the implications of being saddled with lifelong, irreversible side effects from surgery and radiation.

2. They don't have a doctor who wholeheartedly supports the concept of active surveillance. Therefore, they don't receive encouragement to forgo surgery or adequate radiation.

3. Good statistics and probabilities don't provide enough reassurance for patients. With cancer, everyone wants 100 percent certainty. Preconceived ideas about the deadliness of cancer are hard to overcome.

4. Resolution and closure feel good. Cutting out cancer sounds very attractive. Families and friends are frightened as well, and they often insist on treatment.

5. Forgoing treatment frightens uniformed family members and friends who conclude that you have terrible judgment or perhaps you have a death wish. To the uneducated, your

failure to treat your cancer leads to the conclusion that you are in some form of denial.

THE POWER OF A WORD

As Dr. Klotz pointed out in Chapter 9, the medical community fumbled badly in the 1960s, when it labeled Gleason score 6 a "cancer." We now know that Gleason score 3+3=6 never metastasizes. Therefore, Gleason 3+3=6 fails to meet the basic definition of what constitutes a cancer, a capacity to spread. Why is the truth surfacing so slowly? The answer is rather long and involved. Suffice to say that, as of 2017, when this page is being written, doctors are starting to get it right: About 50 percent of men who are eligible for active surveillance end up embarking on a surveillance program. This is genuine progress. In 2007, when active surveillance was first introduced, fewer than five percent of doctors were willing to monitor men with Gleason 3+3=6.

At the first medical conference convened to discuss active surveillance in 2007, it was openly bemoaned that the word "cancer" totally overstates the supposed dangers of *Low-Risk* prostate cancer. The pathology experts who were present, however, shot down the idea of a name change, saying, "Under the microscope it looks like a cancer, so it's cancer." At that time, no one had a rebuttal, so the subject was dropped. Now, we have the benefit of new research showing that Gleason 6 *never metastasizes*. Therefore, even though these cells look like cancer, we now know that they definitely don't behave like cancer.

In retrospect, it's too bad that the conference attendees were unable to rise to the challenge of renaming *Low-Risk* prostate cancer as something else. Back when the makers of 7Up wanted to emphasize the distinctiveness of their product compared with other soft drinks, they came up with the name "The Uncola," a stroke of marketing genius. Since the pathology experts insist that *Low-Risk* disease is a cancer, perhaps we should *un*do the negativity of this word by renaming it: "The Uncancer." Alternatively, the Stages of Blue classification system chose the benign designation of *"Sky"* for *Low-Risk* disease. Calling

Gleason score 6 "cancer" leads everyone to think, "I better be safe and remove the gland."

THE DRAWBACKS OF ACTIVE SURVEILLANCE

As discussed earlier, the biggest concern for men contemplating active surveillance is that the initial random biopsy may have missed a higher-grade tumor lurking somewhere else in the prostate. Most centers address this problem by repeatedly doing random biopsies every couple of years. The problem is that random biopsies are unpleasant, can cause serious infections, increase the risk of impotence, and worsen urinary symptoms. Thankfully, multiparametric MRI is an excellent alternative. Quality studies now show that it is substantially more accurate than random biopsy.[1] Unfortunately, the transition from random biopsy to imaging is happening rather slowly.

New genetic technology is also providing another layer of protection to ensure that men with occult, higher-grade cancers are detected. Genetic tests such as Prolaris, Oncotype DX, ConfirmMDx, and Decipher can be performed on the original biopsy specimen. These tests can identify when a cancer is prone to behave aggressively. The question is what to do when these tests suggest a higher-than-expected risk, when all the other factors meet the criteria for *Basic-Sky*. At this point, most experts recommend proceeding with some form of treatment along the lines of how *Teal* (Section III) is treated.

SHOULD *HIGH-SKY* UNDERGO TREATMENT? IF SO, WHAT TYPE?

Men with *High-Sky* have either a high PSA density (Chapter 2), or Prolaris or Oncotype DX genetic tests pointing to a type of disease that is more likely to behave aggressively. In the latter situation, since so much is riding on the decision about proceeding with treatment versus withholding it, repeating the genetic test from another company might be reasonable. If higher-grade disease is confirmed, the treatments described in Section III for *Basic-Teal* should probably be considered. In general, I treat men with a high PSA density (and normal genetic tests) the same as men who have a normal PSA density, assuming that a diligent search with multiparametric MRI and color Doppler fails to disclose occult disease that was missed by the initial biopsy. Chronic prostate inflammation, "prostatitis," is thought to be the reason that men without higher-grade disease can run higher-than-expected levels of PSA.

DRAWBACKS OF FOCAL THERAPY (CHAPTER 10)

Focal therapy, by "focusing" on the *cancer* rather than treating the whole prostate gland, may be one of the best ways to reduce side effects. The drawback is a higher risk of future cancer relapse compared with radiation or surgery. This is unavoidable. Retaining an intact prostate means that new cancers can crop up in the untreated portion of the gland. The biggest concern with focal therapy, however, is not the later development of a new cancer, *it is the difficult process of finding a superbly talented practitioner you can trust to do the job right.* Focal therapy requires *outstanding imaging skills* to deliver treatment to such a small target within the prostate gland. I have been disappointed by how many "experts" end up missing the cancer with their laser HIFU, cryotherapy or electroporation.

LIVING WITH CANCER

Anxiety and uncertainty about living with untreated "cancer" is also a problem, one that is often magnified by the treating physicians, surgeons, or radiation doctors who are emotionally ambivalent about active surveillance. The half-hearted attitude of the doctors comes from their personal uncertainties about the safety of monitoring untreated cancer. Anxiety from cancer, however, is inescapable. Studies show that men who had surgery or radiation also struggle with anxiety. Even though they had treatment, they know that there is a risk of the cancer returning.

TEACHING OLD DOGS NEW TRICKS

Changing the mind-set of doctors and patients about something called cancer is going to be a slow process. However, men need to realize that survival rates with *Low-Risk* prostate cancer managed with observation are not only extremely favorable, *they are identical to the survival rates of men undergoing immediate surgery.*[2] Men in *Sky* need to vigilantly guard against being rushed into unnecessary treatments that have irreversible side effects.

Having completed this section relating to the *Sky* Stage of Blue, you can now jump to Chapter 46 at the beginning of Section VII and finish the remainder of the book.

References

1. HU Ahmed and others. The PROMIS study: A paired-cohort blinded confirmatory study evaluating the accuracy of multiparametric MRI and TRUS biopsy in men with an elevated PSA. *Journal of Clinical Oncology* 34 suppl: abstr 5000, 2016.

2. FC Hamdy and others: 10-year outcomes after monitoring, surgery, or radiotherapy for localized prostate cancer. *New England Journal of Medicine* 375.15: 1415, 2016.

SECTION III
THE *TEAL* STAGE OF BLUE

Chapter 16
OVERVIEW OF *TEAL*

Mark Scholz, MD

Sometimes you have to choose between a bunch of wrong choices and no right ones. You just have to choose which wrong choice feels the least wrong.

COLLEEN HOOVER

*T*EAL IS VERY CHALLENGING FROM the treatment-selection point of view. The list of treatment options is long (see below). Accurate staging is the key. *Teal* splits into three subtypes: *Low-Teal, Basic-Teal* and *High-Teal*. Treatment is different for each subtype.

THREE SUBTYPES OF *TEAL*
"*Low*"-*Teal* has only one intermediate risk factor, such as a Gleason score of 3+4=7, with all the remaining factors being like those of *Sky*. (PSA less than 10, no nodule or a very small nodule). Men with *Low-Teal* also have favorable biopsy findings: They have Gleason 3+4=7 in no more than two biopsy cores and less than 20 percent of the cancer in the biopsy

core is grade 4. In addition, if imaging with multiparametric MRI shows a tumor, it should be relatively small. Since *Low-Teal* behaves like *Sky*, active surveillance becomes a reasonable consideration, a topic that was covered thoroughly in Section II. A blog posted on the PCRI website discusses active surveillance for *Low-Teal* as well.

Men with *Basic-Teal* have somewhat more extensive disease in their 12-core random biopsy specimen. Up to 50 percent of their biopsy cores may be involved with Gleason 3+4=7. All their other features are like *Sky*. *Basic-Teal* is usually treated rather than monitored.

High-Teal is characterized by one of the following:

1. Two or more intermediate-risk characteristics such as a PSA over 10 *plus* a nodule involving more than two quadrants of the prostate (stage T2b), or

2. A Gleason grade of 4+3=7 (rather than 3+4=7), or

3. Gleason 7 in more than 50 percent of the cores from a 12-core random biopsy.

High-Teal is more likely to metastasize, so staging scans are needed before starting any treatment, especially before starting testosterone inactivating pharmaceuticals (TIP). TIP causes cancer regression and can rapidly erase spots of cancer from the scan, which can lead to misinterpretation of the cancer's actual stage.

The types of scans used for staging are:
- Bone scan (Chapter 6)
- CT scan or MRI of the abdomen and pelvis to rule out enlarged lymph nodes
- A multiparametric MRI (MP-MRI) or color Doppler ultrasound (CDU) of the prostate gland to check for the possibility of extra-capsular disease (Chapters 4 and 5). If unequivocal extra-capsular disease is detected, *Teal* becomes *Azure*.

THE CHALLENGE OF PICKING THE RIGHT TREATMENT

The biggest challenge for *Teal* is sorting through the multiplicity of treatment alternatives. While I have listed 10 choices below, saying there are only 10 choices understates the situation. There are variations within each of these 10 options. For example, for option #1 there are three different types of permanent seeds: iodine, palladium and cesium. When you consider the possibility of varying the dosage and the duration of treatment, the number of options becomes almost infinite.

1. Brachytherapy, permanent low-dose seed radiation

2. High-dose-rate brachytherapy, (i.e., temporary seed radiation)

3. Intensity modulated radiation (IMRT), a type of external beam radiation (EBRT)

4. Brachytherapy combined with IMRT

5. Proton therapy

6. Cyberknife or stereotactic body radiation therapy (SBRT)

7. Focal therapy (in its many forms: Cryo, HIFU, laser, radiation, electroporation)

8. Testosterone inactivating pharmaceuticals (TIP) as a standalone treatment

9. Robotic or open surgery

10. TIP administered for a variable period *in combination* with radiation

USING SCIENTIFIC STUDIES TO COMPARE TREATMENT OPTIONS

Scientific studies are the main basis for evaluating a treatment's effectiveness. Patients naturally tend to rely on their doctor to sort through the studies and determine which are reliable. One generally hopes that the doctors are sophisticated, truth-based scientists, objectively selecting the most accurate studies to guide them in their treatment recommendations. Unfortunately, doctors fall prey to the temptation of quoting the studies that support their preexisting point of view. A study can be found that supports almost any point of view.

The aim of this chapter is to convey one important message—not all scientific studies are created equal. Unfortunately, few people are schooled in how a study's veracity is determined. While there are many potential pitfalls, there are common methods for determining which studies can be trusted. To protect themselves from being misled, patients need to learn how to assess the quality of a study.

An experienced and unbiased expert scrutinizes the value of a study by first looking at its *scientific method*. Did the researchers doing the study ask the right question in the first place? Second, is to consider the *relevance* of the study: Was the study performed with patients with an age and stage of disease like yours? Third, how does the *integrity and the reputation* of the researchers who wrote the study stack up? This criterion is often reflected by the prestige of the journal in which the study is published. Lastly, the *type* of study must be considered.

SCIENTIFIC STUDIES—GOOD, BAD, AND UGLY

Please forgive me if you feel that the logic behind this paragraph is so obvious that I am insulting your intelligence. However, after talking with thousands of patients I have learned that some fail to think things through. Treatment results from studies performed in Petri dishes or on animals have only preliminary value and can be used only for designing future human studies. Over and over, it has been shown that the findings from nonhuman studies are poor predictors of what will happen when that same type of treatment is finally tested in humans. Please don't confuse yourself by considering any nonhuman study in your quest to find optimal treatment.

Another type of untrustworthy study relies on retrospective database queries. The advent of electronic records has opened the door to the possibility of doing all kinds of computerized data searches. One popular methodology relies on searching through the *billing records* of men treated for prostate cancer to estimate the incidence survival and quality-of-life events in the long-term. Recently, one such study received wide press coverage by claiming hormone therapy causes Alzheimer's disease.[1] Unfortunately, there was no press coverage of the backlash from the scientific community, which severely criticized the study's methodology and conclusions.[2,3,4,5]

Prospective studies that compare outcomes by randomly allocating patients into separate treatment groups are by far the best. However, such studies are few and far between because they are so expensive. *Retrospective* studies easily outnumber the randomized studies by more than 100 to 1. As we progress through this section of the book, we will be faced with the need to interpret and compare numerous studies from many different treatment centers, most of them retrospective. Here are a few of the difficulties this presents:

- All retrospective studies are self-reported, so the people writing the study have a major conflict of interest. Who would want to report bad results from their own treatment center?

- In retrospective studies, patients are not of comparable age. Men undergoing surgery are consistently younger than the men who undergo radiation. It is a well-known medical fact that younger patients have better treatment outcomes and fewer side effects than older ones. So how do you accurately compare surgery versus radiation if the patients are different ages?

- The definition of what constitutes a cancer relapse is not uniform between radiation and surgery. Relapses with radiation are detected later. The low levels of PSA from a recurring cancer after radiation are obscured by the background PSA being produced by the prostate gland.

- A time lag occurs with all prostate cancer studies. Cure rates are not finalized until five to 10 years after the treatment. Over this extended waiting period, technology advances.

This is important because radiation technology has greatly improved, whereas cure rates from surgery, even robotic surgery, have remained about the same. Therefore, older radiation studies *understate* the results obtainable with modern techniques.

COMPARING CURE RATES

Despite these difficulties, a broad overview of many studies ever performed can provide a comparative sense of how these different treatments perform. By examining multiple studies, some of the biases and variations between the studies may be averaged out. Reviewing all the retrospective studies of *Teal* ever published is a gargantuan chore, but Dr. Peter Grimm was up to the task. He compiled all studies reporting cure rates with surgery, seed radiation, external beam radiation (EBRT), which in this modern era is usually IMRT, or the combination of seed radiation with IMRT. His landmark conclusions are presented in the following chapter. In that same chapter, a *prospective* trial is also presented that compares cure rates of seed implants combined with IMRT to cure rates of IMRT without seed implants.

SELECTING BETWEEN SO MANY OPTIONS

Most men with *Teal* will need treatment. All the following chapters are authored by world-class experts whom I would personally trust if I needed to undergo treatment for *Teal*. As you review these chapters, please keep in mind that the doctors maintain full independence in their viewpoint. Therefore, it may appear that the book is inconsistent. One doctor may write that a certain treatment is best for a particular class of patients. Another doctor may argue in a totally different direction. All the authors can cite statistics to support their position. The doctors writing these chapters have selected the studies they feel are most relevant to their point of view. As I have tried to convey, this does not mean that all the studies are equally valid.

MY THOUGHTS ON CHOOSING TREATMENT

When *Teal* is managed appropriately, the vast majority of men will be cured. And even if a relapse occurs, most men will live out a normal life expectancy. Therefore, how treatment impacts *quality of life* assumes momentous importance. When comparing the pros and cons of the different treatment options, there is one all-embracing principle that must constantly be kept in mind: *Minimizing side effects* should be the overriding priority. Freeing one's thinking from the "I must survive cancer" mentality and changing it to that of a wary customer shopping for the least-invasive treatment is a difficult, but essential, mental exercise.

All things being otherwise equal, and assuming, as is the case for most men, that there is a strong desire to minimize sexual and urinary side effects, I have placed the following chapters in a rough order of the way I would think when meeting a newly diagnosed man with *Teal* for initial consultation. However, my initial thoughts are often altered by new information once I get to know each patient's situation better. Men have diverse sexual priorities, varying degrees of preexisting urinary function, and differences in overall health status. These factors heavily influence the selection of treatment.

MAKING A FINAL DECISION

Once all the information is gathered and analyzed, the time will come to make a final decision. At that point, I recommend creating a list of all the options still under consideration. Draw a line through your "worst" option and continue to eliminate options until only one remains. The final remaining option might be the best treatment for you. A few more thoughts on these different variables and how they affect the selection of treatment will be presented in Chapter 25, at the end of this section.

References

1.   KT Nead and others. Androgen deprivation therapy and future Alzheimer's disease risk. *Journal of Clinical Oncology* 34.6: 566, 2015.

2. RL Bowen and others. Not all androgen deprivation therapies are created equal: Leuprolide and the decreased risk of developing Alzheimer's disease. *Journal of Clinical Oncology* 34.23: 2800, 2016.

3. M Froehner and MP Wirth. Androgen deprivation therapy and Alzheimer's disease. *Journal of Clinical Oncology* 34.23: 2801, 2016.

4. JJ Leow and others. Association of androgen deprivation therapy with Alzheimer's disease: Unmeasured confounders. *Journal of Clinical Oncology* 34.23: 2801, 2016.

5. C Brady and others. Androgen deprivation therapy and risk of Alzheimer's disease: Importance of holistic geriatric oncology assessment. *Journal of Clinical Oncology* 34.23: 2803, 2016.

Chapter 17

PERMANENT RADIOACTIVE SEED IMPLANTS

Peter Grimm, DO
and
John Blasko, MD

Three Things that cannot long be hidden:
The Sun, The Moon and The Truth.
BUDDHA

BRACHYTHERAPY FOR PROSTATE CANCER, also known as seed implantation, comes in two varieties, permanent and temporary. This chapter addresses permanent seeds. The following chapter covers temporary seeds. Permanent seed implantation involves the insertion of small, carefully spaced, radioactive pellets into the prostate. Three types of permanent radioactive seeds exist: Palladium[103], Iodine[125] and Cesium[137]. They each have slightly different characteristics, but there are more similarities than differences. After implantation the seeds emit, over a period of two months or so, a low but continuous energy that accrues

131

to a large total dose of radiation inside the prostate. The big advantage with seeds is that very little radiation reaches the sensitive surrounding organs such as the bladder and rectum. A well-performed seed implant offers two things that are optimal in the world of radiation treatment: a high dosage of radiation to the prostate and minimal radiation exposure to the surrounding normal tissues.

Modern brachytherapy technique begins by imaging the prostate gland with ultrasound or MRI to create a detailed picture of the gland. From this image, a map for seed placement is created. The seeds are often "strung together" on strands to prevent migration outside the gland. Careful planning of the array of the seeds assures complete coverage of the entire gland, including a small margin around the outside edge of the gland to cover any microscopic spread of the cancer beyond the capsule. Seed implants are performed as an outpatient procedure, which takes about 60 to 90 minutes.

On average, cure rates from seed implants are *superior* to either surgery or external beam radiation therapy such as IMRT (Chapter 19). This

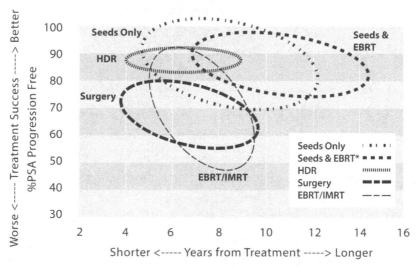

Intermediate Risk Results

www.PCTRF.org   Prostate Cancer Results Study Group

---

* EBRT: See Glossary

bold claim is based on the findings of the Prostate Cancer Results Study Group (PCRSG), a compilation of every reputable study performed that reports cure rates with surgery, EBRT/IMRT, and seed implants. These studies were vetted and scored per prespecified criteria to ensure that they met acceptable research standards such as including an adequate number of patients; utilizing a uniform reporting procedure; and following the patients for a meaningful period after the treatment.

The circles represent an "average" of the cure rates for a single type of treatment. The higher the circle the better the cure rate. Circles extending farther to the right indicate more mature data. Cure rates at 10 or 15 years, for example, carry more weight than cure rates at five years. As can clearly be seen, seed implants or seed implants combined with EBRT/IMRT deliver the highest cure rates. The cure rates with surgery or EBRT/IMRT without seeds are lower. HDR means "high-dose-rate" brachytherapy, otherwise known as temporary seeds. More detailed information on this topic is available at pctrf.org.

As noted above, all the studies in the graph were performed without the benefit of a randomized comparison group. In other words, the studies reported in the graph are *retrospective*. Prospective randomized clinical trials that compare different treatments for prostate cancer are very rare. Recently, however, a randomized study called the ASCENDE-RT trial was completed. The ASCENDE-RT trial compared cure rates between IMRT alone and IMRT *plus* seed implantation for men with both *Teal* and *Azure*. One hundred twenty-two men with *Teal* and 276 men with *Azure* entered the study. Both groups received 12 months of testosterone inactivating pharmaceuticals (TIP) plus whole-pelvis IMRT (Chapter 19). One-half of the men were then randomly assigned to receive additional IMRT to the prostate, while the other half were treated with a seed boost.

RESULTS OF THE ASCENDE-RT TRIAL

The ASCENDE-RT is the *first* randomized trial ever to directly address the question of whether permanent seeds are required to achieve optimal cure rates. As such, it is a landmark trial. Here are the findings:

PSA control rate at 5 years	*PSA control rate at 9 years*
IMRT plus TIP: 84%	IMRT plus TIP: 70%
IMRT plus TIP *plus SEEDS:* 96%	IMRT plus TIP *plus SEEDS:* 94%

An important finding of the ASCENDE trial relates to the shape of the survival curves over time. For the seed-treated patients, after about five years the curve becomes very flat: meaning that *only 2 percent of the men relapsed after five years.* In contrast, the curve for the IMRT-alone group continues to decline all the way out to 10 years. *An additional 14% of the men in the IMRT-alone group relapsed after five years.*

In summary, this randomized study demonstrates a dramatic 24 percent improvement in cure rates in patients who received a seed implant boost compared with those who received IMRT without seeds. Seed implants give the best long-term control rates of prostate cancer.

THE DEFINITION OF SUCCESS

Some critics have argued that PSA control rates are an inferior measure of success. They believe that success should be defined by survival rates. In the ASCENDE trial, survival to this point has been the same. This finding is hardly surprising. It does NOT mean that there is no difference between the treatments. PSA is always the earliest and most accurate indicator of relapse. Everyone familiar with prostate cancer knows that an increasing PSA has a negative impact on quality of life. First, there will be a need for further diagnostic tests. Second, further treatment is needed, usually with TIP and sometimes even with chemotherapy.

Another criticism was that ASCENDE reported a slightly higher incidence of moderately serious urinary complications with seeds. This concern, however, should be tempered by the fact that many seed implant centers have not encountered anywhere near the level of problems reported in the ASCENDE trial. It is anticipated, therefore, that by using an adjustment of the methodology of the seed implant technique used in ASCENDE, especially by reducing the radiation dose to the lower tip of the prostate, this higher incidence of complications will be corrected.

Given all this very positive news about seeds, what is the status of seed utilization in the United States? Shockingly, there has been a dramatic *decrease* in the use of seeds between 2002 and 2010 (the last year for which data is available). In 2002, 17 percent of newly-diagnosed men were treated with seeds. However, by 2010 only 8 percent were treated with seeds. Over the same time interval, the use of surgery increased from 44 percent to 59 percent. This shift appears to coincide with the introduction of new technologies such as robotic surgery, IMRT, and proton therapy. The rapid adoption of these very expensive new technologies has occurred *despite the absence of any comparative data such as the ASCENDE trial to justify their use.* There is no scientifically sound rationale for the increased popularity of these other treatments. Prostate treatment has migrated away from seed implants, not because of science, but because of economics and politics. *These new approaches generate much more revenue for both hospitals and physicians.* Hospital marketing departments take advantage of seductive terms like "robot-assisted" and "proton" to publicly promote their institutions and capture market share. And, in the final analysis, surgeons are more comfortable with surgery, and radiation specialists favor IMRT. That's how they get paid. It's interesting to note that the popularity of brachytherapy is growing rapidly in many other countries where the physicians are paid the same rate regardless of the treatment selected.

Multiple studies over the past 25 years have demonstrated that seeds, either alone or in combination with IMRT, are at least comparable to surgery for *Teal* and almost certainly *superior* to surgery for *Azure*. Short-, intermediate- and long-term quality of life is also better with seeds. Now the ASCENDE-RT prospective, randomized trial also proves that seed implantation provides superior cure rates compared with IMRT. When these excellent clinical outcomes are coupled with proven cost effectiveness, what is there not to like about seed implants?

Chapter 18

HIGH-DOSE-RATE SEEDS

D. Jeffrey Demanes, MD

This above all: to thine own self be true,
And it must follow, as the night the day,
Thou canst not then be false to any man.

WILLIAM SHAKESPEARE

RADIOACTIVITY WAS FIRST DISCOVERED by the French physicist Antoine Henri Becquerel 120 years ago. Becquerel, having accidentally taken radium home in his waistcoat pocket, was diagnosed by a dermatologist, Earnest Besnier, as having a "radium burn." Marie and Pierre Curie purified radium in 1898. Pierre and Earnest were the first people to recognize a possible therapeutic benefit from radium.

Urologists like Pasteau, Degrais, Young, and Barringer were the first to evaluate radium applications directly into the prostate gland in 1913. When radiation is placed directly into the prostate it spares the surrounding body from exposure. In the early 1980s, Dr. Hans Hendrik

Holm revolutionized the process by introducing ultrasound guidance as a method that continues to be used to this day (see the previous chapter). However, with the advent of robotics and computers, engineers such as Eric Vant Hoft and others invented high-dose-rate (HDR) temporary seeds. The use of modern HDR for prostate cancer began in earnest in the late 1980s.

HIGH-DOSE-RATE BRACHYTHERAPY—ACCURACY IS EVERYTHING

HDR is done in four steps, with three chances along the way to refine and improve the accuracy of the sculpted radiation field. The first step is placement, under anesthesia, of small straw-like brachytherapy catheters into and around the prostate using ultrasound guidance. This procedure takes about one hour. Since the prostate is located near the body surface, the catheters can be inserted directly through the skin of the perineum without an incision and are positioned to avoid the highly sensitive neurovascular bundles that control erections.

Once the catheters are in position, the next two steps are called "simulation" and "dosimetry." Simulation involves taking either a CT or ultrasound image of the prostate with the catheters in place. During this imaging process, further adjustments can be made by shifting the position of the catheters to ensure they are in the correct location. A medical physicist then uploads the imaging data into a treatment-planning program that creates a virtual image of the prostate with the catheters in place. Radiation dosing calculations are then made to determine the dosage.

A physicist works with the radiation oncologist to calculate the amount of radiation that will be administered to the tumor, the prostate gland, and a small margin surrounding the gland. The results are displayed graphically for analysis, which affords a third and final opportunity for adjusting and refining the treatment plan. Once the radiation oncologist approves the plan, electronic instructions are sent to a robotic delivery device called an "HDR afterloader." The robotic afterloader controls a *single*, tiny, but very potent radioactive seed attached to the end of a fine cable that is inserted into each of the hollow catheters that were previously positioned in the patient. The robot slides the seed up to the end of each catheter and then slowly withdraws it at a predetermined rate calculated by the computer. The radioactive seed in the straw has no direct contact with body tissue, so there is no residual radioactivity once the treatment is completed. Although the preparations are technically complex, each treatment takes only about 15 to 30 minutes.

ADVANTAGES OF HDR

- The radiation dose accurately conforms to each individual's prostate.
- HDR delivers radiation fast, which may improve the anticancer effect.
- HDR patients are not radioactive after treatment.
- The dose to the surrounding normal tissues is much lower than with intensity modulated external beam radiation therapy (IMRT) or proton therapy.

COMBINING HDR WITH EXTERNAL BEAM RADIATION OR HORMONE THERAPY

HDR can be used in combination with testosterone inactivating pharmaceuticals (TIP) and/or with IMRT. The use of these additional therapies depends on a man's Stage of Blue and his subtype within a Stage of Blue:

1. *Teal:* Men with *Low-Teal, Basic-Teal* and *Sky* can have HDR alone; carefully selected cases may even consider *focal* HDR (Dr. Duke Bahn discusses some of the principles of focal therapy in Chapter 10).

2. *Azure* or *High-Teal—patients generally receive* HDR plus IMRT with or without TIP. (Selected cases of *Azure* with low-volume cancer can consider HDR alone.)

STUDIES REPORTING CURE RATES WITH HDR COMBINED WITH IMRT

Study after study clearly shows that radiation cure rates are improved through administering radiation in higher doses. HDR is probably the most accurate way to deliver ultra-high-dose radiation to the prostate without injuring the bladder and rectum. A general review of all the scientific literature on this topic has been published by B.R. Pieters and colleagues.[1] When he compared all the different ways of giving radiation, he found that IMRT combined with HDR was the most effective. Other studies show that, with HDR brachytherapy plus IMRT, PSA control rates vary from 60 to 90 percent, depending upon the institution, patient characteristics, and the length of follow-up.[2-5] Still other studies indicate that this combination produces cure rates that are consistently better than surgery.[6-9] A randomized clinical trial from England reported that HDR plus IMRT is better than IMRT alone.[10] Finally, a retrospective study from Memorial Sloan Kettering showed that IMRT with HDR had a 98 percent cure rate compared to an 82 percent cure rate using ultra-high-dose IMRT without HDR.[11]

HDR MONOTHERAPY (TREATMENT WITH HDR ALONE)

HDR is often combined with IMRT, but it can be used by itself. The signature studies of HDR alone (monotherapy) began in the mid-1990s with Martinez at William Beaumont Hospital (WBH);[12] Demanes at California Endocurietherapy (CET);[13] and Yoshioka, at Osaka, Japan.[14] Martinez and Demanes conducted a multi-institution study on 298 patients with *Sky* and *Teal* that showed that 97 percent of men treated with HDR alone were disease free after five years of follow up. Mild to moderate urinary complications occurred in 10 percent and more serious urinary complications were uncommon (one percent). There were no major rectal complications and preservation of sexual function was achieved in 80 percent of cases.[12] An updated 10-year follow up study on 448 Demanes patients validated the high cure rates with HDR monotherapy (99 percent of *Sky* patients were cured as were 95 percent of *Teal*) and confirmed the low rate of complications and preservation of sexual function.[15] Disease was controlled in the prostate gland itself in all but one case. The group from Osaka, Japan used HDR monotherapy to treat 190 patients (79 *Teal* and 111 *Azure)* with HDR monotherapy. The PSA disease-free rate after eight years of follow up was 93 percent for *Teal* and 77 percent for *Azure*.[14] Disease was controlled in the prostate in 99 percent of cases. Moderate side effects were noted in 10 percent of cases and more serious complications in only 1 percent.

Other groups[16] have confirmed these findings. One example is R.L. Rogers and colleagues, who reported on 284 *Teal* patients treated with HDR monotherapy. In their study, 94 percent of patients were free of disease at five years, 100 percent of cases had disease controlled in the prostate, and 83 percent maintained potency at two years after treatment. Zamboglou,[17] from Germany, published a large outcomes study of 718 patients. The five-year PSA disease control was 95 percent for *Sky*, 93 percent for *Teal*, and 93 percent for *Azure*. Complications that were severe enough to require treatment were uncommon (3.5 percent urinary and 1.6 percent rectal) and long-term severe complications occurred in less than 1 percent. Potency preservation was 81 percent. These excellent results with HDR monotherapy are so similar to combination therapy with HDR plus IMRT that it raises the serious question as to whether the IMRT portion of the treatment provides any additional benefit, especially in cases in which the pelvic lymph nodes are not treated with radiation.

SIDE EFFECTS

Temporary urinary side effects are expected to last one to two weeks then taper off. Prostate swelling or urinary bleeding immediately after the procedure occasionally (less than one in 10 cases) requires a temporary urinary catheter. In about 10 percent of men, urinary irritation or impaired flow may be more prolonged, particularly in men who have preexisting prostate problems. Medications to relax the bladder neck (alpha blockers like Flomax) are often helpful. In most cases, long-term urinary function is like what it was before treatment. A complication such as urinary incontinence typically occurs in less than one percent of the cases whereas impaired urinary flow due to scarring (this is called "stricture") may occur in one to five percent of cases. Stricture can usually be managed with dilation, but in some cases a surgical procedure through the penis is needed to open the channel. The most severe and rare (0.2 percent) complication is a fistula (an abnormal connection between the urethra and the rectum that requires a urinary diversion or ileostomy). Such events may occur when the patient undergoes transurethral resection (TURP) after brachytherapy. *Anyone who has had previous radiation of any type should never undergo a urological procedure with any but the most experienced urological surgeons.* Healing after corrective surgery in men who have had previous radiation is greatly retarded. Ill-advised surgery can cause a tough situation to become worse. Occasional patients who have had HDR may develop unexplained difficulty with urination and will need to perform self-catheterization, at least temporarily. These patients (those without an obvious mechanical obstruction or narrowing) should delay or postpone surgery as long as possible. The delayed effects of the radiation will eventually cause the prostate to shrink, which will lead to a natural resolution of the symptoms.

Some prostate cancer patients have preexisting urinary symptoms from benign prostate hyperplasia (enlargement), or BPH. If a surgical intervention such as a TURP is contemplated to improve urine function, it is best to perform the procedure *before* brachytherapy. In these cases, brachytherapy should be delayed for three to six months, to allow normal tissue healing. When managed in this way, even patients with BPH can have a good outcome with HDR brachytherapy. It bears repeating that surgical interventions after brachytherapy are generally discouraged and only a specially trained urologist should operate on men who are experiencing complications from after radiation.

Rectal bleeding or other gastrointestinal symptoms are noticeably less common after brachytherapy than after external radiation. Most men who are sexually functional before HDR will be functional afterward. The prophylactic use of erectile dysfunction medications during a period of weeks to months after brachytherapy is recommended to maintain genital blood flow and improve erectile function; such treatment can be helpful in preventing or reducing long-term erectile dysfunction.

SUMMARY AND CONCLUSIONS

Additional summary and review articles in the medical literature about HDR brachytherapy with and without EBRT[18-20] are referenced below. HDR is a highly versatile technology, sufficiently adaptable so that any prostate target (partial or complete) can be treated either with HDR monotherapy, or as part of a larger treatment strategy using IMRT and/or TIP. The successful outcomes documented with HDR can be attributed to this technique's unique capacity to deliver very high doses of radiation extremely accurately. Published studies demonstrate that tumor control in the prostate occurs in greater than 95 percent of patients. Long-term disease control occurs in 95 percent of men in *Sky*, 90 percent in *Teal*, and 70 to 80 percent in *Azure*.

References

1. BR Pieters and others. Comparison of three radiotherapy modalities on biochemical control and overall survival for the treatment of prostate cancer: A systematic review. *Radiotherapy and Oncology* 93.2: 168, 2009.

2. Y Yamada and others. Favorable clinical outcomes of three-dimensional computer-optimized high-dose-rate prostate brachytherapy in the management of localized prostate cancer. *Brachytherapy* 5: 157.3, 2006.

3. TP Phan and others. High dose rate brachytherapy as a boost for the treatment of localized prostate cancer. *Journal of Urology* 177.1: 123, 2007.

4. DJ Demanes and others. Excellent results from high dose rate brachytherapy and external beam for prostate cancer are not improved by androgen deprivation. *American Journal of Clinical Oncology* 32.4: 342, 2009.

5. RM Galalae and others. The 15-year outcomes of high-dose-rate brachytherapy for radical dose escalation in patients with prostate cancer—A benchmark for high-tech external beam radiotherapy alone? *Brachytherapy* 13.2: 117, 2014.

6. TM Do and others. High-grade carcinoma of the prostate: A comparison of current local therapies. *Urology* 57.6: 1121, 2001.

7. M Manoharan and others. Outcome after radical prostatectomy with a pretreatment prostate biopsy Gleason score of ≥ 8. *BJU International* 92.6: 539, 2003.

8. SA Boorjian and others. Impact of prostate-specific antigen testing on the clinical and pathological outcomes after radical prostatectomy for Gleason 8-10 cancers. *BJU International* 101.3: 299, 2008.

9. F Audenet and others. Oncologic control obtained after radical prostatectomy in men with a pathological Gleason score ≥ 8: A single-center experience. *Urologic Oncology: Seminars and Original Investigations* 29.6: 602, 2011.

10. PJ Hoskin and others. Randomised trial of external beam radiotherapy alone or combined with high-dose-rate brachytherapy boost for localised prostate cancer. *Radiotherapy and Oncology* 103.2: 217, 2012.

11. I Deutsch and others. Comparison of PSA relapse-free survival in patients treated with ultra-high-dose IMRT versus combination HDR brachytherapy and IMRT. *Brachytherapy* 9.4: 313, 2010.

12. AA Martinez and others. High-dose-rate prostate brachytherapy: An excellent accelerated-hypofractionated treatment for favorable prostate cancer. *American Journal of Clinical Oncology* 33.5: 481, 2010.

13. DJ Demanes and others. High-dose-rate monotherapy: Safe and effective brachytherapy for patients with localized prostate cancer. *International Journal of Radiation Oncology, Biology, Physics* 81.5: 1286, 2011.

14. Y Yoshioka and others. High-dose-rate brachytherapy as monotherapy for intermediate- and high-risk prostate cancer: Clinical results for a median 8-year follow-up. *International Journal of Radiation Oncology, Biology, Physics* 94.4: 675, 2016.

15. H Hauswald and others. High-dose-rate monotherapy for localized prostate cancer: 10-year results. *International Journal of Radiation Oncology, Biology, Physics* 94.4: 667, 2016.

16. CL Rogers and others. High dose brachytherapy as monotherapy for intermediate risk prostate cancer. *Journal of Urology* 187.1: 109, 2012.

17. N Zamboglou and others. High-dose-rate interstitial brachytherapy as monotherapy for clinically localized prostate cancer: Treatment evolution and mature results. *International Journal of Radiation Oncology, Biology, Physics* 85.3: 672, 2013.

18. GC Morton. High-dose-rate brachytherapy boost for prostate cancer: Rationale and technique. *Journal of Contemporary Brachytherapy* 6.3: 323, 2014.

19. Y Yoshioka and others. High-dose-rate brachytherapy as monotherapy for prostate cancer: Technique, rationale and perspective. *Journal of Contemporary Brachytherapy* 6.1: 91, 2014.

20. DJ Demanes and MI Ghilezan. High-dose-rate brachytherapy as monotherapy for prostate cancer. *Brachytherapy* 13.6: 529, 2014.

Chapter 19
IMRT FOR *TEAL*

Zachary Zumsteg, MD
and
Howard Sandler, MD

People almost invariably arrive at their beliefs not on the basis of proof but on the basis of what they find attractive.
BLAISE PASCAL

In our reasonings concerning matters of fact, there are all imaginable degrees of assurance, from the highest certainty to the lowest species of moral evidence. A wise man, therefore, proportions his belief to the evidence.
DAVID HUME

WHAT IS INTENSITY-MODULATED RADIATION THERAPY?

Other than the discovery that hormonal therapy and radiation can act synergistically to eradicate prostate cancer, the development of modern radiotherapy techniques such as intensity-modulated radiation therapy

(IMRT) represent what is arguably the biggest advance in prostate cancer radiation therapy over the last 25 years. IMRT refers to a special type of computerized radiation that can deliver extraordinarily precise dose distributions to any organ, regardless of shape, at any location in the body. This allows higher radiation doses than were previously achievable, thereby decreasing the risk of recurrence while simultaneously decreasing the likelihood of short- and long-term side effects by limiting the radiation dose to nearby normal tissue.

HOW IMRT FUNCTIONS

IMRT is a specialized form of external beam radiotherapy. A device called a linear accelerator is used to administer high-energy photon beams to the tumor. These beams are identical to the radiation beams used for Xrays and CT scans, except that they have much higher energy. The beams cannot be seen by the human eye or felt by a patient. Additionally, the instant the linear accelerator beams are turned off, there is no radiation left in the patient's body, so patients do not need to be concerned about being around young children or pregnant women; nor do they face issues related to security screening when traveling, as is the case with permanent seeds.

IMRT is delivered with high precision in small, daily doses over a course of seven to nine weeks. There is another type of external radiotherapy, known as stereotactic body radiotherapy (SBRT), which is reviewed in Chapter 22. The main difference between IMRT and SBRT is that SBRT delivers beam radiation in a few very large doses, usually four or five treatments over one to two weeks.

WHY IS IMRT GIVEN OVER SEVEN TO NINE WEEKS?

The reason radiotherapy is effective in eradicating cancer is that tumor cells are much more susceptible to radiation than noncancerous tissues. There are several reasons for this. First, in order to become a cancer cell, with the capacity for essentially unlimited growth, a cell has to give up certain standard functions that normal cells use for self-regulation. *One of these lost functions is the capacity to repair damage from outside sources, such as radiation.* This defective repair machinery in cancer cells is one reason for their continued spread and growth to other locations in the body. The good news is that this reduced capacity for repair is an Achilles heel that makes them more susceptible to radiation. A related reason that cancer cells are more susceptible to radiation is that they typically divide more quickly than normal cells; their rapid proliferation cycles allow less time to repair damage caused by radiation. Thus, because tumor cells have both a lower capacity and less time to repair damage from radiation, they are not able to withstand radiation in the same way that the adjacent normal tissues can.

Although the explanation above is a useful simplification of a complicated reality, it helps explain why, for many decades, almost all cancers have been treated with small daily doses over multiple weeks. If radiotherapy was given in one very large dose, the damage to the normal tissue would be so substantial that it would overwhelm the capacity of the normal tissue to repair itself. However, if small doses of radiation are delivered each day, the normal tissues have time to completely repair the damage before the next day's treatment, whereas tumor cells, lacking adequate repair capacity, are permanently destroyed.

With the extraordinary precision of modern radiation therapy, there may be less need to deliver the radiation in small increments, given that the surrounding normal tissues are exposed to a much smaller degree than when they were using older radiation technology. This fact, in combination with other biologic considerations, has formed the impetus for an investigation of SBRT (Chapter 22). However, SBRT has not yet been evaluated in a head-to-head comparison trial with IMRT for *Teal*. Whether the efficacy and toxicity of SBRT are equivalent to IMRT is still unknown. "Short-course" IMRT administered over four to six weeks is a "half-way" measure between standard IMRT given for eight to nine weeks and SBRT. Preliminary studies using short-course IMRT are showing promise. Patients should discuss the pros and cons of all these different treatment options with their radiation oncologist.

THE PROCESS

When undergoing IMRT, it is imperative that the patient be in the exact same position for each radiation treatment, so a lot of attention is paid to ensuring this. Thus, the first step in IMRT is a mapping session known as a "simulation." Prior to simulation, bowel preparation is sometimes used to eliminate any stool in the rectum. A comfortably full bladder may be requested to ensure optimal imaging. The purpose of simulation is to position the patient, typically lying flat on a table, in the exact physical alignment that he will assume for treatment each day. The radiation therapist, working with the radiation oncology technicians, adjusts the alignment of the patient several times to ensure that the patient is in the optimal position for radiation delivery. Next, a customized immobilization device, often referred to as a mold, is created to guarantee unvarying position day to day. This mold usually fits around the pelvis and upper legs. The patient then undergoes a scan while he remains in this exact position, providing a map that the radiation oncologist can use to design the proper radiation distribution. At the end of the simulation, several small, permanent markings, about the size of a pencil tip, are placed on the patient's body. These tattoos are aligned with lasers in the treatment room each day, to make sure that the patient is in the exact position for accurate treatment.

IMRT is often given with "image guidance" to ensure that variations in patient anatomy due to changes in bladder and bowel filling don't impair accuracy. This process relies on an Xray or CT scan built into the treatment machine that determines the exact position of the prostate each day. Image guidance may require the placement of permanent markers, such as gold seeds (which are easily visualized on Xray or CT). Alternatively, electromagnetic transponders can be implanted that act like a GPS system, providing a real-time position of the prostate during treatment. Image guidance allows the radiation therapist to design a target field with smaller, more precise margins, maximizing radiation to the tumor and minimizing radiation to surrounding organs, like the bladder and rectum.

Following the planning process, patients are administered treatment daily, usually Monday through Friday. Treatments usually take only a few minutes. At the end of his course of treatment, the patient will typically follow up with his radiation oncologist every three to six months for the first few years after treatment, and then yearly. The exact follow-up protocol after therapy is described in detail by Dr. Jeffrey Turner in Chapter 46.

IS TIP NECESSARY FOR *TEAL* PATIENTS RECEIVING IMRT?

The benefit of TIP combined with radiation for *Teal* and *Azure* is arguably the most well-validated treatment strategy in all prostate cancer.[1] It is indisputable that combining TIP and radiation decreases the risk of distant metastases and death from prostate cancer. It improves the overall survival for *Azure* prostate cancer patients in comparison to either treatment alone. This fact has been demonstrated consistently and repeatedly in virtually every large, well-designed, randomized clinical study on the topic over the past 30 years.

Similar data exists for *Teal* as well. Two clinical trials, mostly including *Teal* patients, compared outcomes for patients undergoing radiation therapy with TIP for four to six months to outcomes for patients treated with radiation without TIP.[2,3] Despite some differences in the enrollment criteria, duration of TIP, and radiation technique, both trials show that the addition of TIP to radiation prolonged survival and decreased the risk of prostate cancer recurrence.

Nevertheless, the applicability of this data to modern patients is heavily debated, given that the studies were conducted prior to the development of modern IMRT and therefore used much lower radiation doses than those we currently use in modern radiation oncology. Therefore, some physicians believe that with higher radiation doses TIP may no longer provide a significant benefit for *Teal*, although scientific evidence for this presumption is lacking. Other physicians still strongly advocate for the use of TIP in all men in *Teal*, pointing out that the addition of TIP to radiation has consistently improved survival in prostate cancer, whereas an increased radiation dose has shown only to decrease recurrence rates, not survival. A third group of physicians, recognizing that *Teal* is a widely varying disease, favor the selective use of TIP only in *Teal* that has unfavorable features, thereby sparing the favorable group of patients from this treatment.[4] The following chapter addresses this role for TIP in much greater detail.

WHAT TYPE OF TIP IS GIVEN WITH RADIATION FOR *TEAL?*

If TIP is recommended, most patients require only a short course of four to six months of treatment. Typically, patients will be given a daily pill (Casodex) for a few days, followed by a series of intramuscular injections every one to three months. Some physicians continue the daily Casodex for an entire four to six-month period, whereas others discontinue the Casodex after about two weeks and continue with hormonal injections only (Chapter 27). Usually, TIP will be given for two to three months prior to starting radiation, then continue for the duration. Adverse side effects from TIP include fatigue, hot flushes, decreased sex drive, swollen and painful breasts, mood changes, muscle loss, weight gain, diabetes and decreased red blood counts (see Chapter 30). However, given the short-term nature of hormonal therapy used for *Teal*, these side effects are completely reversed in the vast majority of cases once treatment is completed. Other more serious conditions associated with long-term TIP, such as osteoporosis and, debatably, cardiovascular disease, are much less likely to be significant for patients undergoing a short-term course of TIP.

CURATIVE OPTIONS AFTER IMRT

A common misconception is that, if prostate cancer recurs following treatment, patients treated first with surgery can be cured with radiation, whereas patients treated upfront with radiation have no curative options. In fact, prostatectomy, cryotherapy and additional internal radiation, such as high-dose-rate brachytherapy, are potentially curative options following the recurrence of cancer confined to the prostate after IMRT.

WHAT SIDE EFFECTS CAN RESULT FROM IMRT?

Radiation side effects can be separated into side effects that occur during and immediately after treatment, and side effects that may occur many months or years later. Most short-term side effects gradually build over the course of treatment, then dissipate one to two weeks following treatment completion. For instance, for reasons that are not entirely clear, radiation therapy can cause patients to feel tired during treatment. This fatigue is typically mild, does not require treatment, and does not interfere with a patient's normal activities of daily living or work.

Other than fatigue, the three main groups of side effects associated with any curative treatment for prostate cancer are symptoms influencing urination, bowel movements, and sexual function. During a course of radiation, increased frequency and urgency of urination is possible, due to irritation of the bladder. Additionally, increased stool frequency, loose stool, or even diarrhea may occur during treatment. These side effects usually resolve a few weeks after treatment. The most common long-term side effects experienced by some, but not all, men after IMRT include irritation of the bladder, decreased erectile function, and decreased ejaculate volume. However, other long-term side effects that are possible, albeit rare, include blood in the urine, blood in the stool, and changes in bowel habits. The leakage of urine or stool due to IMRT is also exceptionally rare.[5] It is also extremely rare to have long-term toxicity, requiring hospitalization or other major intervention following IMRT. Dr. Henry Yampolsky reviewed the potential side effects of radiation in greater detail in Chapter 14.

Cancers induced by radiation are theoretically possible following treatment. The risk of radiation-induced cancers is well established for young patients, such as those with Hodgkin lymphoma. However, whether there is a similar risk of radiation-induced cancer in the older population that develops prostate cancer is unclear. It is important to note that clinical trials randomizing patients to either receive or not receive radiation have not demonstrated any increased risk of cancer in the radiation subgroup.[6] Therefore, although an increased risk of other cancers following IMRT cannot be entirely ruled out, if such risk exists, it is low enough that it is completely undetectable in modern clinical trials.

WHY WOULD MEN IN *TEAL* CHOOSE IMRT IN LIEU OF OTHER TREATMENT OPTIONS?

Patients with *Teal* have many options for treatment, and the process of selecting a treatment approach can often feel overwhelming. Part of the reason for this is simply that there are so many available options, including prostatectomy, IMRT, SBRT, and brachytherapy with or without supplemental external radiation, all of which provide excellent and seemingly comparable cure rates. The primary differences in treatment options are related to how they are administered and the risk of side effects. Also, it is important to understand that very few definitive studies exist that compare these treatments head to head in a randomized prospective fashion. Ultimately, the decision to undergo a specific modality will depend on both patient preference and physician recommendation.

IMRT offers several advantages over other available treatments. For example, in contrast to surgery, IMRT is noninvasive, with no need to make a single cut or remove an entire organ from the body. Because of this, IMRT has a much lower risk of bleeding, pain, and infection than surgical approaches. Furthermore, given that the urethra runs through the prostate, surgical removal of the prostate requires removal of part of the urethra, then stitching the cut ends back together, leading to risk of urinary leakage that may require wearing pads throughout the day. Surgery can also lead to shortening of the penis.[7] By contrast, IMRT has a much lower risk of urinary leakage and essentially no risk of penis shortening.

IMRT also has some advantages in comparison to other radiation modalities, such as SBRT and brachytherapy. It is indisputable that external beam radiotherapy given in small, daily doses, such as used in IMRT, has the longest track record and the largest supporting body of evidence in the scientific literature. Essentially, every randomized clinical trial published to date involving radiation for prostate cancer has used standard fractionated external radiation therapy. Thus, external beam radiation approaches, such as IMRT, represent a tried-and-true treatment for *Teal*. Additionally,

IMRT can treat a larger border around the prostate than either SBRT or brachytherapy, which is advantageous for *High-Teal* patients who are at risk for the cancer spreading outside of the prostate. In some clinical studies IMRT has also been suggested to have lower toxicity than SBRT or combined external radiation and brachytherapy.[8]

There are disadvantages with IMRT as well. IMRT is given over the course of seven to nine weeks; so this is potentially inconvenient. Perhaps some patients would prefer to just "get it over with." However, each daily dose of radiation takes only a few minutes, patients can drive themselves to and from appointments, and almost all can continue to work if they choose. Additionally, in comparison to surgery, IMRT has a higher risk of bothersome bowel symptoms, although this risk is still very low. In patients with extremely large prostates, surgical removal of the prostate may result in better long-term urinary function than IMRT. Additionally, some patients may require four to six months of hormonal therapy, which is typically not necessary for patients undergoing surgery. Lastly, early results from a recent randomized trial that enrolled patients with both *Teal* and *Azure* showed a lower chance of recurrence, as assessed by posttreatment PSA levels, when brachytherapy was combined with IMRT (Chapter 20). The combined group, however, had more side effects. Since this study mixed patients with *Teal* and *Azure* together, it is not entirely clear that this new information is applicable to *Teal* patients exclusively.

CONCLUSIONS

IMRT is an excellent option for *Teal*, capable of curing the clear majority of men with a very low risk of short- and long-term toxicity rates. However, other good options are also available, and patients should talk with their urologist and radiation oncologist to decide if IMRT is the best treatment choice for their individual situation.

References

1. ZS Zumsteg and MJ Zelefsky. Short-term androgen deprivation therapy for patients with intermediate-risk prostate cancer undergoing dose-escalated radiotherapy: The standard of care? *Lancet Oncology* 13.6: e259, 2012.

2. CU Jones and others. Radiotherapy and short-term androgen deprivation for localized prostate cancer. *New England Journal of Medicine* 365.2: 107, 2011.

3. AV D'Amico and others. Androgen suppression and radiation vs radiation alone for prostate cancer: A randomized trial. *Journal of the American Medical Association* 299.3: 289, 2008.

4. ZS Zumsteg and others. A new risk classification system for therapeutic decision making with intermediate-risk prostate cancer patients undergoing dose-escalated external-beam radiation therapy. *European Urology* 64.6: 895, 2013.

5. MG Sanda and others. Quality of life and satisfaction with outcome among prostate-cancer survivors. *New England Journal of Medicine* 358.12: 1250, 2008.

6. M Bolla and others. Postoperative radiotherapy after radical prostatectomy for high-risk prostate cancer: Long-term results of a randomised controlled trial (EORTC trial 22911). *Lancet* 380.9858: 2018, 2012.

7. A Parekh and others. Reduced penile size and treatment regret in men with recurrent prostate cancer after surgery, radiotherapy plus androgen deprivation, or radiotherapy alone. *Urology* 81.1: 130, 2013.

8. JB Yu and others. Stereotactic body radiation therapy versus intensity-modulated radiation therapy for prostate cancer: Comparison of toxicity. *Journal of Clinical Oncology* 32.12: 1195, 2014.

Chapter 20

COMBINATION THERAPY FOR INTERMEDIATE-RISK

Sean McBride, MD
and
Michael Zelefsky, MD

Do as much as possible FOR the patient,
and as little as possible TO the patient.
Dr. Bernard Lown

BACKGROUND

The best treatments are tailored to the severity of the disease and the needs of the patient; excess treatment in the pursuit of a cure can lead to the hollowest of successes. More than most malignancies, this is true of prostate cancer, because prostate cancer, especially *Intermediate-Risk*, has a comparatively indolent nature. Therefore, practitioners must carefully match their treatment to the task with which we are charged: the elimination of the cancer with the minimization of morbidity.

Work done by our own group, now validated by others, showed that there are various subtypes of *Intermediate-Risk*.[1,2] The treatment we recommend at our own institution, and the role of combination therapy, is dependent upon which sub-group a patient's cancer falls under. *Favorable Intermediate-Risk* behaves more akin to *Low-Risk* (Chapters 8, 9 and 15). *Favorable Intermediate-Risk* has, at most, only one *Intermediate-Risk* factor. In addition, no more than 50 percent of the biopsied cores can have cancer, and the dominant Gleason pattern must be 3 (e.g., a man with a PSA of 5.6, the tumor in less than 25 percent of the gland and Gleason 3+4=7 in three cores out of 12 sampled). Patients with two *Intermediate-Risk* factors (e.g., a man with Gleason 3+4=7 *and* PSA of 12), patients who have cancer in more than 50 percent of the sampled biopsy cores, or patients with Gleason 4+3=7 are classified as *Unfavorable Intermediate-Risk*; these cancers tend to behave more like *High-Risk*, and it is these men we recommend adding seed radiation to the external beam radiation (i.e., combination therapy).

THE TREATMENT

Seed therapy, also known as brachytherapy, is the temporary or permanent insertion of radioactive pellets into the prostate (Chapters 17 and 18). At most institutions, the seeds are inserted via needles placed during a semisurgical procedure performed under general anesthesia. The distinction between the permanent and temporary seeds lies in the rate at which radioactivity is deposited into the prostate: the temporary seeds (i.e., high-dose-rate) deposit a large amount of radiation within minutes; the permanent seeds (i.e., low-dose-rate) deposit a low dose of continuous radiation over many weeks.

At our institution, for low-dose-rate (LDR) seeds, we use Palladium[103] seeds inserted via needles through the perineum under ultrasound guidance in a two to three-hour operative procedure. Men then go home the same day with seeds in place. The lion's share of the radiation from these seeds is discharged into the prostate during the first month after the procedure. Little in the way of precautions for loved ones is necessary with Palladium[103] seeds, because the radiation stays contained within the prostate.[3]

For high-dose-rate (HDR) temporary seeds, we use Iridium[192] seeds. Needles are inserted through the perineum under ultrasound guidance. Iridium[192] seeds are then funneled into the hollow-bore needles using a robotic-assisted, computer-controlled device. In a matter of a few minutes, an ultrahigh dose of radiation is delivered in a highly conformal manner. This means that the radiation conforms to the shape of the targeted area reducing radiation exposure to the healthy surrounding tissue. Dr. Jeffrey Demanes describes the process in greater detail in Chapter 18.

We find that men with prostate volumes less than 60cc and those with only mild to moderate preexisting trouble with urination make the best brachytherapy candidates. While there are various arguments, both biological and logistical for the preferential use of one type of brachytherapy over the other, for *Unfavorable Intermediate-Risk* we tend to use LDR therapy because of the relative ease of delivery. There is no evidence that either type of seed implant (LDR versus HDR) is superior to the other in terms of cancer cure rates.

Intensity Modulated Radiotherapy (IMRT) is the beaming of small doses of radiation from an outside source into the prostate over several weeks (Chapter 19). With advanced computer-based planning (used in IMRT) and the placement of small markers into the prostate (used in image-guided IGRT), the radiation beams can be aimed at the prostate with incredible, millimeter-level precision. When combined with brachytherapy, the IMRT is usually delivered over approximately four to five weeks and may commence several weeks prior to or after the brachytherapy. There is no data to suggest that any particular order of the IMRT and brachytherapy offers an advantage in terms of tumor eradication or toxicity reduction.[4] At Sloan-Kettering our preference is to perform the brachytherapy prior to the external beam radiation. The entirety of the combined therapy (IMRT and brachytherapy) is usually completed over the course of two months.

THE RATIONALE AND DATA

Compared with either type of radiotherapy alone (seeds versus beam), there is a two-fold rationale for using them in combination: 1) external beam radiotherapy in conjunction with seed radiation allows for the delivery of a significantly higher dose of radiation to the tumor within the prostate when compared with treatment with external beam radiotherapy alone; 2) compared with seeds alone, the addition of IMRT to seed placement allows for the treatment of microscopic amounts of prostate cancer that might exist outside, but still nearby, the prostate.

For these reasons, it was surmised that the appropriate application of this combination therapy in patients with *Intermediate-Risk* would reduce the probability of prostate cancer recurrence. This has been borne out in a variety of *prospective* studies (the gold standard of medical evidence) and retrospective studies. Studies from the United Kingdom and Canada demonstrated that, when compared with external beam radiotherapy alone, the combination of HDR brachytherapy and external beam radiation reduces the chance of the prostate cancer's return in patients with *Intermediate-Risk*.[5,6] In our own institutional experience, recently reported, we found that, when compared with high-dose IMRT alone, the combination of IMRT plus seeds reduced the risk of any recurrence and, more specifically, the risk of prostate cancer spread to distant sites (e.g., the bones).[7]

Unfortunately, the above studies did not divide patients into *Intermediate-Risk* subcategories. However, a recently published paper by Dana-Farber Cancer Institute has shown that in a group of patients with *Favorable Intermediate-Risk,* there were no deaths from prostate cancer in those treated with IMRT alone.[2] This suggests that the lower doses delivered with IMRT (or seeds alone) are, by themselves, sufficient to achieve cure in this favorable group. At Sloan-Kettering, in patients with *Favorable Intermediate-Risk* who are eligible, we tend to prefer permanent seed implants alone. However, in the Dana-Farber study, those with *Unfavorable Intermediate-Risk* had a risk of dying from prostate cancer that approached that of patients with *High-Risk*. Because of this, we recommend combination therapy for *Unfavorable Intermediate-Risk*.

One outstanding question in the field of combination therapy in *Intermediate-Risk* prostate cancer is whether the addition of testosterone inactivating pharmaceuticals (TIP), also known as androgen deprivation therapies, decreases recurrence and, ultimately, saves lives. We know from multiple studies that when treating with IMRT alone, adding a short course of TIP, typically four to six months, improves overall survival. This is likely because testosterone helps prostate cancer cells to repair radiation-induced damage.[8] Thus, with any given radiation dose, when we reduce testosterone or block its effects, we increase the percentage of prostate cancer cells killed. In addition, if small amounts of cancer have spread outside the prostate to distant locations, a brief period of testosterone starvation might eliminate them.

Although there is no data to guide us, the modern radiation doses used with combination therapy might be high enough that the added boost from TIP may no longer be necessary. However, because combination radiation therapy does not target prostate cancer that has spread outside the prostate, a certain proportion of patients with *Unfavorable Intermediate-Risk*—those who have microscopic and thus undetected prostate cancer cells that have traveled to distant sites—may still benefit from this short period of testosterone deprivation. It is for this reason that we will consider four to six months of TIP in *Unfavorable Intermediate-Risk* patients receiving combination therapy. What would trigger such a recommendation in these patients? We routinely obtain an MRI of the prostate, and should that detect a larger-sized tumor that is pushing through the prostate capsule or into the seminal vesicles, we would typically recommend TIP.

Ultimately, if the toxicities of combination therapy were excessive, we could not in good conscience recommend using seeds and beam radiation together if the cure rates were only marginally better. However, the data from the aforementioned studies suggest that combination therapy provides a 20 percent improvement in cure rates. The side effects of seeds and beam radiation are increased in the short-term and are marginally increased in the long-term. The risk of serious disruptions to urinary and bowel function, however, is equivalent to either seeds or beam alone and, more importantly, quite low. The rates of urinary incontinence (the inability to control urine flow) are dramatically less than the rates that are typical after prostatectomy.

SUMMARY OF RECOMMENDATIONS

In eligible patients with *Unfavorable Intermediate-Risk,* our routine radiotherapy recommendation is the combination of brachytherapy and external beam radiotherapy. We will also consider a short course of TIP in patients when results from their MRI raise a concern. Ultimately, however, it is the radiation oncologist who is best able to determine whether a patient's particular prostate cancer is best suited to this combined therapy approach.

References

1. ZS Zumsteg and others. A new risk classification system for therapeutic decision making with intermediate-risk prostate cancer patients undergoing dose-escalated external-beam radiation therapy. *European Urology* 64.6: 895, 2013.

2. FK Keane and others. The likelihood of death from prostate cancer in men with favorable or unfavorable intermediate-risk disease. *Cancer* 120.12: 1787, 2014.

3. LT Dauer and others. Assessment of radiation safety instructions to patients based on measured dose rates following prostate brachytherapy. *Brachytherapy* 3.1: 1, 2004.

4. N Bittner and others. The time gap between Pd-103 prostate brachytherapy and supplemental beam radiation does not impact on rectal morbidity or likelihood of cure. *American Journal of Clinical Oncology* 31.3: 231, 2008.

5. J Sathya and others. Randomized trial comparing iridium implant plus external-beam radiation therapy with external-beam radiation therapy alone in node-negative locally advanced cancer of the prostate. *Journal of Clinical Oncology* 23.6: 1192, 2005.

6. PJ Hoskin and others. Randomised trial of external beam radiotherapy alone or combined with high-dose-rate brachytherapy boost for localised prostate cancer. *Radiotherapy and Oncology* 103.2: 217, 2012.

7. DE Spratt and others. Comparison of high-dose (86.4 Gy) IMRT vs combined brachytherapy plus IMRT for intermediate-risk prostate cancer. *BJU International* 114.3: 360, 2014.

8. WR Polkinghorn and others. Androgen receptor signaling regulates DNA repair in prostate cancers. *Cancer Discovery* 3.11: 1245, 2013.

Chapter 21

PROTON BEAM THERAPY

Carl Rossi, MD

Any new technology tends to go through a 25-year adoption cycle.
MARC ANDREESSEN

WHAT IS A PROTON?

A proton is a subatomic particle found in the nucleus of every element. Proton therapy involves simply using a beam of protons to deliver precision radiation therapy.

Modern proton beam therapy is administered in a specialized facility in which a single proton accelerator (either a cyclotron or a synchrotron) serves anywhere from one to five separate treatment rooms. In a fashion identical to intensity-modulated radiation therapy (IMRT), patients are treated daily on an outpatient basis, utilizing image guidance. A typical treatment session lasts 15 to 20 minutes, with most of that time devoted to patient positioning. The treatment delivery—beam-on-time—is usually less than 60 seconds.

PROTONS VERSUS PHOTONS

Protons appeal to doctors who give radiation because, unlike the photon radiation used in IMRT, protons come to an abrupt stop at their target point within the body. Photon radiation is a more energetic version of the standard Xray, the same Xray that is used to create images as they pass straight through the body to the other side. Photons, and thus IMRT, expose a larger volume of healthy tissue outside the target area, just like Xrays do. Therefore, protons have a fundamental advantage over photons—*protons stop at the target.* It is this property of protons that has led to the development of dedicated proton therapy centers.

THE PATHWAY TO ENHANCED RADIATION TECHNOLOGY

Any form of radiation can kill in an indiscriminate fashion. Practically speaking, there is no "safe dose" of radiation. So, clearly, there is no benefit to unnecessary exposure of normal tissue to radiation. However, the surrounding normal tissue is invariably exposed whenever radiation is used. The technological advances in radiotherapy over the last 20 years, including the development of IMRT and proton beam therapy, have primarily been the result of attempting to reduce radiation exposure to surrounding normal tissue. This reduced exposure is the essential concept when discussing radiation technology enhancements. For example, after IMRT was invented, it was rapidly introduced into clinical use because it reduced normal tissue exposure more than its predecessor technology (three-dimensional conformal radiation therapy). And proton beam therapy likewise reduced exposure even more than that of IMRT.

Men who are considering therapy for prostate cancer have many options, including seed implants, surgery and IMRT. However, the men who are considering IMRT should probably be considering proton therapy instead. The difference between proton beam therapy and IMRT in the treatment of prostate cancer is not so much a difference in the total dose of radiation that can be delivered to the prostate. Rather, it is a difference in the amount of radiation the normal tissue surrounding the prostate receives, which is euphemistically called "low-to-moderate" radiation. With IMRT, the dose of radiation to the surrounding tissues is not low at all. It is the equivalent of several thousand diagnostic CT scans or tens of thousands of dental Xrays.

HISTORY OF PROTON THERAPY

Like many innovations in medicine, the idea of using protons to deliver precision radiation therapy was not originally proposed by a physician. In 1946, physicist Robert Wilson published a short paper entitled "Radiological Use of Fast Protons." Wilson pointed out that the physics of the proton, the way protons interact with human tissue with a low entrance dose, a maximum dose at depth, and no dose beyond the maximum dose point, would potentially make protons an ideal radiation modality. The only problem was how to localize the target. (Remember, this was decades before imaging with CT scans and MRIs was available.) Instead, at that time the best available technology for targeting was two-dimensional Xrays. Despite this handicap, beginning in the late 1950s physicians and physicists at the Harvard Cyclotron Laboratory and in Sweden could successfully treat patients with protons. As the technology and experience improved, treatment was gradually expanded to other parts of the body, and in 1977 prostate cancer was first treated with protons. This was done on a very limited basis—essentially a "proof of concept"—in patients with *Azure*. The technology employed, although antiquated by today's standards, was sufficient to establish baseline levels of safety and efficacy.

The world's first clinical proton beam treatment center opened at Loma Linda University Medical Center in 1990. The Loma Linda center continues treating patients to this day. At present, there are 15 proton treatment centers operating throughout the United States, with another dozen centers in the planning phase or under construction.

RECENT ADVANCES

Most contemporary proton centers deliver protons with a technology known as "passive–scatter" proton therapy. With passive-scatter, a small beam of protons is physically "spread out" or scattered so that the entire beam covers the desired target with a single uniform dose. This technique is relatively simple to plan and deliver and has produced excellent results. Indeed, the clear majority of proton patients whom I have treated were treated with just such a method.

However, passive-scatter proton therapy has disadvantages. Each beam requires the manufacture of a set of patient-specific lead blocks to "sculpt" the treatment field or target area of the proton beam. Each lead block must be calibrated, uniquely identified, and tracked. Any change in the treatment plan requires a whole new set of blocks. The physical size and weight of the solid lead blocks can limit the size of the treatment field. For example, at some institutions pelvic nodes cannot be treated, since the size of the required radiation field is larger than the largest achievable proton field.

A recent development in proton treatment is the development of *intensity modulated* technology for protons—IMPT. With IMPT a pencil-sized beam (with typical diameters ranging between four and eight mm) is electromagnetically manipulated so that radiation can be "painted" throughout the prostate as a series of layers. This process is analogous to a three-dimensional printer creating solid objects; and, like a three-dimensional printer, the layers of dose can be varied. Intensity modulated proton therapy, therefore, permits the coverage of large complex targets like the pelvic lymph nodes, and lends itself handily to simultaneously boosting the dose to intraprostatic nodules while sparing normal structures. The Scripps Proton Treatment Center, which opened in San Diego in 2014, is the first center in the United States to use IMPT.

EARLY CLINICAL TRIALS

When proton beam therapy first started at Loma Linda, virtually all prostate cancer patients were treated with a combination of a *proton* beam "boost" directed at the prostate, followed by *photon* therapy of the prostate and pelvis. This was done in part to attempt to duplicate the published results from the Harvard Cyclotron Laboratory, and in part to maximize the use of the protons at a time when they were a very scarce resource. Initial clinical data published in 1994 confirmed the safety and efficacy of proton beam therapy. A subsequent publication that looked at over 1,200 prostate patients treated between 1991 and 1994 was published in 1997, revealing that proton beam therapy could achieve cure rates equal to that of radical prostatectomy with a lower rate of toxicity.

After demonstrating that proton beam therapy was effective and safe, investigators at Loma Linda and Harvard decided to embark on an ambitious clinical trial to test the hypothesis that *increasing the radiation dose to the prostate* would further improve cure rates. While this hypothesis had been tested previously, one major difference was that when a higher dose was used, there was a point of diminishing returns, with increased normal tissue injury, primarily in the rectum.

Between 1996 and 2000, 383 men with *Sky*, *Teal* and *Azure* were randomly assigned to one of two treatment groups (called "arms" in medical lingo). The *standard arm* consisted of a total radiation dose of 70.2 Gray, with 19.8 Gray being given by protons. The *investigational arm* received a total radiation dose of 79.2 Gray with 28.8 Gray delivered by protons. Note that all patients received 50.4 Gray of Xray therapy to a small field that included the prostate plus a two cm margin. Hormonal therapy was not administered. With a median follow-up of just under nine years, dose escalation from 70.2 to 79.2 Gray showed improved cure rates. Equally important, dose escalation did not result in increased toxicity. This study validated that higher doses of radiation could be safely delivered without excess toxicity.

CONCLUSION

Recent technical advances in proton beam therapy delivery have made widespread clinical use of intensity-modulated *proton* therapy (IMPT) available. Using IMPT, greater dose specificity and better normal tissue sparing can be achieved over the results achievable with the older passive-scatter proton techniques. Modern proton therapy is similar to IMRT but uses the safer protons instead of IMRT's photons. IMPT stands to revolutionize proton therapy in the same way that IMRT revolutionized Xray therapy. IMPT permits customized dosing, opening the door to the treatment of pelvic lymph nodes. Like virtually all previous advances in radiation, IMPT's advantage over its predecessors is grounded in greater sparing of radiation exposure to normal tissues, a result that is achieved due to the superior physical characteristics of protons as compared with Xrays.

Chapter 22

STEREOTACTIC BODY RADIATION THERAPY (SBRT)

Michael Steinberg, MD

The only source of knowledge is experience.
ALBERT EINSTEIN

A BRIEF HISTORY

The story of SBRT for prostate cancer is a classic example of the convergence of technology and biology. *Technology* has improved through image guidance and the development of "shapeable" radiotherapy beams. These breakthroughs enable the safe delivery of much higher doses of radiation, quite a noteworthy technical innovation. Likewise, the ability to deliver a higher dose of radiation led to a surprising *biologic* result: It seems that higher doses of radiation *improve* the anticancer effect of the radiation. SBRT delivers a much larger dose per patient visit (per "fraction") than other external beam therapies, such as IMRT. In addition to the convenience of fewer doctor visits (compared with IMRT), preliminary studies suggest that radiation given in larger fractions may stimulate an anticancer immune reaction (see below).

SBRT treatment for prostate cancer began in 2003.[1] Subsequent studies confirmed what the initial study found: SBRT is an effective way of delivering curative radiotherapy. However, as in most human matters, one size does not fit all, and so it is with radiotherapy for prostate cancer. SBRT is a very good option for men with an aversion to invasive treatment and who prefer a shorter course of therapy.

SBRT technology is relatively new. Thus, clinical trials comparing it with other therapies are emerging. Despite this, with over 10 years of clinical experience,[1] SBRT is an accepted form of radiotherapy which meets the National Comprehensive Cancer Network "standard of care" guidelines for prostate cancer treatment.[2] The longest clinical experience evaluating the effectiveness of SBRT is for *Sky* and favorable *Teal*.* SBRT for *Sky* and *Teal* is becoming more routine (see editor's note, below). For *Azure,* ongoing trials are in motion to gather further evidence to document its efficacy.

SBRT VERSUS IMRT

All forms of ionizing radiation therapy result in molecular damage to vital elements within cells, such as DNA, RNA and proteins. If the damage is sufficient, it becomes lethal to those cells. While all cells can repair damage to some degree, it appears that cancer cells are much less

---

* Editor's note: The selection of treatment for prostate cancer is changing quickly. Merely nine years ago, *Sky* was considered life-threatening and 100% of men were advised to undergo curative treatment. Back then, in 2008, practically no one was managed with active surveillance. Now the industry is changing, albeit slowly. For example, in 2015 it is estimated that 50% of men in *Sky*, which amounts to approximately 50,000 men, were placed on active surveillance. Another 50,000 men in *Sky* underwent curative treatment with surgery or some form of radiation.

How can treatment for *Sky* be justified in this modern era? The argument can be framed as follows: "Since a well-performed, random, 12-core needle biopsy misses higher grade disease 20-30% of the time (when the initial Gleason grade is reported to be 6), some men may feel uncomfortable with active surveillance. As a precaution, they may prefer to undergo curative treatment. The counterargument to treating men with *Sky* is that imaging with MP-MRI can detect higher-grade disease missed by random biopsy.

efficient at this than normal cells. Consequently, radiation does more harm to cancer cells than to normal cells. IMRT exploits this difference between cancer cells and normal tissues by delivering radiotherapy in small fractions of daily treatment using small daily doses (1.8 to 2 Gray) over eight to nine weeks to allow normal tissue repair and recovery between treatments.

However, some studies indicate that the way prostate cancer responds to radiation may be different from other cancers. This is a relatively new discovery. We are starting to learn that prostate cancer cells are more susceptible to *large-dose* fractions (such as those delivered by SBRT) than what was previously believed. The underlying biology of why prostate cancer cells behave differently is not fully known. The current thinking is that it may be related to a unique cascade of immunologic responses triggered by large radiation doses.

SBRT TECHNOLOGY

The two key components in the delivery of SBRT are accurate targeting with image-guidance (IGRT), and treatment fields that closely match the outer borders of the prostate gland (conformal treatment). Accurate targeting is essential for the safe administration of such large doses. The targeting techniques most commonly relied upon are:

- The placement of gold seeds into the prostate, so it can be seen with Xrays

- Precise localization of the prostate using an Xray localization technique

- The placement of radio-frequency beacons (Calypso)

- Specialized CT scan-targeting techniques with Cone Beam CT (CBCT)

- Image guidance with transabdominal ultrasound of the prostate

All these targeting technologies are acceptable in experienced hands.

SHAPING THE RADIATION BEAM TO CONFORM TO THE PROSTATE

Images of the patient's internal anatomy are obtained with a special CT scan and an MRI scan. The prostate, bladder, rectum, seminal vesicles, small bowel and penile bulb are identified on the images and tight margins (three to four mm) are selected around the gland to minimize radiation exposure to surrounding tissue. This is called the "planning target volume," to which five fractions of high-dose radiation are administered, usually every other day, or sometimes, on consecutive days.

There are several different radiation therapy devices used for the delivery of SBRT which may include robotic features in the treatment table or delivery arm. Newer platforms use "volumetric modulated arc technique" (VMAT) with CT image guidance on state-of-the-art conventional linear accelerators. Other technologies, including proton therapy can, in principle, also be used.

CURE RATES AND SIDE EFFECTS

Based on a multi-institutional study of 1,100 patients[3] five-years after therapy, the PSA relapse-free survival rates are 95 percent for *Sky*, 84 percent for *Teal*, and 81 percent for *Azure*. These cure rates are generally equivalent to other forms of radiation or surgical treatment. There is controversy about whether a short course of TIP should be added. So far, preliminary studies indicate that cure rates are similar with or without TIP.

Side effects from SBRT are in the same ball park with IMRT or brachytherapy. They are usually of two kinds, early or late: Early side effects occur within the first three months of treatment and then dissipate. These are less of a concern than late side effects, which can last months or sometimes years after treatment. The most common early side effects are urinary issues, such as urinary frequency (e.g., getting up at night a few times), urgency, and slight urinary burning. Incontinence, or lack of bladder control, is very rare with any form of radiotherapy. Rectal issues include occasionally loose bowel movements, more frequent movements, or occasional bleeding from preexisting hemorrhoids. Bowel incontinence is very rare with any form of radiotherapy.

Standardized scales have been developed to quantify side effects. On these scales, Grade 0 corresponds to no side effects at all. Grade 1 includes minimal side effects that are noticeable but do not need treatment. Grade 2 includes moderate problems that need dietary changes and occasionally medications, such as Flomax or Imodium. Grade 3 includes significant side effects serious enough to require stronger medications or intervention (such as a temporary Foley catheter). Grade 4 side effects are considered severe enough to require some form of invasive intervention (such as cauterization).

Overall, patients are satisfied with their quality of life after SBRT treatment. In a study of 304 patients, the side effects were mostly Grade 1. Specifically, 4.7 percent of the patients had early Grade 2 genitourinary toxicity. Nine percent and 2 percent developed late Grade 2 and 3 genitourinary toxicity, respectively. In regard to gastrointestinal side effects, 3.5 percent of the men had early Grade 2 toxicity and 5 percent experienced late Grade 2 toxicity. In terms of erectile dysfunction, SBRT is just as risk-prone as any other form of radiotherapy. A systematic review of the published literature showed that SBRT leads to erectile dysfunction roughly 50 percent of the time after five years.[4] This is essentially the same rate as for brachytherapy or IMRT.

From the patient's own perspective, regarding urinary function, (using validated questionnaire tools), a minor decreased in urinary quality of life was reported to briefly follow SBRT at around three months after completion; quality of life subsequently recovered to baseline by six months and remained so out to five years and beyond.[5] Urinary quality of life complaints, should they occur, can be compensated for by reducing caffeine and adding medications such as Flomax.

PATIENT ACCESS AND COST

Medicare and the VA Health System provide coverage for SBRT for prostate cancer. Presently, there are still a few private insurers that choose not to cover it, although over the past few years most insurers now do cover SBRT. Ironically, SBRT is substantially less expensive (up to about 35 percent less) than a standard nine-week course of IMRT (which is covered by all insurers). With equivalent outcomes, much less time commitment for the patient and less cost, SBRT represents a high value treatment alternative for prostate cancer.

CONCLUSIONS

Clinical studies show that SBRT is equally successful and just as safe as the other treatment options. Patients are confronted with multiple options for treating their prostate cancer. (All the chapters in this book that discuss *Teal* are adequate proof of that.) The main advantage of SBRT for prostate cancer is that it is noninvasive (no anesthesia, no needles, no catheters, no hospitalization) and the treatment course is one week, as opposed to nine weeks for IMRT.

References

1. CR King and others. Stereotactic body radiotherapy for localized prostate cancer: Interim results of a prospective phase II clinical trial. *International Journal of Radiation Oncology, Biology, Physics* 73.4: 1043, 2009.

2. National Comprehensive Cancer Network (NCCN) 2016 Guidelines.

3. CR King and others. Stereotactic body radiotherapy for localized prostate cancer pooled analysis from a multi-institutional consortium of prospective phase II trials. *Radiotherapy and Oncology* 109.2: 217, 2013.

4. EA Wiegner and CR King. Sexual function after stereotactic body radiotherapy for prostate cancer: Results of a prospective clinical trial. *International Journal of Radiation Oncology, Biology, Physics* 78.2: 442, 2010.

5. CR King and others. Health-related quality of life after stereotactic body radiation therapy for localized prostate cancer: Results from a multi-institutional consortium of prospective trials. *International Journal of Radiation Oncology, Biology, Physics* 87.5: 939, 2013.

6. AJ Katz and others. Stereotactic body radiotherapy for localized prostate cancer: Disease control and quality of life at 6 years. *Radiation Oncology* 8.1: 118, 2013.

Chapter 23

TIP ALONE AS PRIMARY THERAPY FOR *TEAL*

Mark Scholz, MD

*Life is like riding a bicycle. To keep your
balance, you must keep moving.*
ALBERT EINSTEIN

PROSTATE CANCER IS THE ONLY TYPE of cancer that is exquisitely sensitive to hormonal blockage. It's true that breast cancer patients derive some benefit from estrogen blockade, but estrogen blockade works only about 20 percent as well in treating women with breast cancer as TIP works for men with prostate cancer. Prostate gland cells are exquisitely sensitive to testosterone deprivation because the prostate gland itself, the fountainhead of prostate cancer, doesn't develop in the body of a maturing male until testosterone levels rise at puberty. Prostate *cancer* cells, therefore, will only grow and proliferate when testosterone is present; they are so dependent on testosterone for their survival that when testosterone is removed they shrivel and die.

Compared with other treatments like chemotherapy, TIP has greater anticancer efficacy while at the same time being substantially less toxic. After TIP is started, a sharp decline in PSA almost always occurs.[1] If the doctor could feel a bump of cancer in the prostate by digital rectal examination prior to TIP, the bump usually disappears after three to four months of therapy. Historically, TIP was reserved only for men with metastatic cancer. In the 1990s, however, TIP was found to be effective for disease that had relapsed after surgery or radiation (*Indigo*), inducing remissions lasting for an average of 10 years. Now, even more recently, studies show that radiation plus TIP cures more men than radiation alone in men with *High-Teal* and *Azure*.

In the early 1990s, Dr. Stephen Strum and I hypothesized, that since TIP is so powerful in advanced disease, it should be even more effective against early-stage disease. Our initial experience bore out these suppositions. Don Outland, a local high school coach in Southern California was an early beneficiary. He came to us in 1992 for his newly diagnosed prostate cancer. His PSA was 34. Biopsy showed Gleason 6. Even though his scans were clear, his high PSA made us concerned about the possibility of microscopic cancer outside the prostate. Using primary TIP in that era was highly unorthodox. Nevertheless, we decided to proceed, encouraged by the knowledge that treatment could be reversed, if necessary.

After two months, Don's PSA was down to 0.3. A repeat prostate biopsy in June 1993 showed no evidence of any residual cancer! We decided to stop his TIP in February 1994 and by June of 1995 his testosterone blood levels were back to normal. In 2016 Don, by then age 85, continued surveillance alone without ever requiring any additional therapy. His PSA has remained stable between 4 and 5.

Over the years, we have seen hundreds of men with newly diagnosed disease experience similar excellent responses to TIP. We published an article reporting the 12-year outcome for 73 men who embarked on TIP as primary therapy in the mid-1990s. Their average age and PSA were 67 and 9 respectively. The average Gleason was 7. In most of the men participating, the cancer could be felt by digital rectal examination prior to treatment. After treatment, all 73 men recovered a normal testosterone level. Twenty-one of these men (29 percent) never needed further therapy. Twenty-four men (33 percent) required periodic retreatment with TIP to keep their PSA levels under 5. Twenty-eight men (38 percent), rather than continuing intermittent TIP, decided to have local therapy such as surgery, seeds or radiation treatment was administered an average of five-and-a-half years after the first cycle of TIP. Of these 28 men who underwent delayed local therapy, only three developed a PSA relapse, and none have developed metastasis.[2]

In another study, we described factors that predict for a better response to TIP. Longer remissions occurred in older men and in men who were treated with a BPH medicine called Proscar. Less durable remissions were seen in men starting with higher PSA levels and higher Gleason scores. Resistance to TIP has been extremely rare, only occurring in men with large palpable tumors at the initiation of therapy.[3]

Numerous studies have made clear that while TIP radically reduces the number of cancer cells (up to 99.9 percent reduction in some studies), TIP does not completely eradicate every prostate cancer cell. Microscopic evaluation of surgically removed prostate glands after eight months of TIP show that total eradication of cancer occurs in only a small minority of cases. However, studies done in our office show that after 12 months of TIP, the amount of residual cancer is usually so small that a biopsy targeted to the area in the prostate where the cancer was previously located is almost always clear.[4] In other words, TIP dramatically downsizes the tumor. For prostate cancer, which tends to be slow growing, remissions after TIP can last for many years.

One of the advantages of TIP is how easily the results of treatment can be monitored with PSA and scans (Chapters 2, 4 and 5). The PSA will decline to less than 0.05 in more than 95 percent of men within eight months of starting therapy.[1] The rare cancer that produces PSA above a threshold of 0.05 after six months of TIP should probably be treated with radiation or surgery, since it is a sign that a more aggressive cancer variant is present. Primary TIP, therefore, is a good way to smoke out the rare but serious type of prostate cancer that needs aggressive treatment up front.[1]

So, what is the catch? TIP sounds like a wonderful and decidedly superior type of treatment, especially because the side effects (Chapter 30) are reversible. Even though the disease is not arrested altogether, it postpones progression for many years. And men who select TIP always have the choice of jumping ship and doing radiation or surgery if they are so inclined. Forgoing immediate surgery or radiation, with their potentially *irreversible* side effects (Chapters 11, 12, 13 and 14) is attractive when considering the rapid improvements occurring in the medical world. In this environment, postponing irreversible treatment for even five years could lead to a whole array of new treatment options.

Basically, there are two catches. The first is that it may be hard to find a qualified doctor who is familiar with giving TIP in a way that minimizes its potential side effects (Chapter 30). The second problem is that even though TIP's side effects are manageable, they are not trivial.[5] Briefly, without careful attention to diet, notable weight gain occurs. Without regular resistance training, significant muscle weakness will ensue. And perhaps most important of all, while on treatment, most men have a total loss of sex drive! A loss of sex drive is different than impotence. With medications such as Viagra and Cialis, most men on TIP can have erections sufficient for intercourse.[6] The problem is apathy, a low interest in sex, (i.e., no libido). Sex can be enjoyed, but it is not sought after with the usual male verve. Unfortunately, there is no known way to consistently ensure the rejuvenation of libido other than by stopping TIP.

There has been no incentive among surgeons and radiation therapists to support research into the viability of using TIP as a treatment option for *Teal*. After all, TIP competes directly with their preferred approach—surgery and radiation. TIP is rarely presented, or even discussed, as a viable treatment alternative. TIP, like all forms of prostate cancer treatment, has undesirable side effects. However, at least with TIP, men have an opportunity to "test the water" and determine its effectiveness and tolerability without risking *irreversible* life-long impotence or incontinence. If, after starting treatment, a man feels that the side effects of TIP are excessive, therapy can be stopped and another form of treatment implemented.

Some patients express concern that cancer will progress unless "real" treatment, like surgery or radiation, is given. They forget that surgery and radiation only eradicate the "friendly" types of prostate cancers, the ones that remain entirely contained within the prostate. The real danger from prostate cancer lies in the risk of occult (hidden) microscopic spread *outside* the prostate. Radiation and surgery can't cure cancer that has already spread. Only TIP circulates throughout the whole body, attacking potential micrometastasis in the lymph nodes or bones. That is why TIP is considered a standard treatment for *Azure* and is universally relied upon for *Indigo* and *Royal*.

Since there is a broad expert consensus about the benefits of TIP with radiation (Chapter 20), it seems hypocritical to overlook the potential use of TIP as a standalone therapy in men who have a good initial decline in PSA after starting treatment. Certainly, the advantage of being able to forgo immediate radiation or surgery should count for something! TIP appears to be an eminently reasonable treatment option for *Teal*. If biopsy-positive *Sky* can be safely monitored on active surveillance, why not use the same surveillance techniques to monitor men with *Teal* who have become biopsy-negative after being treated with TIP?

References

1. M Scholz and others. Prostate cancer-specific survival and clinical progression-free survival in men with prostate cancer treated intermittently with testosterone inactivating pharmaceuticals. *Urology* 70.3: 506, 2007.

2. M Scholz and others. Primary intermittent androgen deprivation as initial therapy for men with newly diagnosed prostate cancer. *Clinical Genitourinary Cancer* 9.2: 89, 2011.

3. M Scholz and others. Intermittent use of testosterone inactivating pharmaceuticals using finasteride prolongs the time off period. *Journal of Urology* 175.5: 1673, 2006.

4. M Scholz and others. Primary androgen deprivation followed by active surveillance for newly diagnosed prostate cancer: A retrospective study. *Prostate* 73.1: 83, 2013.

5. BW Guess and others. Preventing and treating the side effects of testosterone inactivating pharmaceuticals in men with prostate cancer. *Seminars in Preventative and Alternative Medicine* 2: 76, 2006.

6. M Scholz and SB Strum. Re: Recovery of spontaneous erectile function after nerve-sparing radical retropubic prostatectomy with and without early intracavernous injections of alprostadil: Results of a prospective, randomized trial. [Letter]. *Journal of Urology* 161.6: 1914, 1999.

Chapter 24

ROBOTIC RADICAL PROSTATECTOMY

Timothy Wilson, MD

It is better to be lucky than good—but luck favors the skilled player.
DONALD G. SKINNER, MD

BEFORE JUMPING INTO AN immediate discussion of surgery, let me share a very brief overview. Finding optimal treatment requires an overall perspective. Prostate cancer is the most common cancer (other than skin cancer) and the second leading cause of cancer death among men. It represents 11 percent of all new cancer cases in the United States[1] and, therefore, its management consumes a significant portion of the national healthcare budget.

The selection of treatment is very controversial. Even expert opinions about PSA screening are divisive. However, by the early 2000s, after screening was instituted in the early 1990s, five-year survival rate had improved from 75 percent (in 1985) to 99.8 percent.[2] Widespread screening has changed prostate cancer in a way that can be likened to the way overfishing changes wildlife. Take lobster fishing, for example. The easiest lobsters to find are the large ones. If unrestricted fishing is allowed, within a few years only small lobsters remain. The "overfishing" of prostate cancer has led to something doctors call "stage migration." Now, after close to 30 years of overfishing, almost half of the men are "overdiagnosed." They have small, slow-growing tumors that can be monitored without immediate treatment.[3]

It is only recently (over the last five to 10 years or so) that doctors have begun to realize the radical extent to which the screening process has resulted in this overdiagnosis of indolent, slow-growing disease.[4] New FDA-approved genetic testing helps determine which men need treatment and which can undergo active surveillance.[5] Even so, disagreements persist. Once diagnosed, it's important to seek opinions from different specialists—the urologist, the radiation oncologist, and the medical oncologist. These doctors who specialize in prostate cancer will each have a slightly different perspective. In the process of researching options, patients must remember one very important principle—that newly-diagnosed prostate cancer rarely requires "emergency" or immediate treatment. For the cancers that need treatment, it is generally agreed that treatment can be safely delayed for up to six months. Men with newly-diagnosed prostate cancer have plenty of time to decide about what treatment may be right for them.

My biography at the end of the book hints at the profound depths of my personal involvement in the technological evolution of new improvements in the way prostate cancer is treated, especially with robotic surgery. My view is that surgery has several advantages over radiation therapies and other nonsurgical options such as focal cryosurgery or HIFU:

These advantages are:

1. Examination of the surgically removed prostate allows for accurate staging, which enables us to make rational decisions regarding immediate treatment right after surgery.

2. Surgery provides relief of obstructive voiding symptoms (like getting up at night and having a slow urinary stream).

3. Overall side effects of surgery are no worse than those of radiation.

4. Hormone therapy with testosterone inactivating pharmaceuticals (TIP) will not be necessary (unless after the operation a new, unsuspected degree of cancer spread is detected).

5. Surgery provides the best cure rate.

6. The accuracy of PSA monitoring for relapse is much greater after surgery than after radiation and other nonsurgical options.

7. Salvage radiation (for recurrence) is well tolerated and relatively easy to do.

I will address each of these points in greater detail below. And, at the end of the chapter, I will give a brief description of the surgical procedure itself and discuss some of the potential side effects.

ADVANTAGE 1: ACCURATE STAGING

Removing the entire prostate, seminal vesicles and surrounding lymph nodes is the best possible way to learn the cancer's true extent. With the entire prostate to look at (rather than tiny needle samples), pathologic review improves the accuracy of the Gleason score and detects microscopic spread outside the prostate (not visible on scans) and into the seminal vesicles or the lymph nodes. Microscopic review of the surgical specimen by a pathologist is by far the most accurate way to predict if the disease is cured. In addition, a genetic test called Decipher, recently approved by the FDA, provides additional information about whether a patient will benefit from immediate radiation (beginning three to four months after surgery).[6] Based on the pathology, we can also determine if short-term or long-term hormone therapy is needed.

The cure rates of men who select radiation rather than surgery are only revealed over an extended period, if the PSA begins to rise. These relapses are often unapparent for many years. At that juncture, when the PSA does begin to rise, scans will be ordered. If the scans fail to detect the location of recurrent cancer, a prostate biopsy may be performed to determine if persistent or recurrent cancer is still present in the prostate. This late detection of persistent cancer in men who have radiation has been proposed by some experts to be the explanation for the improved cure rates with surgery compared with radiation, conclusions that have been reported in some studies (see below).

ADVANTAGE 2: RELIEF OF OBSTRUCTIVE VOIDING SYMPTOMS

As men age, they frequently develop prostate-related urinary issues: slow stream, urinary urgency, poor emptying of the bladder and frequent urination at night. This may be due to an enlarged prostate or a small prostate that is misshapen. While urinary symptoms often get worse with radiation, they are generally relieved by surgery. *Surgery gets the prostate out of the way of the bladder.*

ADVANTAGE 3: SIDE EFFECTS OF SURGERY ARE NOT WORSE THAN RADIATION

Radiation oncologists often use the argument that surgery has worse complication rates. Quality of life studies do show that surgery patients take a bigger hit initially. However, after a year, quality-of-life scores are essentially identical to those of men treated with external radiation or brachytherapy.[7] It is true that with surgery most men typically lose their continence and erections, but the vast majority will recover these over the first year. If we consider that radiation usually requires TIP, the quality-of-life argument in favor of surgery becomes even stronger.

Furthermore, there are other important and significant side effects of radiation. A recent study from Ontario, Canada[8] compared the relative frequency of *delayed* problems between surgery and radiation. Men who had surgery had no increased risk of requiring a subsequent readmission to the hospital, a subsequent anal or rectal procedure, development of a secondary cancer, or an additional open surgical procedure. The rates of delayed problems from the radiation group were two to 10.8 times higher than the general population (see chart below).

Comparative Risk of
Complications after Treatment
(Hazard Ratio)
Lancet Oncology 2014

	Surgery	Radiation
Number	15,870	16,595
Age	61.5	69.4
Hospital Admission within Five Years	1	10.8
Rectal or Anal Procedure	1	2.72
Second Cancer	1	2.08
Open Surgical Procedure within Five years	1	3.68

ADVANTAGE 4: PRETREATMENT WITH TIP IS NOT NEEDED

It has been known for many years that *High-Teal* and *Azure* patients are best treated with TIP before, during and after radiation.[9] TIP increases the effectiveness of the radiation and increases the cure rate. However, it also causes erectile dysfunction, hot flashes, and decreased energy—to name the most common side effects. Several randomized trials were conducted in the 1990s in which men received three to four months of TIP prior to surgery. There was no improvement in the cure rate.[10]

ADVANTAGE 5: SURGERY HAS A BETTER CURE RATE

A recent study from Sweden[11] reported the overall survival and cancer-specific survival in men treated for prostate cancer between 1996 and

2010. Ninety-eight percent of all men treated for prostate cancers in Sweden were studied. The study compared 21,533 men treated with surgery and 12,982 men treated with radiation. Median follow-up was 5.37 years. In all groups, surgery was significantly more effective in reducing death from prostate cancer and death from any cause. This is not the only study to come to this conclusion.[12,13,14,15] A study published in *European Urology* in 2011[7] reviewed 404,000 men treated for prostate cancer and found that the 10-year cancer-specific mortality was five times worse (29.2 percent vs 6.1 percent) in men treated with radiation as compared with those treated with surgery.

ADVANTAGE 6: PSA MONITORING FOR RELAPSE IS MORE ACCURATE

After prostatectomy, the PSA becomes undetectable within about six weeks. If the PSA rises, we know the cancer is relapsing. With radiation, somewhere between 15 percent and 25 percent of patients undergo a "PSA bounce," a rise in PSA that is due to delayed radiation prostatitis—inflammation in the prostate caused by the radiation. This is very unnerving for patients and doctors alike, because there is no ironclad way to determine if the PSA elevation is from prostatitis or recurrent cancer. The uncertainty cannot be resolved even with a prostate biopsy, because biopsies within two years of radiation are inaccurate.

ADVANTAGE 7: SALVAGE RADIATION IS EFFECTIVE AND SAFE AFTER SURGERY

Of all the men who've had a prostatectomy, about 25 percent[16] have a subsequent rise in the PSA value. A subsequent rise in PSA is often treated with external beam radiation to the previous location of the prostate, known as the "prostate bed." This is referred to as "salvage radiation." Arnold Palmer, the famous professional golfer, is the best public example of how delayed radiation after surgery is sometimes necessary to mop up residual cancer cells.

Mr. Palmer underwent surgery in January of 1997. Subsequently, his PSA started rising. In the fall of 1998, radiation was administered to the prostate bed. He was disease free until he passed away from other causes at the age of 87. PSA recurrence after surgery is very manageable and, salvage radiation often solves the problem with minimal complications. Conversely, managing a PSA rise after radiation is more difficult. Treatment options will include hormone therapy and local therapy such as cryosurgery (freezing the prostate) and salvage radical prostatectomy. Salvage prostatectomy can be done safely and robotically by expert surgeons, but healing afterward is severely impaired due to the surrounding radiation damage to local tissues. The risk of long-term problems with bladder control and sexual function is much higher. If a patient is likely to need two major treatments, such as surgery and radiation, it is much better to have the surgery first.

STATE-OF-THE-ART ROBOTIC SURGERY FOR PROSTATE CANCER

Robotic surgery (Robot Assisted Radical Prostatectomy—RARP) was approved by the FDA for prostate cancer treatment in 2001. A long history of experience with this technique has accumulated.[17] Compared with open surgery, blood loss is less, hospitalization time is shorter, and men tend to recover physically much more quickly—allowing them to resume their normal activities in just a few weeks. In addition, they tend to recover their bladder control and sexual function more quickly and to a better degree.

In my opinion, RARP improves accuracy, reliability and reproducibility of surgery compared with the prerobotic era. However, the experience of the surgeon makes a significant difference. For men who are considering surgery, it is wise to make sure that the surgeon who is hired is the most experienced in the patient's geographical area. If a patient can afford to travel, it may be worth it. He should ask the surgeon about his personal results and how many procedures the surgeon has performed per year. Like anything else about life, *the more you do something, the better you get at it.*

GENERAL INFORMATION AND RECOVERY AFTER SURGERY

Let me close with a brief presentation of what surgery is like from a patient's perspective. In experienced hands, RARP generally takes between 1.5 and 3.5 hours. Differences in operative time will vary, depending on the size and shape of the prostate and the size and shape of the patient's body. An additional 30 to 60 minutes are required when the lymph nodes are removed. After the operation is completed, men wake up with a catheter that protects the new connection (known as the anastomosis) between the urinary bladder and the urethra. This should only cause mild discomfort. In addition, some surgeons place a small plastic drainage tube through the skin into a small bulb that collects serum. Usually the drain is removed the day after surgery. However, in my practice I do not routinely place a drain.

Most men will be able to go home from the hospital the following day. The catheter is removed a week later. Most can return to work within two to three weeks. About 25 percent of my patients experience the immediate return of complete bladder control. About 50 percent are essentially dry and have no need for pads by six weeks; 85 percent are dry by three months; 90 to 98 percent by one year. These results are influenced by a patient's age, preoperative bladder control, prostate size and the nerve-sparing technique used by his surgeon. Men under 65 who have good erections prior to surgery have about an 85 percent chance of having erections that are sufficient for intercourse within a year.

Preventive measures improve the likelihood of recovering erectile function. I recommend regular doses of Viagra. In addition, I recommend at least one dose (100 mg) of Viagra on the third day prior to surgery. There is preliminary evidence that this decreases the shock to the nerves. Six weeks after the operation, if men are getting at least partial erections, then continuing Viagra or a similar drug is probably fine. For men who want to be proactive and for men who are having zero erections, I recommend starting injection therapy. We teach our patients how to inject a small amount of medicine with a tiny needle directly into the penis. It is analogous to diabetics giving themselves insulin. With the correct dose, a full erection will result within about 10 to 15 minutes and last about an hour. This is repeated two to three times weekly at home. It keeps the penis healthy while the nerves are waking up. It will also allow the patient to have intercourse.

It is important to know that surgery for prostate cancer does not affect the *sensation* of the penis (the way it feels to touch), or the ability to achieve orgasm. Approximately 95 percent of my patients can achieve an orgasm within the first month of surgery—though this may be without an erection. This will seem odd to most men, because we typically associate the two things—erection and climax—together. In fact, they involve two different nerve systems. Of additional importance, after surgery, men will experience a dry climax because the organs (prostate and seminal vesicles) that make semen have been removed.

Men will follow up with the surgeon every three months for the first year following surgery and every six months after the first year. At each follow-up visit, a PSA blood test is performed and the urologist will assess overall health, bladder function and sexual function. In the few men who do not regain satisfactory bladder control (urinary continence), medical therapy can sometimes be successful (see Chapter 13).

CONCLUSION

Prostate cancer is a common disease that cannot be ignored. It is the second leading cause of cancer death in men in the United States. Screening should be done in healthy men and in men who have symptoms potentially caused by prostate cancer. Treatment decisions are dependent on the aggressiveness of the cancer, the symptoms, and the overall health of the patient. When curative treatment is indicated, surgery is best done by an experienced surgeon using the robotic technique (RARP). Though other options like radiotherapy, cryosurgery and high-intensity focused ultrasound (HIFU) exist, the highest cure rates are with surgery. There are multiple advantages of surgery, which are discussed above. Most men who have RARP recover completely over a few months and go on to live full and productive lives. Death from prostate cancer after RARP is rare, and those men who do have a cancer recurrence after RARP can commonly be treated successfully with radiation.[18]

References

1. Surveillance Epidemiology and End Results *https://seer.cancer.gov/data*, 2014.

2. Surveillance Epidemiology and End Results *https://seer.cancer.gov/data*, 2006.

3. I Thompson and others. Guideline for the management of clinically localized prostate cancer: 2007 update. *Journal of Urology* 177.6: 2106, 2007.

4. JJ Tosoian and others. Active surveillance program for prostate cancer: An update of the Johns Hopkins experience. *Journal of Clinical Oncology* 29.16: 2185, 2011.

5. MR Cooperberg and others. Validation of a cell-cycle progression gene panel to improve risk stratification in a contemporary prostatectomy cohort. *Journal of Clinical Oncology* 31.11: 1428, 2013.

6. RJ Karnes and others. Validation of a genomic classifier that predicts metastasis following radical prostatectomy in an at risk patient population. *Journal of Urology* 190.6: 2047, 2013.

7. WR Lee and others. A prospective quality-of-life study in men with clinically localized prostate carcinoma treated with radical prostatectomy, external beam radiotherapy, or interstitial brachytherapy. *International Journal of Radiation Oncology, Biology, Physics* 51.3: 614, 2001.

8. RK Nam and others. Incidence of complications other than urinary incontinence or erectile dysfunction after radical prostatectomy or radiotherapy for prostate cancer: A population-based cohort study. *Lancet Oncology* 15.2: 223, 2014.

9. M Bolla and others. Neoadjuvant hormonal treatment combined with external irradiation in the management of prostate cancer. *Bulletin du Cancer* 93.11: 1101, 2006.

10. MS Soloway and others. Randomized prospective study comparing radical prostatectomy alone versus radical prostatectomy preceded by androgen blockage in clinical stage B2 (T2bNxM0) prostate cancer. *Journal of Urology* 154.2: 424, 1995.

11. P Sooriakumaran and others. Comparative effectiveness of radical prostatectomy and radiotherapy in prostate cancer: Observational study of mortality outcomes. *British Medical Journal* 348: g1502, 2014.

12. F Abdollah and others. A competing-risks analysis of survival after alternative treatment modalities for prostate cancer patients. *European Urology* 59.1: 88, 2011.

13. MR Cooperberg and others. Comparative risk-adjusted mortality outcomes after primary surgery, radiotherapy, or androgen-deprivation therapy for localized prostate cancer. *Cancer* 116.22: 5226, 2010.

14. KG Nepple and others. Mortality after prostate cancer treatment with radical prostatectomy, external-beam radiation therapy or brachytherapy in men without comorbidity. *European Urology* 64.3: 372, 2013.

15. P Stattin and others. Outcomes in localized prostate cancer: National Prostate Cancer Register of Sweden follow-up study. *Journal of the National Cancer Institute* 102.13: 950, 2010.

16. FJ Bianco and others. Radical prostatectomy: Long-term cancer control and recovery of sexual and urinary function ("trifecta"). *Urology* 66.5: 83, 2005.

17. TG Wilson and others. Best practices in robot-assisted radical prostatectomy: Recommendations of the Pasadena Consensus Panel. *European Urology* 62.3: 368, 2012.

18. CR Pound and others. Natural history of progression after PSA elevation following radical prostatectomy. *Journal of the American Medical Association* 281.17: 1591, 1999.

Chapter 25

COMPARING TREATMENTS
FOR *TEAL*

Mark Scholz, MD

Better to trust the man who is frequently in error
than the one who is never in doubt.
Eric Sevareid

ONE OF THE REASONS FOR WRITING this book is to ensure that patients will hear all their options. Flee from doctors or friends who offer black-and-white pronouncements about any single best way to treat *Teal*. Simplistic statements are a sign of ignorance and one of the best indications that you are getting counsel from the wrong source. Also, in your quest for the best treatment, don't make the amateur mistake of giving all information equal weight.

WHERE ARE THE PROSTATE CANCER EXPERTS?
Unfortunately, almost all prostate cancer specialists are either radiation therapists or surgeons. Their views tend to be slanted because they

give one type of treatment. Patients are vaguely aware of the potential for bias but they grossly underestimate the size of the problem. Over time, these doctors develop very polished presentation skills by giving the same speech over and over. They can read people and modify their presentations accordingly.

The shortage of full-time prostate cancer oncologists struck me powerfully when I attended the 2014 American Society of Clinical Oncology, Genitourinary (ASCO GU) Symposium, an annual meeting that has been held since 2004. When I arrived, I saw my name listed on large posters around the meeting hall, along with the names of about 30 other physicians. The hosts of the meeting were honoring the tiny number of doctors who had never missed a meeting. It's not surprising that out of 2,500 attendees, only 30 doctors were selected for mention. Only 30 doctors were on the list because *very few medical oncologists* consistently attend meetings focused on prostate cancer. The prostate cancer world is run by urologists, not oncologists. I tend to assume that all my patients understand that I am a medical oncologist rather than a urologist. However, when I speak to patients, I discover that they operate under the mistaken belief that doctors are generally similar. Here is a brief description of the differences between how medical oncologists and urologists are trained:

MEDICAL ONCOLOGISTS:

1. Assume leadership of a medical team comprised of doctors of various specialties, such as surgeons, radiation therapists, pathologists and radiologists.

2. Are trained to manage all types of cancer.

3. Supervise the integration of multiple therapies in one patient (surgery and radiation and immune, hormonal and chemotherapy).

4. Are board certified in internal medicine as well as medical oncology.

5. By observing patient outcomes, learn first-hand, by experience, which surgeons and radiation doctors are the most skilled. Oncologists are the "primary care" doctors of the cancer world.

6. Are trained in how to administer multiple medications—both for cancer treatment *and* for overall health needs.

7. Have no innate preference for surgery over radiation, as they perform neither.

UROLOGISTS:

1. Are trained first and foremost as surgeons.

2. Are trained to care for numerous *noncancerous* maladies of the genitourinary tract (kidney stones, erectile dysfunction, bladder infections, prostate enlargement, vasectomies, repair of congenital anomalies, urinary leakage, etc.) in addition to prostate cancer.

3. Have minimal training in internal medicine, which is the medical management of a man's general health and wellbeing.

4. Have a rudimentary understanding of cancer treatment (outside of doing surgery).

Most patients are surprised when they learn that university programs (like USC, where I studied) offer no training in their medical oncology program about how to manage early-stage prostate cancer. That role is reserved for the urologists. Although over two million prostate cancer survivors live in the US, fewer than 100 medical oncologists specialize in prostate cancer. Almost all of them work in academia, doing clinical or laboratory research, focusing on men who have advanced, metastatic prostate cancer (*Royal*). Outside of academia, there are fewer than 10 medical oncologists in the whole United States who specialize full-time in treating prostate cancer.

Two of those 10 medical oncologists practice with me in Marina del Rey—Dr. Richard Lam (Chapters 35 and 40) and Dr. Jeffrey Turner (Chapters 39 and 46). The three of us compiled a table comparing the pros and cons of all the different treatment approaches for *Teal*, from a medical oncology perspective. Our viewpoint is based on two sources: 1) Review of the countless published studies, many of which have been performed by doctors whose reputations we know. Therefore, we have inside knowledge as to which clinical trials can be trusted. 2) Direct observations from patients, reporting on how they have fared after being treated by some of the finest doctors in the United States. We learn from experience because our policy is to refer exclusively to outstanding doctors.

The table summarizes our experience. Favorable aspects of a treatment are signaled by plus (+) signs, with a single plus being the least favorable positive aspect and multiple pluses signaling the most favorable. Negative problems are likewise reported with minus (–) signs, also ranging between one (least negative) to four.

The Pros and Cons of Various Treatment Options for *Teal*

	Favorable Aspects		Unfavorable Aspects			
Type of Treatment	Cure Rates	Convenience	Discomfort of the Procedure	Technical Difficulty	Short-Term Side Effects	Long-Term Side Effects
Permanent Seeds	++++	++++	– –	– – –	– –	– – –
Temporary seeds	++++	+++	– – –	– – –	– –	– – –
IMRT	+++	+++	– –	– –	– –	– – –
IMRT/Seeds	++++	+++	– – –	– – –	– –	– – –
Proton	+++	+++	– –	– –	– –	– – –
SBRT	+++	+++		– –	– –	– – –
Surgery	+++	+	– – – –	– – – –	– – – –	– – – –
TIP	+	++	–	– –	– – –	–

Some additional issues should be mentioned:

- Previous operations or radiation in the pelvic area increases the risk of side effects from radiation and surgery. Men who had treatments of this sort should obtain multiple expert opinions before embarking on treatment.

- Unusually large prostate glands (over 100cc) can present a problem for men considering radiation. Dosing the large target area will require a substantially higher dose of radiation for complete coverage. Sometimes the prostate gland size can be shrunk with three to four months of TIP, but this is not always successful.

- Advanced age must also be factored into the treatment-selection equation. In simplistic terms, treatment intensity should be knocked down to a lower Stage of Blue in very elderly or frail men with multiple health problems. For example, to an elderly man with *High-Teal*, I might suggest active surveillance rather than multimodality therapy with TIP, IMRT, and seeds.

COMPARING THE SIDE EFFECTS OF SURGERY AND SEED IMPLANTS

As noted in the opening chapter of this *Teal* section of the book, cure rates for *Teal* are excellent. Therefore, factoring in side effects is more important with *Teal* than it is for other Stages of Blue. Permanent loss of sexual and urinary function has huge consequences, affecting the capacity for intimacy, going to the core of a man's identity. Doctors in the industry often gloss over potential side effects, implying that the risks are just about the same with every option. *Quality studies do not support this conclusion.*[1] Surgery is consistently associated with a higher incidence of permanent urinary and sexual side effects. There is one exception to this blanket statement. When men have notable preexisting urinary issues, these symptoms can sometimes become worse after radiation, but they may improve after surgery.

To provide some concrete prospective scientific support for the proposition that surgery has more side effects—a viewpoint that many radiation therapists are afraid to voice due to a fear of offending their referring doctors, the urologists—let me present the results of a patient survey from the University of Virginia[2] in which 785 men were given survey questions about their sexual and urinary function every six months for up to three years after treatment with either surgery or seed implantation.

The study reported that *one-half* of the men who received seed implants recovered their sexual function to *the same* level as prior to treatment. However, of the men who had surgery, only *one-fifth* reported that their sexual function recovered to *the same* level as prior to treatment. Regarding recovery of *urinary* control, about *four-fifths* of the men were "back to normal" after radioactive seed implants, whereas only about *one-half* of the men recovered to normal after surgery. With stats like these, neither treatment is attractive. However, radiation is clearly the lesser of two evils.

What is important about this study was how the researchers framed their questions to the patients. Most surveys of sexual function after treatment ask the somewhat ambiguous question, "Are you functioning to some degree?" This type of methodology presents a very low bar for measuring success. Many patients do have *some* degree of preserved function, but recover nothing close to what they had experienced before treatment. The Virginia study was designed to pose the question in a totally unambiguous manner: "Do you function the same as before treatment?" This forces an unequivocal "yes" or "no" answer. Asking the question this way to hundreds of men undergoing different types of therapy provides meaningful information about how the side effects from these different treatments compare.

TREATMENT SELECTION BASED ON SUBTYPE

Men with *Low-Teal* should review Section II, because active surveillance or focal therapy may be their best option. Men with *Basic-Teal* can undergo treatment with just *one* type of therapy (Seeds, IMRT, protons, SBRT, TIP or surgery) with a good expectation for a favorable outcome. The best cure rates for men with *High-Teal* are achieved with combination therapy using seeds, IMRT and TIP.

TIME TO STOP AND THINK

Optimal treatment selection for *Teal* first requires an awareness of all the options. The next step is to get thoroughly educated about each option. In this section, eight different treatment approaches were presented. Multiple world-class experts offered a concise presentation of each type of treatment so that the options can be compared side by side. To close this section on *Teal*, let me reiterate the advice I shared at the end of Chapter 16:

> "For *Teal*, there is no single treatment option that is particularly attractive. However, some treatments come out better by comparison. When the time comes to decide, once all the shopping is finished, a list of the options remaining under consideration should be created. Once this is done, you should draw a line through the worst option and continue eliminating options until there is only one left. The last option remaining on the list is probably the right treatment for you."

Since we have discussed the many treatment alternatives and realize that there are three subtypes of *Teal*, it is easily understood why simplistically claiming, "One treatment is best for everyone" offers a major disservice to men with *Teal*. Putting in the time to do the necessary research is your best insurance against making an irreversible mistake.

Having completed this section relating to the *Teal* Stage of Blue, you can now jump to Chapter 46 at the beginning of Section VII and finish reading the remainder of the book.

References

1. JL Donovan and others. Patient-reported outcomes after monitoring, surgery, or radiotherapy for prostate cancer. *New England Journal of Medicine* 375.15: 1425, 2016.

2. JB Malcolm and others. Quality of life after open or robotic prostatectomy, cryoablation or brachytherapy for localized prostate cancer. *Journal of Urology* 183.5: 1822, 2010.

SECTION IV
THE *AZURE* STAGE OF BLUE

Chapter 26
OVERVIEW OF *AZURE*

Mark Scholz, MD

A ship is always safe at the shore—
but that is not what it is built for.

JOHN SHEDD

*A*ZURE QUALIFIES AS A MORE serious type of prostate cancer. Approximately 30,000 men are diagnosed annually with *Azure*. The 10-year mortality rate ranges between three percent and 15 percent depending on the subtype of *Azure*, the patient's age, and the quality of the medical team. The official medical terminology used by doctors for *Azure* is "*High-Risk.*" When patients hear "*High-Risk,*" they assume this means a high risk of dying. Actually, this is not the case. There is, however, a greater risk of *relapse* after surgery or radiation compared with *Teal*. Technically speaking, "*High-Risk*" should probably be called "*Higher-Risk*" due to the somewhat lower *cure rate* for *Azure* compared with *Teal*. This higher-risk is primarily due to a greater likelihood of metastases being present (see below).

Let's first review the specific criteria for a man to be *Azure*:

1. No previous treatment with surgery or radiation

2. Bone scans without metastasis

3. One or more of the following three risk factors:

   a. PSA above 20 and less than 100, or

   b. Gleason score above 7, or

   c. A prostate tumor felt by digital rectal exam extending across the midline of the gland or outside the capsule

4. Any cancer detected on a scan *outside* the prostate, up to and including the pelvic lymph nodes but nothing beyond the pelvic nodes. Any man with metastases detected outside the pelvic nodes is classified as *Royal*

THREE SUBTYPES OF *AZURE*

Once accurate staging is completed, *Azure* is divided into three subcategories (*Low, Basic,* and *High*). *Low-Azure* is when PSA is under 10 and only small amounts of grade 8 tumor are present in one or two biopsy cores.[1] Men with *Low-Azure* need to be evaluated with a MP-MRI (Chapter 4) to confirm that the tumor is relatively small and without any evidence for extra-capsular extension or seminal vesicle invasion. The treatment options for *Low-Azure* are the same as the treatments for *High-Teal* as described in Section III.

High-Azure is indicated by a Gleason score of 9 or 10 and/or a very large tumor. (A "large" tumor is present when more than half of the biopsy cores contain cancer.)[2] *High-Azure* is also signaled by a PSA over 40, a detectable PSA at the completion of radiation,[3] or when the cancer invades the seminal vesicles, the bladder, the rectum, or the pelvic lymph nodes. Treatment for *High-Azure* is discussed in Chapter 28 and 29. *Basic-Azure* is defined as neither *Low* nor *High* (Appendix I and II).

Standard treatment for *Basic-Azure* is the triad of seed implantation, testosterone inactivating pharmaceuticals (TIP) for 18 months,[4] and intensity-modulated radiation therapy (IMRT) to the prostate and possibly the pelvic nodes, if node metastases are present or if the estimated risk of node metastases is over 15 percent (Chapter 28).

THE IMPORTANCE OF MICROSCOPIC METASTASIS

The presence or absence of microscopic metastases powerfully influences the chances for cure; when "micromets" are absent, treatment will almost always be curative; if they are present and untreated, cancer recurrence is almost inevitable. Micromets are *invisible* to the best scans. Unless detected through surgery, their presence can only be *surmised* from the Gleason score, biopsy findings, and PSA. The presence or absence of micromets can therefore only be *estimated*. When the likelihood of micromets is high, systemic therapy with TIP is administered to improve the chance for cure.

This is a good time to mention surgical lymph node removal. In my many discussions with men with *Azure*, the question of surgically removing potentially cancerous pelvic lymph nodes with the goal of improving cure rates is frequently raised. While surgical removal of the pelvic lymph nodes may be useful for *detecting* microscopic metastases, surgical removal is not an effective method of improving cure rates. The problem is that the surgeon can remove only a relatively small percentage of the many nodes that are located in the pelvis. So, performing surgery to diagnose micromets is inaccurate as well.

It is logical to use TIP in men whose risk of micromets is higher, and clinical trials prospectively comparing treated and untreated men validate improved outcomes. Many such trials have been performed, the results of which will be discussed in much greater detail later in this section.

While micromets can be aggressively pursued with TIP and other therapies, these treatments should only be administered on an "as-needed" basis, due to their side effects, expense, and inconvenience. They should be withheld from men who are unlikely to have micromets. The goal is to use the mildest possible therapy when the risk of micromets is lower and reserve the more intensive combinations of treatment for the men who are most likely to have micromets. Therefore, in the following chapters, much attention will be paid to understanding the methods doctors use to predict the likelihood of micromets.

TIP: EARLIER TREATMENT IS BETTER

TIP works better against *microscopic* disease than it does against *macroscopic* disease (cancer visible on a scan).[5] Medical oncologists learned decades ago that improved results can be obtained by starting treatment while the cancer is still microscopic. The validity of using "early" treatment (the official term is "adjuvant") was first tested in the 1970s in women with breast cancer. Women who were newly diagnosed received "prophylactic" chemotherapy (or hormone therapy with Tamoxifen) immediately after mastectomy, even though their body scans were completely clear. Well-designed prospective studies comparing chemotherapy right after surgery to surgery alone showed higher cure rates with immediate chemotherapy.[6] That was 40 years ago, a time when the subspecialty of medical oncology was just getting started. Prior to that, all cancer care was supervised by surgeons. It is not all that long ago that surgery was the only type of treatment available.

I started my cancer career at the tail end of that exclusively surgical era. I can still recall the disdain surgeons would express toward medical oncologists while I was training at USC in the mid-1980s. For surgeons, the idea of "medicines for cancer" was crazy. They would warn their patients, "Stay away from those dangerous medical oncologists who want to give you chemotherapy." Back then the oncologists and the surgeons were fighting a pitched turf war over who would supervise the management of breast cancer patients. In the realm of breast cancer, the oncologists ultimately won. These days, oncologists, not surgeons, supervise breast cancer care.

History is now repeating itself. The urologists (who are also surgeons) find it difficult to believe that hormonal treatment for microscopic disease will have a significant anticancer benefit. Let me be clear: I have nothing against treating cancer contained within the prostate with radiation or surgery. Even so, we must never forget that *the microscopic cancer located outside the gland is the biggest danger.* Metastases are the component of cancer that leads to relapse in the future. Treatment protocols that fail to incorporate a strategy for the treatment of micrometastases will fail.

Throughout this section of the book and the next section on *Indigo,* we will be continually revisiting the question of how to deal with potential micromets. Specifically, we will discuss all the different treatment modalities—TIP, radiation to pelvic lymph nodes, or chemotherapy—and when to use them. The goal is *preemptive* eradication of microscopic disease at an early stage, at a point when the disease is more likely to be curable. In the following chapter, we will introduce all the different ways TIP can be utilized, depending on the Stage of Blue and circumstances of each individual patient.

References

1. V Muralidhar and others. Definition and validation of "favorable high-risk prostate cancer": Implications for personalizing treatment of radiation-managed patients. *International Journal of Radiation Oncology, Biology, Physics* 93.4: 828, 2015.

2. AU Kishan and others. Clinical outcomes for patients with Gleason score 9–10 prostate adenocarcinoma treated with radiotherapy or radical prostatectomy: A multi-institutional comparative analysis. *European Urology* 71.5: 766, 2017.

3. AK Narang and others. Very high-risk localized prostate cancer: Outcomes following definitive radiation. *International Journal of Radiation Oncology, Biology, Physics* 94.2: 254, 2016.

4. A Nabid and others. Duration of androgen deprivation therapy in high-risk prostate cancer: A randomized trial. *Journal of Clinical Oncology* 31.18 suppl: LBA4510, 2013.

5. EM Messing and others. Immediate hormonal therapy compared with observation after radical prostatectomy and pelvic lymphadenectomy in men with node-positive prostate cancer. *New England Journal of Medicine* 341.24: 1781, 1999.

6. G Bonadonna and others. Combination chemotherapy as an adjuvant treatment in operable breast cancer. *New England Journal of Medicine* 294.8: 405, 1976.

Chapter 27
TESTOSTERONE INACTIVATING
PHARMACEUTICALS (TIP)

Mark Scholz, MD

*People are always looking for the single magic bullet that will
totally change everything. There is no single magic bullet.*
Temple Grandin

H ORMONE THERAPY IS A MAINSTAY for *Azure, Indigo,* and
Royal. Prostate cancer dies when it is deprived of testosterone. This
"Achilles, heel" of prostate cancer was discovered in the 1940s, when
surgical removal of the testicles was shown to cause regression of prostate cancer. Subsequently, in 1985, an injectable medicine called Lupron,
which induces the durable suppression of testosterone, was FDA-approved.
Surgical removal of the testicles has been declining in popularity ever since.

Hormone blockade is extremely potent. Consider, however, that
testosterone also supports the normal body functions of libido, potency,
strength, endurance, and emotional stability. Therefore, the side effects

of TIP can be notable. Countermeasures for reducing TIP's side effects are reviewed in Chapter 30.

The testosterone inactivating pharmaceuticals fall into three general categories:

1. **Lupron-like** medications that work by blocking "luteinizing" hormone. Luteinizing hormone (LH) originates from the pituitary gland at the base of the brain. LH stimulates the testicles to increase testosterone production. When LH levels are reduced, testosterone levels drop.

   There are two types of injectable drugs that block LH, the "agonists" and "antagonists." The agonists are called Lupron, Eligard, Trelstar, and Zoladex. There is only one antagonist, Firmagon. Each of these agents eliminate most, but not all, of the testosterone in the blood. The adrenal glands produce small amounts of testosterone and are unaffected by the Lupron-like medications.

2. **Anti-androgen** pills "block" testosterone *activity* without eliminating it from the blood. Anti-androgens have fewer side effects and are occasionally substituted for Lupron-like drugs in frail or elderly men (Chapter 41). However, they are less potent. The trade names of the FDA-approved antiandrogens are Casodex, Flutamide, and Nilutamide. The generic names are bicalutamide, eulexin, and nilandron, respectively.

   The most common role for the anti-androgens is to counteract the testosterone "flare" that lasts for 10 days or so after the first injection of an LH-blocking drug such as Lupron (Firmagon does not cause a testosterone flare). Many doctors choose to stop the antiandrogens after a month, once the flare period has passed. Other doctors believe that the antiandrogens provide additional anticancer efficacy and should be continued for the duration of the hormonal therapy in order to block the small amounts of testosterone produced by the adrenal glands.

3. **Zytiga** and **Xtandi** are FDA-approved medications for hormone-resistant disease *(Royal)*. Prostate cancer cells with resistance to the Lupron-like drugs *manufacture their own testosterone* (instead of feeding on testosterone in the blood). Zytiga works inside the cancer cell to block the synthesis of testosterone. Xtandi also works inside the cancer cell. It prevents testosterone from activating the androgen receptor that turns on cell growth. The side effects of Zytiga and Xtandi, with some exceptions, are very similar to that of the Lupron-like drugs (Chapter 30).

The anticancer effects of TIP are enhanced with more prolonged treatment. So are the side effects. Therefore, TIP's duration is adjusted in accordance with the individual patient's circumstances. The following list presents eight different ways that TIP is commonly used:

1. Men with *High-Teal* who are undergoing radiation often begin TIP two months before starting radiation and continue for a total of four to six months of therapy.[1] Treatment for *Low-Azure* is the same as for *High-Teal*.

2. Men with *Basic-Azure* and *High-Azure* who are undergoing radiation are typically treated with TIP for 18–24 months. Treatment starts two months before radiation and continues during and after the radiation.[2]

3. Men with relapsed disease (*Indigo*) often receive *intermittent* TIP. This means that an initial course is continued for six to 12 months and then stopped. During the off-period, PSA levels are monitored every three months. A second cycle of TIP is initiated when the PSA rises up to a prespecified level, usually in the range of 3 to 6.[3,4]

4. With occasional exceptions, men with *Royal* remain on TIP indefinitely.

5. Men with *Royal* who become resistant to Lupron are usually administered Xtandi[5] or Zytiga.[6] Treatment with Xtandi or Zytiga is continued until there is clear evidence of new metastases on a bone scan or body scan. A rising PSA by itself, without new metastatic lesions, is an insufficient rationale to stop Xtandi or Zytiga.

6. TIP has a role, aside from its anticancer effects, for shrinking an enlarged prostate gland prior to a radioactive seed implant. Otherwise, some men with excessively large prostates would be ineligible for seed implantation.[7]

7. TIP can be used as a primary therapy instead of surgery or radiation to treat men with *Teal* (Chapter 23).[8,9]

8. TIP can be used *after surgery* in men with *Azure*.[10] This is controversial. Some older studies performed with *Teal* showed no improvement in cure rates. However, these studies used a mere three months of TIP. Subsequent studies in *Azure* using TIP for a longer duration show improved survival (Chapter 29).

As can be seen from this introductory list, TIP is administered in a selective fashion and given for a specified period of time, depending on a patient's Stage of Blue. TIP's specific and varied roles will be elaborated further throughout the remainder of the book.

References

1. M Bolla and others. EORTC trial 22991: Results of a phase III study comparing 6 months of androgen suppression and irradiation versus irradiation alone for localized T1b-cT2aN0M0 prostate cancer. *Journal of Clinical Oncology* 34.2 suppl: 22, 2016.

2. A Nabid and others. High-risk prostate cancer treated with pelvic radiotherapy and 36 versus 18 months of androgen blockage: Results of a phase III randomized study. *Journal of Clinical Oncology* 31.6 suppl: 3, 2013.

3. L Klotz and others. Intermittent androgen suppression for rising PSA level after radiotherapy. *New England Journal of Medicine* 367.10: 895, 2012.

4. TM Beer and others. Enzalutmide in metastatic prostate cancer before chemotherapy. *New England Journal of Medicine* 371: 424, 2014.

5. JS De Bono and others. Abiraterone and increased survival in metastatic prostate cancer. *New England Journal of Medicine* 36421: 1995, 2001.

6. R Kucway and others. Prostate volume reduction with androgen deprivation therapy before interstitial brachytherapy. *Journal of Urology* 176.6: 2443, 2002.

7. M Scholz and others. Primary androgen deprivation followed by active surveillance for newly diagnosed prostate cancer: A retrospective study. *Prostate* 73.1: 83, 2013.

8. M Scholz and others. Primary intermittent androgen deprivation as initial therapy for men with newly diagnosed prostate cancer. *Clinical Genitourinary Cancer* 9.2: 89, 2011.

9. TB Dorff and others. Adjuvant androgen deprivation for high-risk prostate cancer after radical prostatectomy: SWOG S9921 study. *Journal of Clinical Oncology* 29.15: 2040, 2011.

Chapter 28

THE *AZURE* STAGE OF PROSTATE CANCER

Mark Scholz, MD

Knowledge is the antidote to fear.
RALPH WALDO EMERSON

TREATMENT SELECTION FOR *Azure* is actually somewhat *less* controversial than for *Teal*. First, everyone agrees that *Azure* requires therapy—active surveillance can only be considered for the very aged or infirm. Second, conclusive studies show that testosterone inactivating pharmaceuticals (TIP) given in combination with radiation give higher cure rates than radiation alone or TIP alone. Finally, as we will demonstrate, TIP plus radiation produces better results than surgery. Mainstream therapy for *Azure*, therefore, should consist of seed implantation *plus* IMRT *plus* TIP. This chapter will provide detailed scientific support for this conclusion.

IMAGING STUDIES FOR STAGING

With *Azure,* the first step is to make sure no *detectable* metastases outside the pelvic lymph nodes can be discovered by a bone scan, CT, or MRI of the abdomen and pelvis. Scanning technology to detect metastases outside the prostate is far from perfect. Even the best imaging centers can render ambiguous reports, commenting on shadows or lesions that may or may not originate from cancer. A questionable abnormality detected on a bone scan, for example, can be further evaluated by a standard MRI (not MP-MRI) focused specifically on the questionable area. An MRI may be able to determine if a questionable abnormality has a cancerous cause or is due to some other benign process. If the MRI fails to resolve the uncertainty, a CT-directed needle biopsy of the lesion may be considered. Suspicious lesions in the pelvic lymph nodes can be further evaluated with specialized PET scans, as described in Chapter 6. Alternatively, laparoscopic surgery can be considered to remove an enlarged lymph node and examine it for the presence of cancer. Suspicious MP-MRI scans that suggest cancer invasion outside the capsule into the seminal vesicle can be further evaluated with a color Doppler ultrasound-directed biopsy (Chapter 5). Accurate assessment of the extent of disease and the location of the cancer in the body is essential for arriving at an optimal treatment plan.

Since cure is a top priority with *Azure,* let's jump to the bottom line and identify the best treatment. Numerous studies purport to address this important issue, but there is a problem: randomized studies comparing different treatments head-to-head are few. Multiple centers publish the cure rates, but only for one type of therapy. Studies from different centers are not directly comparable. They have different types of patients with different age ranges, different treatment styles, and different research methodology. Comparing cure rates between centers can be like comparing apples to oranges. It is well known, for example, that younger men have better treatment outcomes. But retrospective reports comparing young, surgically treated men with older, radiation-treated men are published all the time. Such studies can be highly misleading.

Though there are limitations to relying on any single retrospective study to determine the best treatment for prostate cancer, does this mean that they are all worthless? Perhaps each single study, as a standalone, would be suboptimal. However, after examining *multiple* studies, trends begin to emerge. The Prostate Cancer Results Study Group, founded by Dr. Peter Grimm, compiled *all* the studies that report cure rates for *Azure*.[1] Dr. Grimm uses a graphical format to present *cure rates* for a multitude of studies.

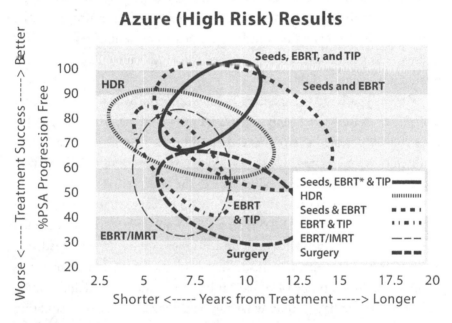

Azure (High Risk) Results

Worse <----- Treatment Success -----> Better

%PSA Progression Free

Seeds, EBRT, and TIP

Seeds and EBRT

HDR

EBRT & TIP

EBRT/IMRT

Surgery

Seeds, EBRT* & TIP	▬▬▬
HDR	▪▪▪▪▪▪▪
Seeds & EBRT	▪ ▪ ▪ ▪
EBRT & TIP	▪ ▪ ▪ ▪ ▪
EBRT/IMRT	▬ ▬ ▬
Surgery	▬▬ ▬▬

Shorter <----- Years from Treatment -----> Longer

www.PCTRF.org   Prostate Cancer Results Study Group

*EBRT – See Glossary; HDR = High-Dose-Rate Seeds

Don't be overwhelmed by the graph's apparent complexity. A massive amount of important information is being conveyed through this format. The large circles convey the *average* cure rate from many different treatment centers for a single type of treatment, be it surgery, radiation, or seed implantation. The circle located closest to the top of the graph has the highest cure rate. As can be seen, either seed implants or seed implants plus IMRT, on average, provides higher cure rates compared with IMRT alone or surgery, *even though surgically treated patients in these studies have the advantage of being much younger.*

For the studies with a longer observation period after treatment, the circles extend farther to the right on the graph. So, the *circles* give a visual "average cure rate" for each type of therapy and a sense of the studies' maturity. The only studies Dr. Grimm excluded from this comprehensive analysis were the ones that were too small (less than 100 patients), failed to use the D'Amico staging methodology to describe their patient participants, or were too immature, (i.e., the patients in the study had not undergone posttreatment observation for an adequate period of time). For more information on this landmark presentation see pctrf.org.

Recently, a large prospective *randomized* trial was completed that comes to the same conclusion as Dr. Grimm's analysis. This trial, called ASCENDE-RT, tested the premise that adding a seed implant to IMRT would improve cure rates over IMRT alone.[2] The details of this important trial are expounded further in Chapter 17. The bottom line is that the cure rate for men treated with IMRT was only 63 percent whereas 83 percent of the men who received IMRT *plus* a seed implant boost were cured, a 20 percent improvement in cure rates! Higher cure rates with seeds are hardly surprising when you consider how radiation functions. Cure rates go up as the total dosage of radiation increases and seeds deliver much higher doses of radiation than what can be achieved with beam radiation (IMRT). The results of the ASCENDE-RT trial confirm that seed implants should be the standard of care for the treatment of *Basic-Azure.*

Seed implants (brachytherapy) come in two forms: Low-dose-rate permanent seeds and high-dose-rate temporary seeds. Chapters 17, 18, and 20 provide detailed reviews of these two approaches. For *Azure,* there is no absolute rule about one type of brachytherapy being superior to the other. However, if there is spread through the capsule or into the seminal vesicle, temporary seeds may provide better coverage.

WHY WOULD SEEDS WORK BETTER THAN SURGERY?

One would think that the surgical removal of the gland would be the most definitive treatment approach possible. The problem is the proximity of the bladder and rectum. These sensitive structures are only millimeters from the prostate. The surgeon's ability to cut a sufficiently wide margin is severely constrained. Incomplete cancer removal is a frequent problem. The official terminology for cancer left behind after surgery is a "positive margin." Sadly, positive margins occur in about *half* of the men who undergo surgery for *Azure*.[3] Incomplete cancer removal means that radiation will be necessary to "sterilize" the residual cancer. The problem is that radiation right after surgery presents a dilemma. Cancer cure rates are best the sooner it is performed while, radiation-related side effects can be reduced by postponing. To avoid this dilemma and avoid the need for undergoing both surgery *and* radiation, it is better to simply do the radiation and skip the surgery altogether.

As Dr. Grimm's analysis clearly shows, seed implants have higher cure rates than surgery anyway. Seed superiority to surgery initially seems counterintuitive. Cutting the gland out sounds so definitive. However, when you understand that the seeds implanted near the capsule of the prostate emit *radiation that extends over the edges of the gland,* you can see why the chances for disease control are improved. The radiation covers a larger area around the gland than what can be achieved with surgery. Better cancer coverage leads to a higher cure rate.

One possible exception to the general rule of avoiding surgery for men with *Azure* is for the stage of men who have *Low-Azure* in conjunction with an extremely large prostate gland. Large glands are often associated with notable, preexisting urinary symptoms. Such men are at a higher risk for developing long-term urinary side effects after radiation, as described by Dr. Tim Wilson in Chapter 24. If surgery is skillfully performed without creating incontinence, urinary flow may be improved by surgery, since it removes the obstructing gland.

CURE RATES WITH SURGERY

Cure rates with surgery for *Azure* are quite disappointing as almost everyone eventually relapses. In a large study of 9,300 men undergoing surgery for *Azure* at Johns Hopkins, the Mecca of prostate surgery, the reported relapse rates were incredibly high.[4] These patients seemed like reasonable candidates for cure with surgery. They had a median PSA of 7.5 and digital rectal examinations that were judged to be free of extra-capsular extension. Despite these hopeful presurgical indicators, pathologic evaluation of the prostate after it was surgically removed showed that *70 percent of the men had extra-capsular extension.* Over the next 15 years, *80 percent* of them developed recurrent cancer.

As long as surgeons continue in the role of diagnosing men with prostate cancer (via the random biopsy performed in their medical office), surgery will invariably come up for discussion. There is a popular saying among urologists, "A chance to cut is a chance to cure." But from my viewpoint as a nonsurgical prostate expert, when considering treatment for men in *Azure*, the only time when surgery might be a consideration is in men with *Low-Azure*.

PROPHYLACTIC TREATMENT OF THE PELVIC NODES WITH RADIATION

Azure is associated with a substantially higher risk of *microscopic* cancer spreading to the pelvic nodes, cancer that is invisible on standard scans such as CT or MRI. It is logical, therefore, to consider "prophylactic" radiation to the pelvic lymph nodes, even when the scans appear normal. However, prophylactic node radiation can be controversial for two reasons. First, the studies are contradictory. The best study documenting improved cure rates was conducted by Dr. Mack Roach at UCSF.[5] A smaller study by Pascal Pommier,[6] however, suggested that pelvic radiation may only have a minimal impact on cure rates. Dr. Pommier's study, though, had major weaknesses. Far fewer patients were evaluated compared with Dr. Roach's study. Also, *half* of the participants in Dr. Pommier's study were at very low risk for having microscopic metastases to begin with. How would a study be able to show an improvement in cure rates with radiation to the pelvic nodes if there is no cancer in the pelvic nodes to begin with?

WHAT ABOUT SIDE EFFECTS FROM PELVIC RADIATION?

The second reason that pelvic node radiation has been controversial is related to concerns about side effects, especially intestinal dysfunction—a frequent complication of older radiation technology. As recently as 10 years ago, pelvic node radiation technology was imprecise and unfocused. Permanent damage to the surrounding bowel occurred very frequently. However, with modern IMRT, bowel damage is extremely uncommon. For example, Dr. Curtiland Deville compared radiation to the prostate alone with radiation to the prostate *plus* additional pelvic node radiation using IMRT. In two separate studies, the incidence of side effects, with or without pelvic node radiation, was the same.[7,8]

In cases in which the risk of cancer spread to the nodes is low, pelvic radiation should be withheld. Therefore, men need to be able to estimate the likelihood of occult microscopic pelvic node metastases. This risk can be calculated using the following equation:

$$\text{Probability of metastasis (in \%)} = (GS - 5) \times \left(\frac{PSA}{3} + 1.5 \times T\right)$$

GS is the Gleason score and T is the clinical stage estimated by digital rectal examination. T = 0 for stage T1c, 1 for T2a, and 2 for T2b or T2c (see Chapter 1 for an explanation of how to assign the clinical stage). Dr. Mack Roach, chief of radiation at UCSF, recommends that only men with a calculated risk above 15 percent should undergo node radiation. When using this equation to estimate the risk of nodal metastases, it is important to note that the formula does not account for the number of positive biopsy cores or for the extent of the tumor detected by MP-MRI or color Doppler ultrasound imaging. Therefore, the estimated risk of node metastases provided by the formula above should be adjusted upward in men with multiple positive cores or unfavorable MP-MRI findings, such as extracapsular extension or seminal vesicle invasion.

Before we leave this important theme of lymph node radiation, we also have to consider that not all radiation therapists are created equal. Dr. Colleen Lawton of the Medical College of Wisconsin has taken surveys from multiple radiation oncologists with expertise in genitourinary oncology and found that there is significant disagreement among GU radiation oncology specialists about the optimal methodology for performing pelvic nodal radiation therapy.[9] To address this, Dr. Lawton convened a meeting of experts to reach a consensus. The results are published on the American Society of Therapeutic Radiation Oncology (ASTRO) website. Guidelines for pelvic node radiation were also published by Dr. Victoria Harris.[10] It should be emphasized that the treatment methodology for applying pelvic node radiation continues to evolve. Optimal results require that treatment be administered by radiation experts with extensive experience and skill.

TESTOSTERONE INACTIVATING PHARMACEUTICALS (TIP) ADDED TO RADIATION

TIP is the third leg of the *Azure* treatment triad. The most famous study evaluating the benefit of TIP was performed by Dr. Michael Bolla in Europe. Dr. Bolla prospectively evaluated the survival rates of hundreds of men who were treated with radiation combined with TIP for 36 months, versus those treated with radiation without TIP.[11] Ten years after the radiation was completed, the mortality rate from cancer in the men treated with TIP was only 10 percent, compared to 30 percent in the men who did not receive TIP.

In another study, Dr. Bolla compared short-term TIP with long-term TIP. The study evaluated 970 men with an average PSA of 18 treated with 50 Gray radiation to the pelvis and 70 Gray to the prostate gland.[12] Half of the men in the study were treated with hormone therapy for six months and the other half were treated for three years. The five-year mortality with six months of TIP was 19 percent, compared to 15 percent when the TIP was continued for three years, confirming better survival with longer-term TIP. Another similar study, performed by Dr. Eric Horowitz, compared radiation combined with two years of

TIP versus radiation plus TIP continued for only four months.[13] The cancer death rate after 10 years was reduced from 16 percent in the men treated for four months to 11 percent in the men treated for two years. Once again, longer-term TIP gave better results. Of course, these reported survival differences between short- and long-term TIP are not huge, with only about a five percent difference between the two groups. Since the side effects of TIP increase with longer treatment periods, the decision about treatment duration needs to be individualized on a patient-to-patient basis.

One question that frequently arises is whether Lupron should be used alone or in combination with Casodex to increase the TIP's anti-cancer efficacy. (Lupron and Casodex are "trade names" for TIP—see Chapter 27). A study published by Dr. Akash Nanda from Harvard, indicated that adding Casodex to Lupron results in lower mortality rates compared with those for men treated with Lupron alone.[14]

So, for *Basic-Azure* prospective, randomized trials show improved cure rates when TIP is added to radiation. The survival rates are optimal when the duration of TIP is longer and when Casodex is added to Lupron. These men should receive a combination of IMRT, brachytherapy, and TIP. TIP should begin at least two months before radiation[5] and continued for a total of 18 months. IMRT should be administered to the prostate and possibly to the pelvic nodes (when the calculated risk of nodes is greater than 15 percent). A seed implant boost to the prostate should be considered standard, except possibly for men with *Low-Azure* who have unusually severe preexisting urinary symptoms. In the next chapter, we will discuss an even more aggressive treatment approach for *High-Azure* that incorporates Taxotere and possibly "off-label" Zytiga or Xtandi. We will also discuss the latest thinking about giving TIP after surgery.

References

1. P Grimm and others. Comparative analysis of prostate-specific antigen free survival outcomes for patients with low, intermediate and high risk prostate cancer treatment by radical therapy. Results from the Prostate Cancer Results Study Group. *British Journal of Urology International* 109.s1: 22, 2012.

2. WJ Morris and others. ASCENDE-RT*: A multicenter, randomized trial of dose-escalated external beam radiation therapy (EBRT-B) versus low-dose-rate brachytherapy (LDR-B) for men with unfavorable-risk localized prostate cancer. *Journal of Clinical Oncology* 33 suppl 7: abstr 3, 2015.

3. NJ Hartly and others. Comparison of positive surgical margin rates in high risk prostate cancer: open versus minimally invasive radical prostatectomy. *International Braz J Urol* 39.5: 639, 2013.

4. JI Epstein and others. Long-term survival after radical prostatectomy for men with high Gleason sum in pathologic specimen. *Urology* 76.3: 715, 2010.

5. M Roach and others. Phase III trial comparing whole-pelvic versus prostate-only radiotherapy and neoadjuvant versus adjuvant combined androgen suppression: Radiation Therapy Oncology Group 9413. *Journal of Clinical Oncology* 21.10: 1904, 2003.

6. P Pommier and others. Is there a role for pelvic irradiation in localized prostate adenocarcinoma? Preliminary results of GETUG-01. *Journal of Clinical Oncology* 25.34: 5366, 2007.

7. C Deville and others. Clinical toxicities and dosimetric parameters after whole-pelvis versus prostate-only intensity-modulated radiation therapy for prostate cancer. *International Journal of Radiation Oncology, Biology, Physics* 78.3: 763, 2010.

8. C Deville and others. Comparative toxicity and dosimetric profile of whole-pelvis versus prostate bed-only intensity-modulated radiation therapy after prostatectomy. *International Journal of Radiation Oncology, Biology, Physics* 82.4: 1389, 2012.

9. CAF Lawton and others. RTOG GU radiation oncology specialists reach consensus on pelvic lymph node volumes for high-risk prostate cancer. *International Journal of Radiation Oncology, Biology, Physics* 74.2: 383, 2009.

10. VA Harris and others. Consensus guidelines and contouring atlas for pelvic node delineation in prostate and pelvic node intensity modulated radiation therapy. *International Journal of Radiation Oncology, Biology, Physics* 92.4: 874, 2015.

11. M Bolla and others. External irradiation with or without long-term androgen suppression for prostate cancer with high metastatic risk: 10-year results of an EORTC randomised study. *Lancet Oncology* 11.11: 1066, 2010.

12. M Bolla and others. Duration of androgen suppression in the treatment of prostate cancer. *New England Journal of Medicine* 360.24: 2516, 2009.

13. EM Horwitz and others. Ten-year follow-up of radiation therapy oncology group protocol 92-02: A phase III trial of the duration of elective androgen deprivation in locally advanced prostate cancer. *Journal of Clinical Oncology* 26.15: 2497, 2008.

14. A Nanda and others. Total androgen blockade versus a luteinizing hormone-releasing hormone agonist alone in men with high-risk prostate cancer treated with radiotherapy. *International Journal of Radiation Oncology, Biology, Physics* 76.5: 1439, 2010.

Chapter 29

UNORTHODOX THERAPIES FOR *HIGH-AZURE*

Mark Scholz, MD

It is the mark of an educated mind to be able to
entertain a thought without accepting it.
Aristotle

A S THE CANCER BECOMES MORE ADVANCED, the attitude of some doctors can become pessimistic. Pessimism in oncology is certainly understandable. Oncologists must deal with the stark reality of cancer: the fact that people die. Some doctors feel it is dishonest to convey an overly optimistic prognosis. They are concerned about misrepresenting the situation and raising false hopes. Though assessments should be realistic, we professionals also need to stay open to the possibility that certain patients are going to do better than expected. We cannot always determine in advance who might beat the odds. The danger is that negative expectations can become a self-fulfilling prophecy, especially if they lead to a decision to use less-than-maximal therapy.

High-Azure is an indisputably a dangerous type of prostate cancer. The best way to confront the danger is by aiming for a cure by using every available type of effective therapy. A maximal approach is beneficial for most men, even those who are not cured. Maximal therapy is more likely to lead to a prolonged remission. Men who have longer remissions are more likely to live into a future era of new discoveries; discoveries that are coming out faster and faster all the time. So, beyond the basic triad of seeds, IMRT, and TIP that is recommended in the previous chapter for *Basic-Azure*, what additional therapies should be considered for *High-Azure*?

CHEMOTHERAPY FOR *HIGH-AZURE*

In 2015, Dr. Howard Sandler presented an important study at a large cancer meeting suggesting that Taxotere, a popular form of chemotherapy used to treat advanced prostate cancer (see Chapters 35 and 40), is also beneficial for *High-Azure*. (Dr. Sandler is the coauthor of Chapter 19). In this study, Taxotere for six cycles was combined with radiation and TIP in 280 men. Their survival was compared with 281 other men treated with radiation and TIP without Taxotere. *Mortality rates within four years were reduced by 30 percent in the men who received Taxotere.* The rate of new metastases was reduced by 37 percent. The data from this study, called STAMPEDE, was published in *The Lancet* in 2016.[1] Men with either *High-Azure* or with *High-Indigo* were included in the study. A contradictory study from Scandinavia that followed 459 men showed no improvement in cure rates for Taxotere-treated men.[2] The trial design was strange, however, because neither of the two groups were administered any TIP. The relevance, therefore, of the Scandinavian study to real-world care is questionable.

XTANDI AND ZYTIGA FOR *AZURE*

Xtandi and Zytiga are FDA-approved, but only for men with metastatic, hormone-resistant disease *(Royal)*. Studies for *Azure* are ongoing.[3] In the meantime, what should patients do? We know that these agents are more effective than Lupron for *metastatic* disease. Might we therefore conclude that they will be more effective than Lupron for *earlier-stage* disease? My oncology professor at USC, Dr. John Daniels, a successful inventor in his own right, once told me, "Most new inventions are nothing more than repurposed old inventions."

There is no doubt that Xtandi and Zytiga are potent. They induce cancer remissions even after Lupron stops working. As was previously stated, treatments effective in advanced cancer generally prove to be even more effective against earlier-stage disease. This logic is so simple, one might wonder why the doctors in academia feel the need to perform studies to prove it. The real reason comes back to cost. Insurance companies save money by limiting access to new medications. Without a study proving a benefit for *Azure,* they can wriggle out of their responsibility for covering payment.

There is *one* potential argument against using the most active agents for earlier-stage disease: the idea that there may be a benefit to holding a treatment *in reserve* to serve as a "backup" in case standard treatment fails. The problem with this logic is that using effective therapy as a backup plans result in much lower cure rates. The battle against life-threatening cancer should be viewed as all-out war. Delaying effective treatment merely gives the cancer more time to develop resistance. Results are best with immediate, maximal therapy.

Based on these conclusions, if we agree that these agents can enhance cure rates by using them at an earlier stage, what are the potential situations in which Xtandi and Zytiga might be useful? Basically, any situation in which the cure rates with Lupron are less than ideal:

- *High-Azure*
- *High-Indigo,* men with disease relapsed after surgery or radiation who have proven pelvic lymph node metastases
- Basic *Royal* (Chapter 39) men with oligometastatic disease that is undergoing radiation to all metastatic sites

In all three of these situations, Lupron is known to be beneficial. In some cases, studies have shown that adding Casodex further increases the anticancer effect. This is important, because a comparative study shows that Xtandi is clearly far more potent than Casodex.[4] Therefore, substituting Xtandi for Casodex in the situations listed above is likely to improve the anticancer effect.

GENERAL THOUGHTS FOR EXTENDING LIFE IN MEN WITH AZURE

To improve the odds of a longer life, we should eat a good diet (Chapter 47); get annual medical checkups (Chapter 46); do physical exercise (Chapter 48); and get married. Seriously? Yes, it's true; studies show that married men with prostate cancer outlive single men by 25 percent.[5] A less formidable undertaking than marriage is to consider taking certain medications not normally considered for their anticancer effects—aspirin, statins, and metformin. Credible studies indicate that these agents also prolong survival.

ASPIRIN

Two notable studies report that aspirin improves survival in *Azure*. In a 2014 study authored by Dr. Eric Jacobs, low-dose aspirin reduced prostate cancer mortality by 40 percent compared with the men who did not take aspirin.[6] In another study, also published in the *Journal of Clinical Oncology*, aspirin improved the 10-year prostate cancer survival rate from 81 percent to 96 percent.[7]

How can a lowly aspirin make such a big difference? No one knows for sure, but the experts speculate that aspirin interrupts the cancer's ability to metastasize by an inhibitory effect on the body's blood clotting system. The mechanism of how cancer metastasizes is tightly interwoven with the normal coagulation system of the blood. Coagulation contributes to making the blood "sticky" enough for cancer cells floating in the blood to "land" in an area of the body outside the prostate and produce new tumors. In simple terms, aspirin makes the blood vessel walls more "slippery" impeding the circulating tumor cells from landing and forming new tumors.

STATIN DRUGS

The use of statins is another "outside-the-box" anticancer approach to consider. The trade names for these cholesterol pills are Lipitor, Crestor,

Livalo, and Pravachol. In 2015, at the annual urology meeting, Dr. Robert Hamilton reported on 1,364 men with *Indigo* on intermittent TIP.[8] After seven years, statin use resulted in a 35 percent lower mortality rate. Another study presented at the annual meeting of the American Society of Clinical Oncology (ASCO) in 2015 by Dr. Grace L. Lu-Yao evaluated 22,110 *Azure* patients.[9] Statin medications, in this case combined with metformin (see below), resulted in a 43 percent reduction in prostate cancer mortality.

METFORMIN

Another "noncancer" medication with potential anticancer effects is metformin, a generic diabetes medication. Metformin suppresses insulin, which is a good thing from a cancer point of view, because insulin has a stimulatory effect on cell growth that is similar to growth hormone. In one study from Ontario, prostate cancer survival was evaluated in 3,800 patients with diabetes. The patients taking metformin had a 25 percent reduction in mortality compared with patients treated with other types of diabetic medication.[10] Dr. Mark Preston presented another study, the results of a computer query of the Danish Cancer Registry. He compared 12,000 men in northern Denmark who took metformin to 120,000 who did not take metformin. Men on metformin were found to have a 44 percent lower risk for developing prostate cancer, compared with men who never used metformin.[11]

Nothing is without risk. All medications have potential side effects. However, these three medications have been prescribed to millions of people, in most cases without notable problems. General practitioners are quite familiar with the standard strategies for limiting the side effects of these medications. Overall, these agents are generally well tolerated, and the risk of side effects seems justifiable, considering their favorable effects on survival rates.

ADDING TIP TO SURGERY IN MEN WITH *AZURE*

The last unconventional treatment for *Azure* involves the use of TIP after surgery. Surgery for *Azure* is still popular with many surgeons although

I don't advocate it. As discussed by Dr. Tim Wilson in Chapter 24, certain studies using short-course TIP to treat *Teal* showed no benefit. Therefore, adding TIP to surgery is considered ineffective by most urologists. Something, however, is needed to offset the poor cure rates of surgery alone. As can be clearly seen from the multiple studies listed in the table below, relapse rates with surgery alone are very high.

Table 1: Five-Year Relapse Rates After Surgery in Multiple Studies of *Azure*

# of Patients in the Study	110	206	957	712	1179	188	Average
Relapse Rates	55%[12]	48%[13]	32%[14]	35%[15]	53%[16]	29%[17]	42%

The pessimistic view of urologists about using TIP to improve cure rates dates back to trials performed in the 1990s. Those randomized studies only evaluated three months of TIP after surgery and there was no improvement in cure rates. However, other important studies are being overlooked:

1. Dr. Martin Gleave at Vancouver General Hospital compared eight months of TIP after surgery to three months of TIP. Cure rates using eight months were unchanged for *Teal* but improved with *Azure*.[18]

2. In the *New England Journal of Medicine*, Dr. Edward Messing evaluated the effect of immediate, lifelong TIP started right after surgery. The ten-year survival rate was 85 percent in men treated with immediate TIP compared with 60 percent in men whose TIP was started after the cancer progressed.[19]

3. In the *Journal of Clinical Oncology*, Dr. Tanya Dorff reported that two years of TIP, started immediately after surgery in *Azure*, reduced the five-year relapse rate *to less than 10 percent*. This is a remarkable improvement in cure rates compared with what has been reported previously for surgery alone (see Table 1 above).[20] In Dr. Dorff's study, the five-year

relapse-free rate in the men with pelvic node metastases was only 12.6 percent (Table 2). This benefit seen with adding long-term TIP to surgery in men with *Azure* is hardly surprising. *Azure* has a much higher risk of micrometastases compared with *Teal*. TIP is a *systemic* therapy with anticancer effects that treats the cancer wherever it might be in the body.

Table 2: Cure Rates at Five Years with TIP Added to Surgery

	#of Patients	Free from Relapse
All Patients	351	92.7%
Node Positive	64	87.4%
Gleason ≥ 8 or Seminal Vesicle Invasion	199	91.8%
Gleason 7, Margin Positive or PSA >10	88	98.7%

CONCLUSION

The cure rates for *Azure* are actually quite good if appropriately aggressive treatment is used. Treatment selection varies for *Low-*, *Basic-* and *High-Azure*. Men with *High-Azure* are potential candidates for additional treatment beyond the basic triad of IMRT, seeds, and TIP, the standard approach that is used for *Basic-Azure*.

References

1. ND James and others. Addition of docetaxel, zoledronic acid, or both to first-line long-term hormone therapy in prostate cancer (STAMPEDE): Survival results from an adaptive, multiarm, multistage, platform randomised controlled trial. *Lancet* 387.10024: 1163, 2016.

2. G Ahlgren and others. A randomized phase III trial between adjuvant docetaxel and surveillance after radical prostatectomy for high risk prostate cancer: Results of SPCG12. *Journal of Clinical Oncology* 34 suppl: abstr 5001, 2016.

3. ME Taplin and others. Intense androgen-deprivation therapy with abiraterone acetate plus leuprolide acetate in patients with localized high-risk prostate cancer: Results of a randomized phase II neoadjuvant study. *Journal of Clinical Oncology* 32.33: 3705, 2014.

4. DF Penson and others. Enzalutamide versus bicalutamide in castration-resistant prostate cancer: The STRIVE trial. *Journal of Clinical Oncology* 34.18: 2098, 2016.

5. AA Aizer and others. Marital status and survival in patients with cancer. *Journal of Clinical Oncology* 31.31: 3869, 2013.

6. EJ Jacobs and others. Daily aspirin use and prostate cancer–specific mortality in a large cohort of men with nonmetastatic prostate cancer. *Journal of Clinical Oncology* 32.33: 3716, 2014.

7. KS Choe and others. Aspirin use and the risk of prostate cancer mortality in men treated with prostatectomy or radiotherapy. *Journal of Clinical Oncology* 30.28: 3540, 2012.

8. Robert Hamilton and others. MP 73-04 The association between statin use and outcomes in patients initiating androgen deprivation therapy. *Journal of Urology* 193.4 suppl: e930, 2015.

9. GL Lu-Yao. Combination statin/metformin and prostate cancer specific mortality: A population-based study. *Journal of Clinical Oncology* 33.15 suppl: abstr 5018, 2015.

10. D Margel and others. Metformin use and all-cause and prostate cancer–specific mortality among men with diabetes. *Journal of Clinical Oncology* 31.25: 3069, 2013.

11. MA Preston and others. Metformin use and prostate cancer risk. *European Urology* 66.6: 1012, 2014.

12. CT Nguyen and others. The specific definition of high risk prostate cancer has minimal impact on biochemical relapse-free survival. *Journal of Urology* 181.1: 75, 2009.

13. O Yossepowitch and others. Radical prostatectomy for clinically localized, high risk prostate cancer: Critical analysis of risk assessment methods. *Journal of Urology* 178.2: 493, 2007.

14. M Spahn and others. Outcome predictors of radical prostatectomy in patients with prostate-specific antigen greater than 20 ng/mL: A European multi-institutional study of 712 patients. *European Urology* 58.1: 1, 2010.

15. JF Ward and others. Radical prostatectomy for clinically advanced (cT3) prostate cancer since the advent of prostate-specific antigen testing: 15-year outcome. *British Journal of Urology International* 95.6: 751, 2005.

16. A Mattei and others. The template of the primary lymphatic landing sites of the prostate should be revisited: Results of a multimodality mapping study. *European Urology* 53.1: 118, 2008.

17. U Zwergel and others. Outcome of prostate cancer patients with initial PSA ≥ 20 ng/mK undergoing radical prostatectomy. *European Urology* 52.4: 1058, 2007.

18. ME Gleave and others. Randomized comparative study of 3 versus 8-month neoadjuvant hormonal therapy before radical prostatectomy: Biochemical and pathological effects. *Journal of Urology* 166.2: 500, 2001.

19. EM Messing and others. Immediate hormonal therapy compared with observation after radical prostatectomy and pelvic lymphadenectomy in men with node-positive prostate cancer. *New England Journal of Medicine* 341.24: 1781, 1999.

20. TB Dorff and others. Adjuvant androgen deprivation for high-risk prostate cancer after radical prostatectomy: SWOG S9921 study. *Journal of Clinical Oncology* 29.15: 2040, 2011.

Chapter 30

REDUCING THE SIDE EFFECTS OF TIP

Mark Scholz, MD

Character cannot be developed in ease and quiet.
Only through experience of trial and suffering can the soul be
strengthened, ambition inspired, and success achieved.

HELEN KELLER

BLOCKING TESTOSTERONE, the hormone that induces libido, strength, endurance, emotional stability, and potency, creates all kinds of side effects. This chapter briefly outlines the most common side effects of TIP and discusses how to minimize them.[1]

FATIGUE AND LASSITUDE FROM MUSCLE ATROPHY

Fatigue is one of the most troublesome side effects of TIP. Fatigue mostly comes from muscle loss. To a lesser degree, anemia may be a factor. Well-designed and very convincing scientific studies have unequivocally demonstrated that strength training to build muscles counteracts fatigue in a big way.[2] The ideal strength-training program consists of one-hour sessions three times every week that include every major muscle group. Three sets of 10 to 12 repetitions should be performed for each muscle group during each one-hour session, with weights selected to cause muscle failure toward the end of the third set (Chapter 48).

HOT FLASHES

Hot flashes occur in about two-thirds of men. When severe, progesterone injections (Depo Provera) can dramatically reduce the frequency and intensity of hot flashes.

However, some caution should be exercised when considering progesterone. It is a chemical precursor to testosterone, and there is a possibility of "feeding" the tumor. Better alternatives are low-dose Effexor, a medication usually reserved for the treatment of depression, or Neurontin, a medication originally FDA-approved for the treatment of seizures. Another approach that can be effective is acupuncture.[3] Lastly, if these treatments are ineffective, one can consider using a transdermal estrogen patch (Vivelle Dot). Estrogen is very effective at controlling hot flashes. However, with estrogen there is a risk of breast enlargement or nipple tenderness. *Oral* estrogen for men should be avoided, because it can cause blood clots.

BREAST ENLARGEMENT

Breast growth (even without estrogen patches) occurs frequently in men treated with anti-androgens and Xtandi, and, less frequently (approximately a third of the time), in men treated with the Lupron-like drugs. If there is early evidence of breast growth, an estrogen-blocking pill such as Femara should be considered. Alternatively, prior to starting TIP, radiation to the breast area can be administered as a preventive measure. If radiation is delayed until after breast enlargement has occurred, it can only forestall further growth. It cannot cause the regression of the existing breasts.

ERECTILE ATROPHY

While on hormonal therapy, the occurrence of nocturnal erections usually ceases, potentially resulting in permanent shrinkage of the penis. The normal pattern of nocturnal erections can often be reestablished with the regular use of Cialis or Viagra. If these medications fail to restore the normal pattern of nighttime erections, then either a vacuum pump or injection therapy should be considered. Chapter 12 covers this topic in much greater detail.

ANEMIA

Blood is a mixture of red cells and "serum" (water). When the number of red cells is diminished, the condition is termed "anemia." Anemia is detected by checking the "hematocrit" using the Complete Blood Count (CBC) blood test (Appendix III). Hematocrits below the 32 to 34 percent range can be associated with increased fatigue. TIP almost always causes some degree of anemia, though generally only to a mild degree.[4] Because the red cells carry oxygen from the lungs to the rest of the body, more severe degrees of anemia can cause shortness of breath with minimal exercise. Anemia reverses when the hormone therapy is stopped. If anemia is severe, it can be corrected with medications such as Procrit and Aranesp. Iron is not beneficial for this type of anemia.

LIVER CHANGES

Casodex, Flutamide, Nilutamide, and Zytiga can occasionally cause liver abnormalities. Therefore, monitoring with a blood test called the "hepatic panel" (Appendix III) needs to be done routinely in any patient starting these medications (Appendix III). The liver problems usually reverse quickly if it is detected in a timely fashion and the medication is stopped.

MOOD SWINGS AND DEPRESSION

Men on TIP occasionally experience more intense feelings or depressive feelings.[5] Low doses of antidepressant medications such as Zoloft, Celexa, or Paxil are very effective at reversing these unpleasant feelings.

MISCELLANEOUS SIDE EFFECTS OF TIP

Nilutamide can occasionally cause lung problems. Treatment needs to be stopped immediately if shortness of breath or coughing occurs. Xtandi, in rare cases, causes seizures, so men with a seizure history can't use Xtandi. Since Zytiga can lower the level of potassium in the blood, potassium levels need to be monitored and supplemented, if necessary.

WEIGHT GAIN AND HEART PROBLEMS FROM TIP

Questions have arisen about the impact of low testosterone on heart disease. Some studies, mostly retrospective, have shown an increased incidence of heart attacks in men taking TIP. Prospective studies generally show no increased risk of heart disease and, in some cases, show a lowering of the risk of a heart attack.

The best way to explain these conflicting findings is by considering that most of these studies fail to measure the impact of TIP-associated weight gain. TIP slows metabolism (due to muscle loss), so weight gain is common. While TIP may not *directly* increase the risk of heart disease, weight gain does causes diabetes and hypertension, both of which increase the risk of heart disease.

The most extensive study evaluating the risk of TIP-associated heart disease was published in 2011 by Dr. Paul Nguyen in the *Journal of the American Medical Association*.[6] He analyzed 4,100 patients from eight randomized prospective trials, comparing men receiving TIP with those not receiving TIP. He reported that the incidence of cardiovascular mortality was equivalent in both groups. Not surprisingly, overall survival was better in the groups treated with TIP.

OSTEOPOROSIS

TIP causes accelerated calcium loss from the bones. When the degree of calcium loss is severe, it is termed osteoporosis. Untreated bone loss often results in hip and spine fractures. Normal bone metabolism functions through a balance between the rate of bone breakdown and the formation of new bone. When the specific cells, the "osteo*clasts*," which disassemble bone are more active than that of "osteo*blasts*," the cells that build bone, there is a net reduction in bone. Osteoporosis occurs when the rate of bone breakdown exceeds the formation of new bone.

Osteoporosis prevention begins with an exercise program. Supplementation with calcium and vitamin D should also be considered routine. We recommend 250 mg of calcium at bedtime along with 1,000 units of vitamin D. Blood levels of vitamin D should be checked after three months and the dose of vitamin D adjusted up or down to achieve normal blood levels. Medications such as bisphosphonates and denosumab (see below) work by inhibiting the osteoclasts, thus slowing the rate of bone breakdown and allowing the formation of new bone by the osteoblasts.

ORAL BISPHOSPHONATES: BONIVA, ACTONEL, AND FOSAMAX

Bisphosphonates come in both oral and intravenous forms. Absorption of the oral forms into the blood is enhanced when they are administered on an empty stomach. The most common side effect from oral bisphosphonates is stomach or esophageal irritation, which can be minimized by maintaining an erect position for an hour after taking the drug.

INTRAVENOUS BISPHOSPHONATES: ZOMETA

The intravenous administration of Zometa has the advantage of bypassing the stomach, thus alleviating concerns about stomach irritation. Also, with the intravenous approach, 100 percent of the drug gets into the system. The oral preparations are only 1 to 2 percent absorbed. The most common side effect from Zometa is a brief, flu-like muscle soreness lasting a day or so. This does not usually recur after the first infusion. For the treatment of osteoporosis, infusions are repeated every three to six months.

DENOSUMAB INJECTIONS: PROLIA AND XGEVA

Like Zometa, denosumab inhibits the osteoclasts, but by a different mechanism. Denosumab is marketed in two strengths for injection. A half-dose shot, called Prolia, is administered every six months for osteoporosis. A full-dose shot called Xgeva is given monthly to inhibit cancer metastasis in the bone.

SCANNING FOR OSTEOPOROSIS

Unfortunately, the most common scanning technique for diagnosing osteoporosis—the DEXA scan—grossly underestimates the degree of bone mineral loss from the spine in men. Why? Because almost all men over 50 have calcium deposition in the ligaments surrounding the spine. When the DEXA scan is used to measure bone density, the excess calcium in the ligaments causes the bone density to be incorrectly interpreted as "normal."

Fortunately, there is a better technique, called QCT, that measures bone mineral density in the center of the vertebral column. Awareness of the DEXA scans' limitations in men is poorly appreciated by many physicians, even though these limitations have been well documented in a study from Massachusetts General Hospital. In this study, 41 men underwent both DEXA and QCT scanning. QCT detected osteoporosis in 26 of the men (63 percent), but DEXA diagnosed it in only two (5 percent).[7]

OSTEONECROSIS, A MEDICATION-INDUCED JAW PROBLEM

Zometa and Denosumab, and, to a far lesser degree, oral bisphosphonates, can induce damage to the jaw, a condition termed osteonecrosis. The risk of developing osteonecrosis is much higher when a tooth is extracted. When osteonecrosis occurs, the gum tissue recedes, leaving exposed bone that is susceptible to recurrent infections. The risk of osteonecrosis becomes higher as the lifelong cumulative medication dosage increases. In my experience, osteonecrosis reverses after the medication is stopped, albeit slowly.

FINAL THOUGHTS ABOUT TIP-RELATED SIDE EFFECTS

The effects of TIP vary greatly between patients. Side effects can be significantly reduced with many of the measures outlined in this chapter. The biggest priority for minimizing TIP-related side effects is to maintain muscle mass through regular fitness training. Adhering to a disciplined diet comes in a close second. Weight gain and muscle loss are much easier to prevent than they are to treat.

Now that you have completed this section related to the *Azure* Stage of Blue, you can jump to Chapter 46 at the beginning of Section VII and finish the reading remainder of the book.

References

1. BW Guess and others. Preventing and treating the side effects of testosterone inactivating pharmaceuticals in men with prostate cancer. *Seminars in Preventative and Alternative Medicine* 2.2: 76, 2006.

2. JR Gardner and others. Effects of exercise on treatment-related adverse effects for patients with prostate cancer receiving androgen-deprivation therapy: A systematic review. *Journal of Clinical Oncology* 32.4: 335, 2014.

3. TM Beer and others. Acupuncture for hot flashes in prostate cancer patients. *Urology* 76.5: 1182, 2010.

4. SB Strum and others. Anaemia associated with androgen deprivation in patients with prostate cancer receiving combined hormone blockade. *British Journal* Urology 79.6: 933, 1997.

5. KT Dinh and others. Association of androgen deprivation with depression in localized prostate cancer. *Journal of Clinical Oncology* 34.16: 1905, 2016.

6. PL Nguyen and others. Association of androgen deprivation therapy with cardiovascular death in patients with prostate cancer: A meta-analysis of randomized trials. *Journal of the American Medical Association* 306.21: 2359, 2011.

7. MR Smith and others. Low bone mineral density in hormone-naïve men with prostate carcinoma. *Cancer* 91.12: 2238, 2001.

SECTION V
THE *INDIGO* STAGE OF BLUE

Chapter 31
OVERVIEW OF *INDIGO*

Mark Scholz, MD

Drive is considered aggression today; I knew it then as purpose.
BETTE DAVIS

*I believe that present day civilized man suffers from
insufficient discharge of his aggressive drive.*
KONRAD LORENZ

THE QUALIFICATIONS FOR *Indigo* are previous treatment with surgery, radiation or cryotherapy, a clear bone scan, a normal testosterone level in the blood, and one or more of the following:

- A rising PSA that is due to progressing cancer.*
- Residual disease after surgery noted on a pathology report, such as a positive margin or seminal vesicle invasion.

---

* Not all PSA increases come from cancer; see Chapter 36.

- Residual disease after radiation or cryotherapy detected in the prostate by imaging or by a biopsy.

- Surgically detected or scan-detected cancer in the pelvic lymph nodes.

Over 50,000 men relapse after surgery or radiation each year. The dreaded words, "The cancer is back," can shake someone to the core. The original hope for a cure with surgery or radiation has been dashed. With other types of cancer, a relapse foreshadows impending mortality; it's only a matter of time before the battle's lost. Prostate cancer is totally different. *Indigo* men are more likely to die of natural causes than from prostate cancer.[1]

INDIGO'S SHOCKING SURVIVAL RATES

Why is survival so good for relapsed prostate cancer compared with other cancers? Three easy reasons: First, PSA is an amazing blood test. It detects relapses early, while the cancer is microscopic and potentially curable. Second, prostate cancer is less malignant: it grows sluggishly and metastasizes slowly. Third, testosterone inactivating pharmaceuticals (TIP) are supereffective, routinely inducing *10-year remissions* if started while the cancer is still microscopic.[2] Unlike other cancers, for which a relapse usually means death, with *Indigo*, extended remissions are the norm.

THE GOAL FOR INDIGO IS CURE

The *Indigo* stage of prostate cancer can be *controlled* for a decade or more with ongoing TIP. However, if a *cure* is attainable, it offers two distinct advantages over simply controlling the disease with TIP. First, even though mortality from *Indigo* is uncommon and delayed, the risk remains. Cure *eliminates* the risk of dying from prostate cancer. Secondly, attaining a cure improves *quality* of life. Lifelong TIP has a negative impact on quality of life. Cured men can be freed from the need for ongoing TIP, chemotherapy, or radiation.

DIFFERENT SUBTYPES OF *INDIGO* REQUIRE DIFFERENT TREATMENT

Aggressive, multiagent treatment would be inappropriate if cure could be achieved with less aggressive means. Treatment, therefore, needs to be adjusted in accordance with each patient's stage of disease. For example, men who have *regional pelvic lymph node metastases* require a more aggressive approach than men who merely have a *local relapse* in the prostate gland or "prostate fossa" (where the prostate used to be located prior to surgery). Treatment will vary in accordance with each of *Indigo's* three subtypes—*Low-Indigo, Basic-Indigo,* and *High-Indigo.*

Low-Indigo means the residual cancer is located in the prostate (or prostate fossa). Surgery or radiation has failed to completely eradicate it. Potential *Low-Indigo* patients are assessed in terms of their PSA, their original Stage of Blue, and the results from various scans. *Low-Indigo* status is confirmed when these factors indicate that *lymph node metastases are very unlikely.* If all the prognostic factors indicate that the presence of *microscopic* pelvic lymph node disease is more likely, the stage becomes *Basic-Indigo. High-Indigo* means that node metastases are unequivocally confirmed by surgery or by scans.

ESTIMATING THE RISK OF MICROSCOPIC DISEASE

Scans are incapable of detecting microscopic metastases in the lymph nodes. Years of experience have taught us that the *likelihood* of microscopic cancer existing in the pelvic lymph nodes (generally the first area of the body where prostate cancer spreads) can be *estimated* by the PSA, PSA-doubling time, Gleason score of the original tumor, and the original extent of the disease in the prostate. There is a proper process of estimation for accurately assigning men between the *Low* and *Basic* subtypes of *Indigo*. Chapter 33 presents the methodology for how this estimation process is performed. Men in *High-Indigo* have unequivocal node disease, so "estimations" are unnecessary.

STAGING SCANS FOR *INDIGO*

Ascertaining the precise Stage of Blue and subtype is essential for proper treatment selection, and scans play a huge role in this process. When the cancer's location in the body can be determined, treatment can be focused more effectively. The types of scans that may be useful for *Indigo* are:

- C^{11} acetate or C^{11} choline PET scans, which offer the best chance for finding the location of recurrent disease (Chapter 6).

- Color Doppler ultrasound or multiparametric MRI aimed at the prostate area for detecting residual cancer in the prostate gland (in men previously treated with radiation) or in the surgical fossa (in men who'd had a prostatectomy). See Chapters 4 and 5.

- *Pelvic* MRI or CT scans to check for enlarged pelvic lymph nodes. Unfortunately, these scans are rather crude and are usually unable to detect disease unless the PSA is quite elevated.

- Technetium scans, which have long been the standard methodology for evaluating the bones. Unfortunately, they also rarely detect metastases unless the PSA is above the 10-to-20 range.[3] F18 PET bone scans are clearly better than Technetium scans.

- Other new and promising technology:
  - o Axumin PET,[4] which detects cancer's aberrant amino acid metabolism
  - o PSMA[5] labeled with Gallium[68]
  - o MRI combined with a contrast medium called Combidex.[6] Unfortunately, Combidex is only available in the Netherlands.

THE *OLD* WAY *INDIGO* IS TREATED

The standard approach to *Indigo*, commonly in use for the last couple of decades and continuing to this day, follows a one-size-fits-all approach. All men with *Indigo* are treated with the same protocol—a sequential, one-treatment-at-a-time policy—regardless of the patient's subtype. It begins with adjuvant or salvage radiation administered locally to the prostate fossa alone (no pelvic node radiation). Fossa radiation alone leads to a cure in some men. However, when it is not curative and the cancer subsequently resurfaces, the next step is to start TIP. TIP almost always drops PSA to undetectable levels, usually for many years. However, TIP alone is practically never curative. Over time, hormone resistance commonly develops.

THE *NEW* WAY TO TREAT *INDIGO*

Recently, it has become technically feasible to extend the radiation field to cover the pelvic nodes with relative safety. Despite these technical enhancements, pelvic node radiation is only beneficial for selected patients. The goal for *Indigo*, therefore, is to select the type of treatment in accordance with each man's likelihood of having metastasis in the lymph nodes. *Low-Indigo* men who have localized disease are good candidates for the traditional, one-at-a-time treatment approach. Men with *Basic-Indigo* or *High-Indigo* are potential candidates for a more modern approach that relies on extended radiation fields, supplemental TIP, and possibly even chemotherapy.

References

1. JM Crook and others. Intermittent androgen suppression for rising PSA level after radiotherapy. *New England Journal of Medicine* 367.10: 895, 2012.

2. G Duchesne and others. Timing of androgen-deprivation therapy in patients with prostate cancer with a rising PSA (TROG 03.06 and VCOG PR 01-03 [TOAD]): A randomised, multi-centre, non-blinded, phase 3 trial. *Lancet Oncology* 17.6: 727, 2016.

3. S Loeb and others. Prostate specific antigen at the initial diagnosis of metastasis to bone in patients after radical prostatectomy. *Journal of Urology* 184.1: 157, 2010.

4. B Turkbey. Localized prostate cancer detection with ^{18}F FACBC PET/CT: Comparison with MR imaging and histopathologic analysis. *Radiology* 270.3: 849, 2014.

5. T Maurer and others. Diagnostic efficacy of [68]Gallium-PSMA positron emission tomography compared to conventional imaging for lymph nodes staging of 130 consecutive patients with intermediate to high risk prostate cancer. *Journal of Urology* 195.5: 1436, 2016.

6. RH Blum and M Scholz. "Now Playing for a Limited Time Only: The Combidex Follies." *Invasion of the Prostate Snatchers*. Other Press, 2010.

Chapter 32

INTRODUCTION TO RADIATION FOR *INDIGO*

Christopher Rose, MD

A sound man is good at salvage, at seeing nothing is lost.
LAOZI

RADIATION IS A MAINSTAY FOR salvage treatment after surgery. Radiation can also be a salvage option in men relapsing after previous radiation. Radiation therapy can successfully eradicate microscopic or even gross disease in the operative site or regional lymph nodes.* Whether the relapse is after surgery or radiation, cure rates can be further improved in selected patients by adding hormonal therapy or chemotherapy to radiation.

As was outlined in the previous chapter, there are three different subtypes of *Indigo:*

---

* In addition, radiation can sometimes be used for *Royal* when there are relatively few metastases (see Chapter 39 on oligometastases).

I. **Local Disease** *(Low-Indigo):* Cancer cells persist in the vicinity of the prostate after previous surgery or radiation. Sometimes, but not always, this is signaled by a positive margin* noted in the surgical pathology report.

II. **Suspected Regional Metastases** *(Basic-Indigo):* Sometimes lymph node disease is *suspected* due to elevated pretreatment PSA levels or a high Gleason score. Sometimes lymph node disease is suspected because of a rapid PSA doubling time.

III. **Regional Metastases** *(High-Indigo):* Spread of the cancer into the pelvic lymph nodes. This is communicated by the pathology report from the operation or by a scan.

The *timing* of radiation after surgery can vary. It can be given relatively quickly after surgery as a preventive measure while the PSA is still undetectable. This is called "adjuvant" therapy. Alternatively, treatment may be delayed until the PSA begins to rise, which is called "salvage" treatment. This chapter introduces these varied roles for radiation in men who have persistent or recurrent disease after primary therapy.

THE NEED FOR USING THE LATEST RADIATION TECHNOLOGY

Intensity modulated radiotherapy with image guidance (IMRT/IGRT) is a substantial technical improvement over the older "conformal" techniques and should be used in all cases of postsurgical radiotherapy. Both local and regional areas of the body can be targeted for radiation for men in *Indigo*. Expertise in CT-based, target-volume delineation is required to accurately target the prostate bed and regional lymphatics, and limit radiation exposure to the adjacent bladder, rectum, and small intestine. Many of the techniques described in this chapter require

---

* Positive margins occur because the prostate gland is located only millimeters from the bladder and rectum. To preserve the surrounding organs, the surgeon cuts a close circle around the gland. Microscopic amounts of cancer are left behind, but in quantities too small to produce a detectable level of PSA in the blood.

special training to achieve optimal results and limit unnecessary side effects.

ADJUVANT RADIOTHERAPY

Adjuvant radiotherapy can be considered for men who have adverse features identified by the pathologist after examining the surgically removed prostate while the PSA is still undetectable. "Adverse features" include extracapsular extension, seminal vesicle invasion, or tumor cells at the margin of the area where the prostate was cut away, called a "positive margin." The benefit of adjuvant radiation was investigated in two prospective trials involving more than 1,600 patients. In these two studies, the outcome of men treated with adjuvant radiation was compared with men who were merely observed, (i.e., who received no adjuvant radiation), although some of these men did receive *salvage* radiation. In the first study, adjuvant treatment improved the cure rate from 41 percent to 61 percent.[1] In a second study, the 10-year *survival rate* was improved from 66 percent to 74 percent.[2] Therefore, both studies confirmed that adjuvant radiation was beneficial. However, as can be seen from the statistics, only a subgroup of men had improved cure rates, even though all the men had to undergo radiation and its potential risks to achieve this. To maximize the benefit and to minimize the risk, an important *methodology* should be used for selecting which candidates are optimal for immediate or delayed radiation. This methodology will be carefully outlined in the following chapter.

SALVAGE RADIOTHERAPY

Salvage radiotherapy is given to patients whose PSA either fails to become undetectable after primary treatment or if the PSA subsequently rises after previously being undetectable. "Early" salvage radiation is defined as radiation initiated after a rise occurs but before the PSA rises above 0.5. At such low levels, scans such as CT, MRI, or sodium fluoride PET, or even specialized PET scans using C^{11} choline or C^{11} acetate are generally unable to pinpoint the location of the recurrence. The PSA is therefore *assumed* to be originating from microscopic cancer in the prostate bed or perhaps in the pelvic lymph nodes. How to determine if radiation should be directed locally, regionally, or to both areas of the body will be covered in the following chapter as well.

Studies show that *salvage* radiation, like *adjuvant* radiation, can also control cancer. In one large multi-institutional study that included patients with varying PSA levels (above and below 0.5), remission was sustained for six years in one-third of the men. The odds for staying in remission were much better when the radiation was started before the PSA rose above 0.5.[3] Success using salvage radiation is clearly tied to starting treatment at a lower level of PSA.

TIP WITH SALVAGE RADIATION

In some situations, the effectiveness of salvage radiation can be further improved with the addition of TIP. For example, in one prospective study, high-dose Casodex added to radiation improved survival rates, compared with men who were treated with radiation alone.[4] The degree of survival improvement was greatest in men with higher Gleason scores and higher PSA levels (above 0.7). Another prospective study evaluating the impact of adding six months of Lupron to radiation resulted in better cure rates, compared with men who had radiation alone.[5]

WHAT ABOUT TIP WITHOUT RADIATION?

The studies cited above indicate that radiation alone is beneficial. They also indicate that TIP improves the results. But is the converse true? Is it possible that TIP can be substituted for radiation? To address this question, Dr. Firas Abdollah evaluated the eight-year, cancer-specific survival rate with TIP alone and compared it to men who had radiation added to TIP. The survival rate with TIP alone was lower (86 percent) than what was achieved with the combination (92 percent).[6]

In the same vein, at the meeting of the American Urologic Association in 2016, Dr. James Eastham released the results of a retrospective evaluation of 1,338 men with node metastases who received TIP alone, compared with men who were treated with TIP plus radiation. The 10-year mortality rate was reduced by as much as 40 percent in men who received radiation and TIP, compared with TIP alone.[7] Given that the side effects of modern salvage radiation tend to be mild, our center in Beverly Hills will generally administer node radiation in appropriate cases, unless there are medical contraindications such as active inflammatory bowel disease or unfavorable anatomy.

RADIOTHERAPY SIDE EFFECTS

Patients who undergo post prostatectomy radiotherapy have several side-effect-related vulnerabilities, since both urinary and sexual function have been previously diminished by surgery. For patients who achieve a complete recovery of urinary continence after surgery, radiation therapy is not expected to cause incontinence. However, a good outcome depends on delaying radiation until full urinary recovery has occurred. Patients who are incontinent at the time of radiation will usually remain incontinent after completion of radiation. A study evaluating the impact of radiation on erectile function will be discussed in the following chapter, but I can state here—that from the perspective of maintaining good urinary control the longer that radiation can be postponed, the better.

CONCLUSION

The goal for radiation is to maximize cancer control while minimizing the risk of damage to the surrounding organs. Modern technology has dramatically reduced the risk of bladder and intestinal damage that plagued older methods of radiation. These days, customized treatment protocols integrated with specialized imaging enable radiation to safely target sites of disease in the pelvic or lower-abdominal lymph nodes while reducing the risk of collateral damage.

References

1. M Bolla and others. Postoperative radiotherapy after radical prostatectomy for high-risk prostate cancer: Long-term results of a randomised controlled trial (EORTC trial 22911). *Lancet* 380.9858: 2018, 2012.

2. IM Thompson and others. Adjuvant radiotherapy for pathological T3N0M0 prostate cancer significantly reduces risk of metastases and improves survival:

Long-term follow-up of a randomized clinical trial. *Journal of Urology* 181.3: 956, 2009.

3. AJ Stephenson and others. Predicting the outcome of salvage radiation therapy for recurrent prostate cancer after radical prostatectomy. *Journal of Clinical Oncology* 25.15: 2035, 2007.

4. WU Shipley and others. Report of NRG oncology/RTOG 9601, a phase 3 trial in prostate cancer: Anti-androgen therapy (AAT) with bicalutamide during and after radiation therapy (RT) in patients following radical prostatectomy (RP with pT2-3pN0 disease and an elevated PSA. *International Journal of Radiation Oncology, Biology, Physics* 94.1: 3, 2016.

5. C Carrie and others. Salvage radiotherapy with or without short-term hormone therapy for rising prostate-specific antigen concentration after radical prostatectomy (GETUG-AFU 16): a randomised, multicentre, open-label phase 3 trial. *Lancet Oncology* 17.6: 747, 2016.

6. F Abdollah and others. Impact of adjuvant radiotherapy on survival of patients with node-positive prostate cancer. *Journal of Clinical Oncology* 32.35: 3939, 2014.

7. K Touijer and others. MP50-01 Survival analysis of patients with node positive prostate cancer after radical prostatectomy comparing observation vs. adjuvant androgen deprivation therapy alone vs. adjuvant androgen deprivation plus external beam radiation therapy. *Journal of Urology* 195.4 suppl: e672, 2016.

8. WU Shipley and others. Initial Report of RTOG 9601: A phase III trial in prostate cancer: Anti-androgen therapy (AAT) with bicalutamide during and after radiation therapy (RT) improves freedom from progression and reduces the incidence of metastatic disease in patients following radical prostatectomy (RP) with pT2-3, N0 disease, and elevated PSA levels. *International Journal of Radiation Oncology, Biology, Physics* 78.3: S27, 2010.

Chapter 33

INDIGO—CANCER RELAPSE OR PELVIC NODE DISEASE

Mark Scholz, MD

It's a miracle that curiosity survives formal education.
ALBERT EINSTEIN

THE PRESENCE OR ABSENCE of nodal metastases in the pelvis is what defines the different subtypes of *Indigo*. The information gleaned from the scans, the pathology report, the PSA doubling time, and the original Stage of Blue help us assess the likelihood of nodal metastases. Once this assessment is made, *Indigo* is divided into three subtypes: *Low-Indigo, Basic-Indigo,* and *High-Indigo.*

LOW-INDIGO

Low-Indigo can occur after surgery or radiation. *Low-Indigo* means that there is persistent cancer in the prostate (after radiation) or near where the prostate used to be after surgery (in the so-called "fossa"), *and* the likelihood of microscopic spread to the lymph nodes is quite low. The criteria required to qualify for *Low-Indigo* are that all scans be clear, along with all of the following:

1. If the PSA is rising, the doubling time should be over eight months (remember, doubling time calculations are unreliable in men who are in the midst of recovering their testosterone after stopping TIP).*

2. Multiparametric MRI of the prostate (which remains after radiation) shows that seminal vesicle invasion and extra-capsular extension of the tumor are absent.

3. If PSA is rising, it should be less than 0.5 (after surgery) and less than 5.0 (after radiation). The PSA can be higher after radiation, because the prostate gland is still intact and produces PSA (see below).

4. The original Stage of Blue, prior to surgery or radiation, needs to have been *Sky, Low-Teal* or *Basic-Teal*, not *High-Teal* or *Azure*.

LOW-INDIGO AFTER SURGERY

After surgery, *Low-Indigo* may be signaled by a positive surgical margin reported in the pathology report (though no seminal vesicle invasion or lymph node spread is reported). As was noted in the previous chapter, optimal *timing* for administering radiation after surgery is controversial. The advantage of immediate *adjuvant* radiation is debated, because radiation given during this time period leads to decent cure rates but it may also impair sexual recovery. If radiation can be safely postponed or withheld altogether, the chance for maintaining sexual function is improved.

---

* Measurements of PSA doubling time in men who were previously treated with radiation plus TIP can only be accurately calculated *after* the testosterone level has fully recovered into the normal range.

The impact of radiation on sexual and urinary recovery was evaluated in 113 men who had radiation at different time points after surgery.[2] Questionnaires to establish a baseline for sexual and urinary function were given to the men after surgery. The same questionnaire was readministered after the men subsequently underwent radiation. The patients were divided into two groups: men who had adjuvant radiation within a year of surgery (a median of eight months) and men whose salvage radiation was postponed (a median of 28 months). The study found no significant difference in the rate of urinary recovery between the two groups. However, men receiving *adjuvant* radiation had inferior recovery of sexual function, compared with men who had *salvage* radiation.

Since salvage radiation seems to be associated with better rates of sexual recovery compared with adjuvant radiation, what is the impact of delaying radiation on the rate of cancer control? Does *salvage* radiation administered while the PSA is still low, say, less than 0.5, deliver the same cure rates as *adjuvant* radiation? Two recent studies address this question. The first[3] evaluated 596 men with positive margins whose PSA was initially undetectable. The patients were divided into two groups: those who had immediate radiation within six months of surgery while their PSA levels were still undetectable, and men who started radiation after their PSA levels began to increase *but before their PSA rose above 0.5*. In this latter group, 60 percent of the men never had a PSA increase; these men were therefore able to avoid radiation altogether. However, 40 percent did develop a PSA increase and underwent radiation while their PSA was still less than 0.5. Metastasis-free survival at 10 years for the group in which every man got *adjuvant* radiation was 90 percent. For the other group, with either no radiation or *salvage* radiation, it was 89 percent, essentially the same cure rate while avoiding radiation in 60 percent of the men.

In the second study,[4] 422 men with positive margins were divided into four groups: 1) radiation right after surgery; 2) radiation started after a PSA relapse but while the PSA was under 0.5; 3) radiation started when the PSA was over 0.5; and 4) men who never received any radiation whatsoever, no matter how high their PSA had increased. Groups 1 and

2 were 4.3 times *less* likely to develop metastases over the next eight years compared with groups 3 and 4. Importantly, the cancer control rate for groups 1 and 2 were equivalent.

Both studies are retrospective. As we have discussed in previous chapters, the problem with retrospective studies is that unsuspected factors may affect the accuracy of the results. Despite this limitation, we now have two good studies suggesting that men with positive margins whose original Stage was *Sky* or *Teal* can safely forgo immediate radiation if they monitor their PSA levels very closely and initiate radiation at the earliest sign of a PSA relapse, if a relapse occurs.

LOW-INDIGO AFTER RADIATION

Interpreting PSA after radiation can be tricky. Persistent cancer can exist in the prostate gland, even when PSA is still in the "normal" range. There is no ironclad rule that defines a normal PSA level after radiation. A reasonable level to begin considering that a relapse may be occurring is if the PSA rises above 1.0. Even in men who have been cured, the PSA will not be zero (as is the case after surgery), because the benign cells in the prostate gland continue to make some PSA, even after being irradiated. Therefore, if there is a minute amount of PSA being produced by residual cancer in the prostate, this PSA from the cancer cells will be "overshadowed" by the larger amount of "benign" PSA being produced by the gland. Interpreting PSA after radiation is even further complicated, because PSA levels after radiation can be affected by several other noncancerous factors, including the size of the prostate, the degree of testosterone recovery, and the degree of prostate inflammation induced by the radiation. (Chapter 36 further discusses the factors that influence PSA after radiation.)

Persistent cancer after radiation, therefore, can be detected by a rising PSA, by imaging, or from a biopsy. If the PSA is rising, for patients to qualify as *Low-Indigo* the PSA should generally be less than 5.0. For clinical research, cancer relapse after previous radiation to the prostate (without previous surgery) is defined as a rise in PSA by 2 points or more above the lowest PSA attained after radiation. For example, a relapse is deemed to have occurred when a PSA that first dropped to 0.5 has subsequently risen to 2.5. However, as mentioned above, sometimes relapse can be detected without any rise in PSA through an abnormal digital rectal exam, scan findings, or a positive prostate biopsy.

Men who are relapsing after radiation are typically treated with focal therapy, usually cryotherapy. Side effects with *focal* cryotherapy are much milder than when the whole gland is treated with cryotherapy. Focal cryotherapy is also far less likely to cause damaging urinary or sexual problems than surgery.[5,6] Dr. Duke Bahn discusses focal cryotherapy in Chapter 10. Alternatively, men can consider treatment with a salvage seed implantation[7,8] or with intermittent TIP (see below). Men with PSA doubling times over 12 months can also consider observation without any immediate treatment.

Seed implantation for local relapse after radiation is gaining in popularity as a viable form of salvage treatment. In previous years, it was believed that additional radiation after previous external beam radiation would invariably result in devastating, nonhealing radiation burns. Experience has shown that this blanket conclusion is incorrect, especially if the original radiation was administered some time ago. An extended interval between the initial treatment and the time of relapse allows the body to heal from the previous radiation, which reduces the risk of serious side effects from the second treatment. Intermittent TIP to suppress local disease is another reasonable alternative to consider in lieu of focal cryotherapy or salvage seed implantation.

INTERMITTENT TIP

A typical intermittent protocol consists of TIP administered for six to nine months followed by a "treatment holiday." After TIP is stopped, testosterone levels recover back to normal and the PSA begins to rise. A second cycle of TIP is started when the PSA rises back to the original PSA baseline, or up into the 3-to-6 range, whichever is lower.[9,10] Intermittent TIP has been a standard approach for the treatment of a PSA relapse for 20 years. Intermittent TIP is the most logical approach if the predicted side effects of salvage cryotherapy or brachytherapy are excessive, or if a patient is strongly opposed to the use of cryotherapy or radiation.

Patients sometimes question the prudence of using TIP *intermittently*. Why would anyone want to stop a treatment that is effectively controlling the disease? It sounds cavalier. Several clinical trials have investigated this question. In one of them, Dr. Laurence Klotz, the author of Chapter 9, conducted a huge prospective trial involving close to 1,400 men with *Indigo*.[11] The men were divided into two groups: 690 men received intermittent TIP for eight months, and another 696 men were given TIP continuously. Among the men who received TIP intermittently, the PSA could rise up to 10 during the holiday period, after which the next cycle of TIP was started. The study showed equal survival rates between the two groups. Also, the average time to TIP resistance was identical—10 years. The men on intermittent therapy were on "holiday" from TIP 73 percent of the time. As would be expected with *Indigo*, the study confirmed that mortality from advancing age was more common than death from prostate cancer.

BASIC-INDIGO

Men in the *Basic-Indigo* stage, based on various prognostic factors, are judged to be at risk for microscopic metastases in the pelvic lymph nodes, *even though their scan and pathology reports are negative for node metastases.* The factors leading to this conclusion can be any one of the following:

1. A rising PSA above 0.5 after surgery and above 5.0 after radiation

2. An original Stage of *High-Teal* or *Azure*

3. A PSA doubling time of less than eight months

4. A pathology report or a scan showing seminal vesicle invasion

Men in *Basic-Indigo* who underwent previous surgery are typically treated with IMRT to both the prostate fossa and the pelvic lymph nodes.

TIP should be administered as well. As discussed in Chapter 32, two prospective studies show that adding TIP to radiation improves cure rates. *Basic-Indigo* men who underwent previous radiation should receive IMRT to the pelvic lymph nodes plus TIP (assuming node radiation was withheld at the time that the radiation was initially given). Any locally persistent disease detected in the prostate can be managed with focal cryotherapy or a salvage seed implantation, as was discussed above for *Low-Indigo*.

TAXOTERE FOR *BASIC-INDIGO*

Dr. Mary-Ellen Taplin performed a very interesting study in *Basic-Indigo*.[12] Sixty-two men with rising PSA levels were treated with TIP *and* the drug Taxotere *without giving any radiation*. After eight years of observation, 24 percent of the men were in stable remission and thus appear to have been cured. While this is a very small study, in my 20-year experience of giving TIP to hundreds of men with relapsed prostate cancer, I have only observed one single man who was cured by TIP alone without using any radiation. Therefore, this impact of Taxotere on cure rates in men with *Basic-Indigo* appears to be quite notable. The idea of using Taxotere for *Basic-Indigo* is discussed in more detail in the following chapter.

FORGOING TREATMENT ALTOGETHER

It's not uncommon for men to ask, "Doctor, I am concerned about the immediate side effects of TIP. How long will I live if I simply do nothing?" My answer consists of pointing out that eventually everyone does something, usually TIP, when the cancer progresses. The question then is, "What is lost by delaying TIP until cancer symptoms develop?" A randomized study done in Australia, New Zealand, and Canada showed that the risk of mortality within five years is doubled. In this study, 293 men were assigned immediate TIP or delayed TIP. Sixteen men (11 percent) died in the immediate therapy arm, and 30 (20 percent) died in the delayed therapy arm. Five-year overall survival was 86 percent in the delayed therapy arm versus 91 percent in the immediate therapy arm.[13]

HIGH-INDIGO

High-Indigo is characterized by *unequivocal* pelvic lymph node metastases after surgery or radiation. The presence of metastases may be established by surgery, by a biopsy, or with a scan. Scans showing enlarged lymph nodes in the context of a rising PSA are almost always due to prostate cancer. If there is doubt, a CT-directed needle biopsy can be performed for confirmation. Men who have unequivocal pelvic node disease may (or may not) have additional local disease in the prostate or prostate fossa. Their local disease may warrant locally directed treatment in addition to the treatment that is planned for the pelvic nodes.

High-Indigo warrants aggressive multimodality therapy, which includes:

1.   TIP for 12 to 18 months,

2.   IMRT to the pelvic lymph nodes, and

3.   four to six cycles of Taxotere chemotherapy.

The most compelling study substantiating the benefit of using aggressive combination therapy for *High-Indigo* was performed by several luminary researchers, Drs. James Eastham, Peter Scardino, Francesco Montorsi, and Alberto Briganti.[14] They retrospectively evaluated 1,338 men with lymph node metastasis after surgery. The survival of men who were treated with TIP alone was compared with men who were treated with TIP plus radiation. The 10-year mortality rate was substantially reduced with immediate combination therapy. The degree of mortality reduction varied between five percent and 40 percent, depending on the severity of the cancer. The benefit of treatment was largest in the most severe types of cancer.

OLIGOMETASTASES

High-Indigo metastatic disease in the pelvic region—and nowhere else in the body—is a subtype of what is termed "oligometastatic disease." Oligometastatic disease is defined as the presence of fewer than five metastatic sites, though, under the umbrella term "oligometastases," the metastatic sites are not necessarily confined to the pelvic region. Dr. Jeffrey Turner covers the topic of oligometastases in detail in Chapter 39.

TAXOTERE CHEMOTHERAPY

A benefit for using Taxotere chemotherapy for *High-Indigo* is suggested by the results of a large prospective trial called STAMPEDE[15] (Systemic therapy in advancing or metastatic prostate cancer: evaluation of drug efficacy trial). This trial involved almost 3,000 men with extensive local disease or metastatic disease. Half of the men were given Taxotere plus TIP. Their survival rate was compared with men treated with TIP alone. The group of men receiving Taxotere plus TIP had substantially better survival rates, compared with the men who received TIP alone.

TREATMENT CONSIDERATIONS RELATIVE TO AGE

Men with *Indigo* are often in their 70s. Thus, an important question needs to be raised: "Considering my age and health, is all this extra treatment really needed? Should I really be trying to achieve a cure?" Since average survival times for *Indigo* treated with TIP alone easily surpass 10 years, baseline heath status and age needs to be factored into the treatment-selection equation. Maximizing longevity with an all-out-treatment protocol is very logical in younger men. A general rule of thumb is that when life expectancy, apart from prostate cancer considerations, is estimated to be less than 10 years, a less aggressive approach should be considered. For example, healthy men in their 80s and unhealthy men in their early- to mid-70s are generally expected to live less than 10 years. A much milder alternative, using Casodex alone, may keep the disease in check for many years with relatively few side effects.

HIGH PSA NADIR, THE MOST IMPORTANT WARNING SIGN

As discussed above, the different subtypes of *Indigo* are classified by the metrics of PSA doubling time, the original Stage of Blue, and information related to the cancer's location. However, there is one predictive factor that, when encountered, plays an outsized role. That factor is called an "elevated PSA nadir" (the lowest PSA measurement) on TIP. A high PSA nadir is defined by a PSA that fails to drop to less than 0.1 within the first six months of starting TIP using Casodex plus Lupron.[16] A high PSA nadir means that hormone resistance is present, which is a characteristic of *Royal*. Fortunately, a high PSA nadir is relatively uncommon for men in *Indigo*, unless they have already been exposed to TIP for many years.

ULTRAFAST PSA DOUBLING TIMES

Not as serious as a high PSA nadir, but certainly worrisome, is a brisk PSA doubling time of, say, three months or less. Fast doubling times are an indication of a more life-threatening situation. Even though the scans may be clear, treatment should consist of more extended-duration TIP with a consideration of the early implementation of Taxotere.

PUTTING IT ALL TOGETHER

Treatment selection for *Indigo* requires the acquisition of an accurate "profile" of the cancer by taking the original Stage of Blue, the PSA doubling time, the pathology report, and the scan findings into account. Fortunately, a wide variety of treatment options are available, and they are almost always effective when treating *Indigo* at its initial stages. Most men will have their disease controlled on a long-term basis and sometimes even cured.

References

1. B Turkbey and others. Localized prostate cancer detection with ¹⁸F FACBC PET/CT: comparison with MR imaging and histopathologic analysis. *Radiology* 270.3: 849, 2014.

2. G Murphy and others. MP04-11 Comparing quality of life outcomes in men receiving early versus late post-prostatectomy radiation therapy. *The Journal of Urology* 195.4 suppl: e32, 2016.

3. N Fossati and others. Long-term impact of adjuvant versus early salvage radiation therapy on clinical recurrence in pT3N0 prostate cancer treated with radical prostatectomy: Results of a multi-institutional analysis. *European Urology* 71.6: 886, 2017.

4. R Den and others. Efficacy of early and delayed radiation in a prostatectomy cohort adjusted for genomic and clinical risk. *Journal of Urology* 34.2 suppl: 12, 2016.

5. DK Bahn and others. Focal cryotherapy for clinically unilateral, low-intermediate risk prostate cancer in 73 men with a median follow-up for 3.7 years. *European Urology* 62.1: 55, 2012.

6. EH Lambert and others. Focal cryosurgery: Encouraging health outcomes for unifocal prostate cancer. *Urology* 69.6: 1117, 2007.

7. B Lee and others. Feasibility of high-dose-rate brachytherapy salvage for local prostate cancer recurrence after radiotherapy: The University of California-San Francisco experience. *International Journal of Radiation Oncology, Biology, Physics* 67.4: 1106, 2007.

8. RJ Burri and others. Long-term outcome and toxicity of salvage brachytherapy for local failure after initial radiotherapy for prostate cancer. *International Journal of Radiation Oncology, Biology, Physics* 77.5: 1338, 2010.

9. M Scholz and others. Intermittent use of testosterone inactivation pharmaceutical using finasteride prolongs the time off period. *Journal of Urology* 175.5: 1673, 2006.

10. M Scholz and others. Primary intermittent androgen deprivation as initial therapy for men with newly diagnosed prostate cancer. *Clinical Genitourinary Cancer* 9.2: 89, 2011.

11. JM Crook and others. Intermittent androgen suppression for rising PSA level after radiotherapy. *New England Journal of Medicine* 367.10: 895, 2012.

12. M Taplin and others. Docetaxel, estramustine, and 15-month androgen deprivation for men with prostate-specific antigen progression after definitive local therapy for prostate cancer. *Journal of Clinical Oncology* 24.34: 5408, 2006.

13. GM Duchesne and others. Timing of androgen-deprivation therapy in patients with prostate cancer with a rising PSA (TROG 03.06 and VCOG PR 01-03 [TOAD]): A randomised, multicentre, non-blinded, phase 3 trial. *Lancet Oncology* 17.6: 727, 2016.

14. K Touijer and others. MP50-01 Survival analysis of patients with node positive prostate cancer after radical prostatectomy comparing observation vs. adjuvant androgen deprivation therapy alone vs. adjuvant androgen deprivation plus external beam radiation therapy. *Journal of Urology* 195.4 suppl: e672, 2016.

15. ND James and others. Docetaxel and/or zoledronic acid for hormone-naïve prostate cancer: First survival results from STAMPEDE. *Lancet* 387: 1163, 2016.

16. M Scholz and others. Prostate cancer-specific survival and clinical progression-free survival in men with prostate cancer treated intermittently with testosterone inactivating pharmaceuticals. *Urology* 70.3: 506, 2007.

Chapter 34
UNORTHODOX THERAPIES FOR *INDIGO*

Mark Scholz, MD

Fortune is powerless to help one who does not exert himself.
LEONARDO DA VINCI

MANY OF THE UNORTHODOX TREATMENTS that were discussed in Chapter 29 for *Azure*, such as aspirin, metformin, and statins, are also worthy of consideration for *Indigo*. The idea of using Zytiga and Xtandi prior to the onset of hormone resistance is another consideration for *Indigo* and was also discussed in Chapter 29. Treatment with ancillary agents such as these should generally be considered as *additions*, not *substitutions*, to an overall combination protocol that would include the standard treatments such as Lupron and radiation, as was described in the previous chapter. Another "unorthodox" approach is to dial down treatment intensity by using milder hormonal treatment in the elderly (Chapter 41).

In Chapter 31, I stressed that the goal for *Indigo* should be cure whenever possible. While *Indigo* can be *controlled* for a decade or more with TIP, *cure* offers two distinct advantages. First, though mortality from *Indigo* is uncommon and delayed, the risk remains. Second, men who are cured have a better *quality* of life. They have been freed from the need for lifelong, cancer suppressive therapy with TIP.

TAXOTERE FOR *BASIC-INDIGO*

In Chapter 33, based on the results of the randomized clinical trial called STAMPEDE, Taxotere was shown to be beneficial for *High-Indigo*. Evidence was also presented that suggests that Taxotere may improve cure rates for *Basic-Indigo*.

Patients often ask me what I mean by "cure." Cure means that the PSA remains *undetectable* indefinitely in men who have previously undergone surgery after testosterone levels have recovered back into the normal range. A working definition to describe cure for relapsed men whose original treatment was radiation to the prostate is a stable PSA under 1.0.

There are three clinical trials that I am aware of that suggest that Taxotere can cure some men with *Basic-Indigo*. These trials evaluated the cure rates for *Basic-Indigo* in men who were treated with TIP plus Taxotere *but without any radiation*. Since we know that TIP by itself rarely, if ever, cures relapsed disease, attaining and maintaining a zero PSA after treatment with TIP plus Taxotere would certainly indicate that the Taxotere should be given the credit for why men receiving this combination are cured.

Let me briefly summarize these three trials to provide a better understanding for this idea that Taxotere may be able to cure *Basic-Indigo*. The first study, performed at the University of Maryland, was published back in 2005.[1] Thirty-three men with a median PSA of 13 and a PSA doubling time of six months were treated with six cycles of Taxotere followed by 12 to 20 months of Lupron and Casodex. After TIP was stopped, testosterone levels in the blood recovered to normal in all but one of the men. Two years after stopping TIP, the PSA continued to be undetectable in five of the 33 men (15 percent).

The second trial, by the Dana-Farber Cancer Institute, evaluated 62 men who were treated with four cycles of Taxotere.[2] Prior to starting treatment, the median PSA for the whole group was 3.0, and the median PSA doubling time was seven months. A follow-up article on this same group of men *eight years after treatment* reported that 15 of the 62 men (24 percent) were in continuous complete remission (cure).[3] Analysis of the data showed that the men who started treatment with a lower PSA, that is, less than 3.0, were more likely to be in this group of 15 men who achieved continuous complete remission.

In the third trial, 41 men were administered four cycles of Taxotere plus eight cycles of Avastin (an angiogenesis drug that is mentioned in Chapter 40) and 18 months of TIP. All the men in the trial had to have a PSA doubling time of less than 10 months to be eligible to participate. One year after the completion of TIP, 29 men had recovered their testosterone and could be considered evaluable. Of these 29 men, 13 (45 percent) were maintaining undetectable PSA levels. This is an impressive result, but the duration of the follow-up period is short.

COMBINING TAXOTERE, RADIATION, AND TIP

Modern radiation, as was carefully pointed out in the previous chapter, also contributes to durable responses and cures in men with *Indigo*. Since Taxotere may be able to further improve cure rates, the question becomes, "How do we integrate Taxotere, TIP, and radiation together?" There are no trials addressing this question. One approach is to start TIP and Taxotere together. The Taxotere is continued for a total of four cycles. A month or so after the Taxotere is completed, radiation is started. TIP is continued throughout the whole process—before, during, and after the radiation. How long the TIP is extended after finishing the radiation depends on the seriousness of the patient's cancer profile and how well the treatment is being tolerated.

IMMUNE THERAPY FOR *BASIC-INDIGO*

Immune therapy with new drugs such as Yervoy, Keytruda, and Opdivo is being looked at closely for the treatment of advanced prostate cancer.

This is a hot area of study, because these drugs show significant activity in other cancers such as melanoma and lung cancer. They are, as yet, unstudied in *Indigo*. Chapter 42 covers the latest thinking regarding their use for men with advanced prostate cancer. Provenge is a type of immune treatment that is only FDA-approved for *Royal*. Relatively few studies have been performed to evaluate Provenge's effectiveness in men with *Indigo*, mainly for cost reasons. Provenge is expensive and insurance companies refuse coverage.

One study with Provenge that was performed at the University of California, San Francisco did show that Provenge slows the rate of PSA rise in *Indigo*.[5] The rate of PSA rise, (i.e., the PSA doubling time), is well known to provide an accurate estimation of how aggressively the cancer is behaving. One would think that the effectiveness of a specific treatment in *Indigo* could be judged by whether the treatment causes a slowing in the rate of PSA increase. It is an established fact that men with slow PSA doubling times live longer than men with fast doubling times. Therefore, why can't we conclude that a slowing in the PSA doubling time that occurs during treatment is a sign that cancer mortality will be reduced? The problem is that studies observing patients who are monitored over time often show a slowing in the rate of PSA doubling—*even when they are receiving no treatment whatsoever!* This problem with trying to use a slowing of the PSA-doubling rate as a surrogate for cancer survival is well-illustrated by the pomegranate extract fiasco. Initial studies of pomegranate administered to men with rising PSA did indeed show that the rate of PSA rise was retarded.[6] However, a subsequent study that *randomly allocated* men between a pomegranate extract and a placebo showed that the rate of PSA rise was slowed *to the same degree in both groups*.[7] Pomegranate has no more anticancer activity than a placebo.

Despite the problems that arise in determining the meaning of changes in PSA doubling time, what does it mean when the PSA stops rising altogether for an extended period? After all, we know that for most men a rising PSA eventually results in the development of metastases. Logically, one would think that a continuously stable PSA is a sign that the treatment is beneficial. Another clinical trial performed at UCSF is pertinent in this regard. Dr. Eric Small and others administered Leukine (GM-CSF), a medication that is FDA-approved to stimulate the immune system after chemotherapy, to 29 men with *Basic–Indigo*.[8] All of the participants in the trial started Leukine with a PSA that was less than 6.0. The median pretreatment PSA doubling time for the group was eight months. After *five years of therapy*, seven of the men (29 percent) were free of disease progression and maintaining stable PSA levels.

The Prostate Oncology Specialists administered Leukine three times a week, along with low-dose cyclophosphamide (which also has an immunostimulatory effect) to 24 men with *Basic–Indigo*.[9] In this study, a beneficial treatment response was defined as a 100 percent or greater increase in PSA doubling time. The median starting PSA was 8 and baseline PSA doubling time was four months for the 24 men. Treatment was well tolerated, with occasional redness at the site of injection. Fourteen men were judged to have a positive response to Leukine. In these 14 men, their baseline PSA doubling time was five months, which increased to a 24-month doubling time while on treatment.

Generally, treatment for *Basic–Indigo* should consist of TIP combined with state-of-the-art IMRT to the pelvic nodes. When there is locally persistent disease in the prostate or prostate fossa, it can be treated with IMRT, cryotherapy, or brachytherapy. The data presented above, however, would suggest that some men, perhaps those who have very rapid PSA doubling times (less than three months, for example), might be able to improve their cure rates by adding four cycles of Taxotere to their TIP and IMRT. At the other end of the spectrum, perhaps some men with *Basic–Indigo* who have relatively very slow doubling times and who are reluctant to undergo an aggressive combination therapy might want to consider using immune therapy to inhibit progression of the disease on a long-term basis.

References

1. A Hussain and others. Docetaxel followed by hormone therapy in men experiencing increasing prostate-specific antigen after primary local treatments for prostate cancer. *Journal of Clinical Oncology* 23.12: 2789, 2005.

2. ME Taplin and others. Docetaxel, estramustine, and 15-month androgen deprivation for men with prostate-specific antigen progression after definitive local therapy for prostate cancer. *Journal of Clinical Oncology* 24.34: 5408, 2006.

3. M Nakabayashi and others. Long-term follow-up of a phase II trial of chemotherapy plus hormone therapy for biochemical relapse after definitive local therapy for prostate cancer. *Urology* 81.3: 611, 2013.

4. RR McKay and others. Docetaxel, bevacizumab, and androgen deprivation therapy for biochemical disease recurrence after definitive local therapy for prostate cancer. *Cancer* 121.15: 2603, 2015.

5. G Beinart and others. Antigen-presenting cells 8015 (Provenge) in patients with androgen-independent, biochemically relapsed prostate cancer. *Clinical Prostate Cancer* 4.1: 55, 2005.

6. AJ Pantuck and others. Phase II study of pomegranate juice for men with rising prostate-specific antigen following surgery or radiation for prostate cancer. *Clinical Cancer Research* 12.13: 4018, 2006.

7. AJ Pantuck and others. A randomized, double-blind, placebo-controlled study of the effects of pomegranate extract on rising PSA levels in men following primary therapy for prostate cancer. *Prostate Cancer and Prostatic Diseases* 18.3: 242, 2015.

8. BI Rini and others. Clinical and immunological characteristics of patients with serologic progression of prostate cancer achieving long-term disease control with granulocyte-macrophage colony-stimulating factor. *Journal of Urology* 175.6: 2087, 2006.

9. M Scholz and others. Retrospective evaluation of GM-CSF, low-dose cyclophosphamide, and celecoxib on PSA doubling time (DT) in men with prostate cancer and PSA relapse after surgery or radiation. *Journal of Clinical Oncology* 28.10 suppl: abstr e15061, 2010.

Chapter 35

MINIMIZING THE SIDE EFFECTS OF CHEMOTHERAPY

Richard Lam, MD

We must always change, renew and rejuvenate ourselves;
otherwise we harden.

Johann Wolfgang von Goethe

Taxotere and Jevtana are the most active chemotherapeutic agents available for prostate cancer. They have two basic roles. The first is treating metastatic disease. In this role, they can be used as a single agent or combined with other agents such as Carboplatin or Xeloda.

The other use for Taxotere (or Jevtana) is as a *preventive* agent to avert a future cancer relapse. In this regard, testosterone-inactivating pharmaceuticals (TIP) are used as the first line of defense. Adding Taxotere to TIP is termed "adjuvant" chemotherapy. Interestingly, one study that treated men with adjuvant Taxotere, without the addition of any TIP, showed no benefit from the Taxotere.[1] So, there is no basis for the idea of using Taxotere as a substitute for TIP.

TAXOTERE PROTOCOLS CAN VARY

Taxotere and Jevtana are administered intravenously, most commonly every three weeks. Alternatively, smaller doses can be given weekly.[2] Another protocol from Europe uses an intermediate dosage every two weeks.[3] There are advantages and disadvantages to the different schedules. Weekly low-dose infusions are better tolerated, but they require more trips to the doctor's office. Men who are more elderly or frail are often started on weekly treatment at the outset.[5] Since some studies suggest that every three-week protocols might be more effective, we typically use this protocol first.[4] If tiredness is excessive from the three-week protocol, the program can be changed to weekly administrations.

LOW NEUTROPHIL COUNTS

A primary concern when discussing Taxotere-related side effects is the possibility of a low neutrophil count. "Neutrophils" are a subtype of the white blood cell count (WBC). Neutrophils and white blood cells are components of the immune system. The lowering of blood counts after Taxotere usually occurs five to 10 days after treatment. Low blood counts can be dangerous if the neutrophil count drops below 500. At that point, the risk of blood infections sharply increases. In some circumstances, blood infections can be life-threatening.

Medications such as Neulasta and Leukine stimulate the bone marrow to increase the production of neutrophils, compensating for the Taxotere-lowering effects and thereby reducing the risk of infection. Our practice uses these medications routinely whenever Taxotere is administered. Other offices have the policy of only using them if the patient has already encountered an infection. Another preventive policy utilized by some physicians implements prophylactic antibiotics if the WBC drops too low. Low counts are detected by measuring the WBC a week or so after the infusion. If a low neutrophil count is detected, prophylactic treatment with an antibiotic such as Cipro or Levaquin is started and continued until the blood counts recover, usually within a week or so.

LOW RED BLOOD CELL COUNTS—ANEMIA

Anemia is detected by the complete blood count (CBC) blood test as well. The components of the CBC that detect anemia are the red blood count (RBC), hematocrit (HCT), and hemoglobin (HGB). All three of these indicators provide the same information about the presence or absence of anemia. Even prior to starting Taxotere, many men have some degree of preexisting anemia due to hormone therapy. When progressive prostate cancer is in the bone marrow, it may contribute to anemia as well. The effects of hormone therapy, cancer, and chemotherapy on the bone marrow can be additive.

Severe anemia causes shortness of breath. Mild anemia may contribute to fatigue. Anemia from hormone therapy or chemotherapy does not respond to iron supplements. It may respond, however, to medications such as Aranesp and Procrit.[6] If these medications are ineffective, a transfusion may be necessary.

LOW PLATELET COUNTS

Platelets are essential for normal coagulation of the blood. While a normal level is above 100,000, an increased risk of bleeding is unlikely, unless levels drop below 20,000. Chemotherapy lowers platelet counts, but only rarely to a dangerous degree. Platelet counts usually recover if the chemotherapy dosage is reduced or if the next cycle of treatment is delayed. Men with very suppressed platelet counts should stop aspirin and any other anticoagulants. Chronically low platelet counts can also occur after extensive amounts of previous radiation. Spontaneous bleeding caused by a low platelet count should be treated with a platelet transfusion, though transfusions are only a temporary bridge while waiting for the recovery of normal marrow production. Transfused platelets only survive in the blood for a few days.

FATIGUE AND TIREDNESS

Since most men with prostate cancer receiving Taxotere are already on TIP, fatigue is often a preexisting problem. Taxotere causes additional tiredness on a cyclical basis. Fatigue from chemo usually starts a few days after each infusion and lasts anywhere from two days to two weeks. Normal energy levels usually return to baseline before the next cycle of chemo. The tiredness, however, may become cumulative with successive cycles. As is the case with fatigue from TIP, exercise has the potential to make a big difference. In addition, medications or supplements such as prednisone, Provigil, Nuvigil, caffeine, and ginseng may improve energy levels. When fatigue is severe, the chemotherapy dosage may need to be reduced or the treatment time between infusions extended. Some experienced prostate oncologists believe that Jevtana causes less fatigue than Taxotere.

OTHER COMMON SIDE EFFECTS OF TAXOTERE

Other side effects of Taxotere also vary between the one-week and three-week treatment schedules. Hair loss tends to be more severe using the three-week schedule. Hair grows back when the chemo is stopped. Nausea is not very common with either schedule because antinausea medicines are so effective. Taxotere can affect the taste buds, making food taste strange. "Icing the tongue" by keeping ice chips in the mouth during the infusion is advisable to reduce blood flow to the mouth during treatment. This protects the taste buds by reducing the exposure to the Taxotere circulating in the blood during the infusion.

The weakening of fingernails is much more commonly associated with the once-a-week protocol. For this reason, we routinely ice the fingertips during and immediately after the infusion. *Narrowing* of the tear ducts occurs more commonly with weekly Taxotere than with the three-week protocol.[7] This problem is usually diagnosed when men report tears "spilling out of the eyes" because the ducts are not draining properly. We recommend artificial tears during and immediately after each infusion to flush the Taxotere from the surface of the eye to prevent irritation and scaring of the tear ducts. Ophthalmology consultation should be obtained, as some men need to have a small tube placed in the tear ducts to keep them open.

Another side effect of Taxotere is neuropathy. "Neuropathy" is numbness that usually starts in the fingers and toes and can spread into the hands, feet, and up the arms and legs. Generally, these symptoms are mild and slowly reverse over time after the Taxotere is stopped. However, more severe cases of numbness can occur that may require more than a year to recover. Prescription Neurontin, alpha lipoic acid, or high doses of L-glutamine, an amino acid, may have some impact on reducing the unpleasant symptoms. Some experienced prostate oncologists have reported a lower incidence of neuropathy from Jevtana, compared with Taxotere. Other side effects that can be caused by Taxotere or Jevtana are skin rashes, liver inflammation, or diarrhea, though these problems are fairly uncommon.

Taxotere and Jevtana prolong survival. Their beneficial effects are even further enhanced when used prior to the development of hormone resistance. Supportive care as outlined above reduces the side effects of chemotherapy without impairing its anticancer efficacy.

CARBOPLATIN AND XELODA

Both Carboplatin and Xeloda appear to improve the effectiveness of Taxotere and Jevtana. The side effects of these two agents (tiredness and low blood counts) are very similar to those of Taxotere, with slight variations. As might be expected, side effects increase when a higher dosage is used. Xeloda has a higher incidence of mouth sores, skin changes, and pain in the hands and feet ("hand-and-foot syndrome"). Carboplatin has a higher incidence of neuropathy, causes allergic reactions more frequently, and has a greater propensity to lower platelet counts. Prior to the advent of modern antinausea medication, Carboplatin had a reputation for greater nausea. With effective antinausea medications, however, this problem is rarely an issue. Overall, Carboplatin and Xeloda tend to be well tolerated, since they are used in relatively small doses when combined with Taxotere or Jevtana.

References

1. G Ahlgren and others. A randomized phase III trial between adjuvant docetaxel and surveillance after radical prostatectomy for high risk prostate cancer: Results of SPCG12. *Journal of Clinical Oncology* 34 suppl: abstr 5001, 2016.

2. W Berry and others. Phase II trial of single-agent weekly docetaxel in hormone-refractory, symptomatic, metastatic carcinoma of the prostate. *Seminars in Oncology* 28 suppl 15: 8, 2001.

3. P Kellokumpu-Lehtinen and others. 2-weekly versus 3-weekly docetaxel to treat castration-resistant advanced prostate cancer: A randomized, phase 3 trial. *Lancet Oncology* 14.2: 117, 2013.

4. IF Tannock and others. Docetaxel plus prednisone or mitoxantrone plus prednisone for advanced prostate cancer. *New England Journal of Medicine* 351.15: 1502, 2004.

5. M Scholz and others. Low-dose single-agent weekly docetaxel (Taxotere) is effective and well tolerated in elderly men with prostate cancer. *American Society of Clinical Oncology Annual Meeting, abstr 2441,* 2001.

6. J Seidenfeld and others. Epoetin treatment of anemia associated with cancer therapy: A systematic review and meta-analysis of controlled clinical trials. *Journal of the National Cancer Institute* 93.16: 1204, 2001.

7. B Esmaeli and V Valero. Epiphora and canalicular stenosis associated with adjuvant docetaxel in early breast cancer: Is excessive tearing clinically important? *Journal of Clinical Oncology* 31.17: 2076, 2013.

Chapter 36

INDIGO—SITUATIONS IN WHICH PSA IS MISLEADING

Mark Scholz, MD

Misunderstanding is generally simpler than true understanding,
and hence has more potential for popularity.

RAHEEL FAROOQ

PSA CAN BE ELEVATED FROM *noncancerous* causes. Noncancerous elevations in PSA can cause false alarms. These false alarms need to be accurately identified, because there is a danger that treatment may be recommended when it is not needed.

Before addressing the main theme of this chapter, which is *elevations* of PSA due to causes *besides* cancer, let's briefly discuss the opposite situation: Having a *low* PSA can't prove the absence of cancer. PSA can be undetectable while small amounts of cancer persist; the residual cancer may be producing such a small amount of PSA that standard laboratory machines can't detect it. This phenomenon is commonly observed in men who have an undetectable PSA after surgery and subsequently relapse. The cancer was always there, but the cancer cells were too few to produce sufficient PSA to be measurable. After surgery or radiation, the usual policy is to monitor PSA levels on a predetermined schedule for at least 10 years to detect recurrent disease as early as possible, should a recurrence arise. A recommended monitoring schedule is presented in Chapter 46.

A SMALL PSA RISE AFTER SURGERY

Monitoring PSA after surgery, compared with radiation (see below), is straightforward. The PSA, after all, is expected to be zero once the prostate gland has been entirely removed. This means that all the "background noise" from the residual prostate gland should be gone. However, total surgical removal of the gland is not as simple as it sounds. Small chunks of the benign gland (not cancer) can be left behind after the operation. When that occurs, PSA may hover indefinitely in the 0.1 to 0.3 range, even when there is no cancer. Men with these very low levels of PSA after surgery (unless the original Stage was *Azure* or the postoperative pathology report shows positive margins, node disease, or other unfavorable factors) should forgo immediate treatment. Instead, they should monitor their PSA closely, perhaps as frequently as monthly, to determine if there is an upward trend. Treatment can be withheld if the PSA remains stable. The longer that the PSA remains stable, the more likely the PSA is due to persistent prostate gland tissue rather than cancer.

When reflecting on the meaning of a small amount of PSA after surgery, the *original* Stage of Blue must come under strong consideration. If it was *Sky*, then residual PSA produced by benign prostate gland cells left behind by the surgeon is a more likely explanation. However, if the patient was *Azure*, whether there is a detectable PSA or not, the risk of cancer recurrence is high. As was discussed in previous chapters, men in *Azure* should consider an aggressive protocol with radiation and hormones, even if their PSA is low.

In the process of trying to sort through the meaning of a low but detectable level of PSA after surgery, a scan of the prostate fossa with a color Doppler ultrasound or multiparametric MRI is often proposed. If the scan detects a small nodule, this information may be useful for tracking any growth of the nodule. Sequential scans to determine if the nodule is growing may provide some additional information besides PSA to determine if cancer is present. Newer PET scans such as Axumin or C[11] acetate may occasionally suggest local recurrence in the fossa as well. When a nodule is detected, many urologists will recommend a biopsy to *prove* it's cancerous. Unfortunately, accurately targeting a small nodule is difficult, and a negative biopsy won't eliminate uncertainty. A negative biopsy may simply indicate inaccurate targeting of the nodule by the needle. If treatment is being withheld, sequential scans and PSA testing may be a better way to ascertain if cancer is growing. PSA levels that don't rise and nodules that don't enlarge are either due to persistent noncancerous glandular tissue or an extremely low-grade type of prostate cancer that won't require treatment anyway.

A PSA RISE AFTER RADIATION

Noncancerous PSA elevations occur rather frequently after radiation, particularly after seed radiation. The term for these elevations is "PSA bounce." A bounce is believed to result from radiation-induced prostate inflammation, (i.e., prostatitis). With a bounce, the main priority is to distinguish it from a cancer relapse.

THE PSA BOUNCE

The bounce phenomenon was first described by Dr. Frank Critz, an innovator and promoter of seed implant radiation.[1] He reported that *noncancerous* PSA elevations occurred in about one-third of his seed-implanted patients. In some cases, PSA levels would remain elevated for a couple of months. In other cases, the PSA would remain high for over a year. The PSA bounce might occur right after radiation or be delayed three or four years after the radiation was completed. The fact that the PSA rise was not due to a cancer recurrence was easily confirmed in retrospect because the PSA would drop back to its previous baseline with no specific anticancer therapy whatsoever. Dr. Critz's study reported that the occurrence of a PSA bounce had no bearing on the risk of having a future cancer relapse.

Multiple centers have reported the PSA bounce.[2,3] The challenge presented by a PSA bounce is how to distinguish it from a cancer relapse. What a tragedy to treat a rising PSA with TIP when cancer is not the cause! While there is no perfect methodology for distinguishing between a relapse and a bounce, two factors are commonly considered:

- The patient's original Stage of Blue. Since relapses are far more common after *Azure,* a PSA rise is more likely to be from cancer. On the other hand, when men with *Sky* develop a rising PSA, since their risk of relapse is low, they are more likely to be having a bounce than a relapse.

- The intensity of the radiation dose. When the radiation dose is higher, particularly with seed implants, the risk of having a bounce is also increased. However, a bounce can also occur with other types of radiation, including IMRT, SBRT, Cyberknife, and Proton therapy.

Monitoring PSA after radiation can be challenging. PSA produced by the residual prostate gland potentially obscures PSA from an early, recurrent cancer. As a rough starting point, consider a PSA elevation above 1.0 to be "abnormal." There are exceptions, and apart from a bounce, it is possible to have a PSA above 1.0 and still be free of cancer. Here is a list of noncancerous factors that influence the level of PSA after radiation:

- The size of the prostate gland. Bigger glands produce more PSA.

- The time elapsed since radiation. Sometimes PSA levels will not decline to their lowest levels for two or more years after the radiation has been completed.

- The testosterone levels. PSA should be zero if the testosterone is low. However, after testosterone recovers, PSA levels will normally rise after radiation (but generally not higher than 1.0). PSA, therefore, is affected by the degree of testosterone recovery.

The most reliable method for distinguishing a cancer relapse from a bounce is to examine a continuous graph of multiple PSA levels that have been checked over time (while evaluating for a bounce, PSA should be checked monthly). PSA from recurrent cancer tends to manifest as a smooth, unbroken, upward progression. Since a bounce is caused by inflammation, PSA levels tend to wax and wane, oscillating up and down on a graph in a zig-zag, spiking pattern.

PSA is a powerful blood test that is interwoven into the fabric of prostate cancer management. We rely heavily on PSA, so there is always the danger of overinterpreting its significance. In my career, I have observed the unfortunate occurrence of unnecessary radiation and TIP for men with slightly elevated PSA levels that were not due to cancer. A diagnostic approach that delays immediate treatment and relies upon the sequential and frequent monitoring of the PSA over time is the best way to clarify the underlying cause of a PSA elevation.

FINAL THOUGHTS ABOUT *INDIGO*

The main themes for *Indigo* are:

1. Know what you are treating. The subtype of *Indigo* must be determined accurately:

    a. Don't rely on suboptimal scans or on scans read by suboptimal doctors.

    b. Incorporate information from the previous Stage of Blue, PSA doubling rate, and pathology reports.

    c. Be aware that not all rises in PSA come from cancer.

2. Cure, rather than control, should be the initial goal. Chronic intermittent TIP can be used as a backup if the initial attempt to cure is unsuccessful. However, men who achieve a cure enjoy a better quality of life.

3. Cure rates are higher when recurrence is detected early and treated promptly.

4. Higher cure rates are achieved with combination therapy than with monotherapy.

Having completed this section relating to the *Indigo* Stage of Blue, you can now jump to the section midway through Chapter 46 to the subhead "Non-Prostate Cancer Health Issues" and finish the remainder of the book.

References

1. FA Critz and others. Prostate specific antigen bounce after radioactive seed implantation followed by external beam radiation for prostate cancer. *Journal of Urology* 163.4: 1085, 2000.

2. D Reed and others. Clinical correlates to PSA spikes and positive repeat biopsies after prostate brachytherapy. *Urology* 62.4: 683, 2003.

3. S Smathers and others. Temporary PSA rises and repeat prostate biopsies after brachytherapy. *International Journal of Radiation Oncology, Biology, Physics* 50.5: 1207, 2001.

SECTION VI
THE *ROYAL* STAGE OF BLUE

Chapter 37
OVERVIEW OF *ROYAL*

Mark Scholz, MD

However beautiful the strategy, you should
occasionally look at the results.
WINSTON CHURCHILL

MEN IN *ROYAL* HAVE A MORE advanced stage of prostate cancer. *Royal* is defined as the presence of metastases located *outside* the pelvic lymph nodes or, alternatively, the development of Lupron resistance (or any resistance to one of the Lupron-like drugs). Therefore, in comparison to the other Stages of Blue, treatment for *Royal* is aggressive. For example, *Sky* is managed with a "go-slow," surveillance-type approach. Conversely, treatment for *Royal* is all-out. The goal is a complete remission, to attain a PSA under 0.1.

STARTING AS *ROYAL* VERSUS DEVELOPING INTO *ROYAL* OVER TIME
There are two distinctly different pathways to *Royal*. One begins with PSA screening leading to the initial diagnosis of an earlier, less serious

Stage of Blue, which is usually treated with surgery or radiation. After a period, about one-third of these men relapse (*Indigo*) and start treatment with Lupron. When resistance to Lupron later develops, they enter *Royal*. A less common and more abrupt pathway to *Royal* occurs in men who fail to undergo PSA screening. In this scenario, unbeknown to the patients, unmonitored prostate cancer grows silently and spreads to the bones without anyone being aware of its existence. Men finally come to medical attention when they start seeking an explanation for bone pain. Diagnostic scans then reveal the presence of metastatic prostate cancer.

THREE SUBTYPES OF *ROYAL*

Once men "become" *Royal*, three subtypes can be defined: *Low*, *Basic* and *High*. In *Low-Royal*, Lupron resistance exists, but the scans are negative for metastatic disease. *Basic-Royal* occurs when five or fewer *visible* metastases are present on a scan (with or without Lupron resistance), with at least one of the metastases located outside of the pelvic lymph nodes.* "Oligometastases" is the name used for *Basic-Royal* in medical textbooks. *High-Royal* means that there are over five metastatic sites, with at least one located outside of the pelvic lymph nodes.

LOW-ROYAL: LUPRON RESISTANCE WHILE ON LUPRON

"Lupron resistance" is defined as a rising PSA while the testosterone level is under 50. There are various names for Lupron resistance, including androgen independence, hormone resistance and castration resistance. Men evolving out of *Indigo* into *Royal* have often been on Lupron for 10 or more years. The development of a PSA increase while on Lupron should sound alarms, because it signals the development of a more virulent cancer. Unfortunately, the many previous years of quiet success with Lupron often lull doctors and patients into inactivity.

---

* Men with 5 or fewer metastases exclusively in the pelvic nodes are *High-Azure* or *High-Indigo,* depending on whether they have had previous treatment or not, and assuming they are not Lupron-resistant.

They don't realize the urgency of the situation, that there is a need to start additional treatment promptly. Complacency in Lupron-resistant men allows the untreated cancer to grow deeper "roots," making future eradication more difficult.

BASIC-ROYAL: OLIGOMETASTATIC DISEASE

As noted above, *Royal* with five or fewer metastases is called "oligometastases." Multimodality therapy with radiation, hormones, and chemotherapy can induce complete cancer remissions and, in some cases, even a cure. Using aggressive combination therapy for *Basic-Royal* is a relatively new policy. Previously, technology was so poor that the detection of a "few" metastases on a scan would always mean that additional, undetected metastases were invariably present, "flying under the radar." Treating metastases in that era, with radiation, for example, was futile, because other metastases would eventually show up. It was like playing the parlor game "Whack-a-Mole." Due to a marked improvement in scans, which can detect much smaller metastases, patients are now more likely to benefit from radiation to the metastatic sites. The subject of oligometastases is covered in Chapter 39.

HIGH-ROYAL

More than five metastases is designated *High-Royal*. With aggressive systemic therapy, complete remissions (PSA under 0.1) are possible, even in men with widespread metastases. *Systemic* treatments—immunotherapy, second-line hormonal therapy, Xofigo, and chemotherapy—circulate via the bloodstream and attack prostate cancer cells throughout the body. Occasionally, certain metastatic sites are selected to undergo additional spot radiation. Traditionally, each of these treatments is *sequenced*. If the initial therapy proves ineffective, or later becomes ineffective, treatment is stopped and the next most effective option is started.

THE TRADITIONAL SEQUENTIAL APPROACH FOR TREATING *HIGH-ROYAL*

Practically speaking, if the cancer is not rampaging out of control, the first treatment in sequence will often be Provenge. Provenge causes relatively few side effects, and a full course is completed within four weeks. Our policy is to start second-line, hormonal therapy with Xtandi or Zytiga immediately after Provenge. Both Xtandi and Zytiga are convenient, well-tolerated, and effective oral agents (Chapter 40). If, after a period, Xtandi and Zytiga stop working, Taxotere or Xofigo are the next treatment options to consider. Xofigo may be preferred prior to Taxotere, due to fewer side effects. One exception would be when liver metastases are present, since Xofigo is ineffective for liver metastases. When Taxotere is being used, another type of chemo-therapy, called Carboplatin,[2,3] may be added to enhance the anticancer effect. If Taxotere stops working, another type of chemotherapy, called Jevtana, is the usual backup. Other "off-label" agents can be tried after Jevtana or, alternatively, new agents that are only available in clinical trials (Chapters 44).

DETERMINING IF TREATMENT IS WORKING

Continual monitoring to assess the effectiveness of treatment is essential. Staying on an ineffective therapy after it stops working postpones the initiation of a new potentially effective therapy. Treatment delays allow the disease to grow unimpeded. PSA is a good marker for monitoring the efficacy of Zytiga, Xtandi, Taxotere, or Jevtana. Generally, a 30 percent decline in PSA indicates the disease is responding.[4] PSA monitoring after Provenge is irrelevant, because the therapy is completed within four weeks. Xofigo, however, is different. Studies show that Xofigo prolongs survival *even if the PSA is rising*. One study suggests that a better indicator of Xofigo's effectiveness is ALP (alkaline phosphatase).[5] ALP is one of several different blood markers (see table) used in addition to PSA for ascertaining the effectiveness of prostate cancer therapy.

Marker	Full Name	Comments
PSA	Prostate Specific Antigen	Most widely used test
PAP	Prostatic Acid Phosphatase	Less precise but still useful
ALP	Alkaline Phosphatase	Measures disease activity in bone and liver
LDI[6]	Lactate Dehydrogenase	Very sensitive indicator, but not specific for cancer
CTC[7]	Circulating Tumor Cells	Accurate, but often not covered by insurance

In addition to blood testing, doctors regularly question their patients about cancer *symptoms*. A rapid reduction in cancer-related pain after starting a new treatment provides additional confirmation that the treatment is working. Chapter 45 discusses how to distinguish between cancer pain and pain from other causes.

MONITORING FOR DISEASE PROGRESSION WITH SCANS

In addition to blood testing and querying patients about any changes in pain symptoms, scans of the body and bones should be performed at least every six months. "Standard" bone scans rely upon an injection of a radioactive substance called Technetium-99. Newer PET bone scans use a more accurate type of technology called F^{18}, which is preferred when available.[8] Any type of bone scan occasionally yields ambiguous results. An MRI of the area of uncertainty may provide greater detail and help differentiate cancer-related abnormalities from those that are benign.

CT scans of the abdomen and pelvis are the most common type of body scans used to detect lymph node or liver metastases. Sometimes an MRI of the abdomen and pelvis is substituted for CT. New PET scans can detect lymph node metastases at a much earlier stage than has previously been possible (Chapter 6). These scans are radically altering our approach to metastatic disease. When interpreting any scan, comparing the previous scan images alongside the most recent images improves the doctor's ability to determine if the cancer is progressing or regressing.

PARTICIPATION IN CLINICAL TRIALS

Clinical trials are attractive to patients because they provide access to new drugs. The general policy followed by most prostate doctors is to exhaust all the FDA-approved treatment options before embarking on investigational therapy. Clinical trial participation can be challenging. Individual patients may be excluded for being too sick or not sick enough, or for having too many prior treatments or not enough prior treatment. The reality of these tightly specified trial-entry criteria is frustrating but necessary to ensure accurate research. The results of well-performed clinical trials provide the basis for most of the treatment recommendations expressed in this book. The challenge for patients is to find out whether or not the new drug being proposed is likely to help them personally. Chapter 44 addresses the world of clinical trials more fully.

SEQUENTIAL THERAPY VS. COMBINATION THERAPY

Scientists test one new agent at a time. If two drugs are given simultaneously, it's impossible to know which one is working. This one-at-a-time treatment policy continues in the clinic after FDA approval. And due to the absence of combination testing, doctors are worried that unpredictable side effects may occur if a new drug is used with other drugs. There are, however, some compelling arguments for a combination approach:

- Most new therapies are less toxic than older therapies. This creates the possibility of using treatments in combination without causing excessive side effects.

- Attacking the cancer with multiple agents at an earlier stage, before the cancer develops treatment resistance, is likely to increase the effectiveness of the anticancer therapy.

- Two treatments administered together may be *synergistic*. In other words, because of the treatment interactions, the anticancer effect of two agents given simultaneously might be triple instead of double.

The conventional approach has been to treat *Royal* with medications sequentially. This has two advantages. When one medicine is used at a time, there is no difficulty ascertaining the effectiveness of the agent. Its effectiveness is revealed by whether the disease responds or progresses. Single-agent therapy is also likely to be less toxic. Men who are elderly and testosterone-deprived may be unable to withstand the increased side effects of combination therapy. However, the prostate cancer world has recently been blessed with several new, less toxic agents, putting combination therapy on the table for discussion. This important topic of using sequential versus combination therapy will be revisited in the following chapters.

CONCLUSION

Royal is the most potentially life threatening of the Stages of Blue and requires aggressive treatment. The goal is to maximize therapy, attain a complete cancer remission and reduce the PSA to less than 0.1. On the other hand, enthusiasm for aggressive treatment must be balanced against the risk of excessively toxic side effects. The recent advent of less-toxic agents, however, opens the door to the possibility of improving on the traditional, one-at-a-time treatment approach by considering a broader array of therapeutic options, including combinations.

References

1. J Mateo and others. DNA-repair defects and olaparib in metastatic prostate cancer. *New England Journal of Medicine* 373.18: 1697, 2015.

2. RW Ross and others. A phase 2 study of carboplatin plus docetaxel in men with metastatic hormone-refractory prostate cancer who are refractory to docetaxel. *Cancer* 112.3: 521, 2008.

3. CW Reuter and others. Carboplatin plus weekly docetaxel as salvage chemo-therapy in docetaxel-resistant and castration-resistant prostate cancer (drpc). *Journal of Clinical Oncology* 29.7 suppl: abstr 172, 2011.

4. DP Petrylak and others. Evaluation of prostate-specific antigen declines for surrogacy in patients treated on SWOG 99-16. *Journal of the National Cancer Institute* 98.8: 516, 2006.

5. C Parker and others. Alpha emitter Radium-223 and survival in metastatic prostate cancer. *New England Journal of Medicine* 369.3: 213, 2013.

6. J Zhang and others. Prognostic value of pretreatment serum lactate dehydrogenase level in patients with solid tumors: a systematic review and meta-analysis. *Scientific Reports* 5: 9800, 2015.

7. B Hu and others. Circulating tumor cells in prostate cancer. *Cancers* 5.4: 1676, 2013.

8. A Iagaru and others. Prospective evaluation of ^{99m}Tc MDP scintigraphy, [18]F NaF PET/CT, and ^{18}F FDG PET/CT for detection of skeletal metastases. *Molecular Imaging Biology* 14.2: 252, 2012.

Chapter 38

EARLY HORMONAL RESISTANCE: *LOW-ROYAL*

Mark Scholz, MD

The early bird catches the worm.
WILLIAM CAMDEN

Low-Royal IS DESIGNATED WHEN a man who is *Indigo* develops a rising PSA on Lupron and the restaging body and bone scans are clear, showing no metastases. In the clinical research world, patients with clear scans are sometimes labeled stage M0, or "M zero."

THE SEARCH FOR METASTASIS

Recent research reveals that PET scans (Chapter 6) are able to detect metastases at a much earlier stage than standard CT scans or bone scans. Standard CT and bone scans can only detect metastases that are more than a half-inch in diameter.[1] New PET scans can detect disease as small as 3 or 4 millimeters (approximately 1/8 inch) in diameter. Another common reason metastases remain undetected with *Low-Royal* is that doctors simply fail to order *any* scans.[2] This lackadaisical attitude is prevalent but unacceptable. Once the PSA starts rising on Lupron, every effort should be made to find the cancer's location as quickly as possible. If the cancer is located, treatment can be focused more effectively, and insurance coverage for FDA-approved treatments is much easier to obtain.

BARRIERS TO TREATMENT CREATED BY INSURANCE

Payment for medications such as Provenge, Zytiga, and Xgeva (Chapter 40) is usually denied if no metastatic site can be detected. Busy doctors become fatigued by the constant struggle to get insurance companies to pay for new treatments. Many doctors see no harm in starting Casodex, an easily accessible but inferior treatment.* After all, Casodex has been the standard practice for many years. This policy, however, is totally outdated. Better treatments, ones that have been proven to extend life,[3] end up being postponed, and this is dangerous. Fighting cancer is a dynamic process. Multiple studies show that delaying treatment *makes it markedly less effective.*[4,5,6]

UNSUSPECTING DOCTORS AND PATIENTS

Doctors and patients are often unaware of the dangers of postponing effective treatment. Why? Isn't it obvious that the cancer requires immediate treatment? A physician's thinking may be clouded by many years of successful disease control with Lupron. It seems logical to assume that the quiet behavior of the cancer, seen over the previous 10 or so years, will continue indefinitely into the future. Men with *Low-Royal* are in a strange pseudoreality in which only the PSA is rising. It is like the calm before the storm. Unfortunately, doctors fail to realize that the onset of Lupron resistance changes everything. The pussycat is morphing into a tiger.

---

* Sadly, the only treatment for *Low-Royal* currently recommended by the American Urologic Association (AUA) is Casodex or ketoconazole (Chapter 40). By the time a large group of doctors (the AUA) finally gets around to agreeing on how to treat some aspect of prostate cancer, their policy is usually out of date. Insurance companies love to cite these outdated recommendations. It gives them justification for withholding payment on new drugs.

DON'T TEMPORIZE, FIGHT!

Lupron resistance is a reliable sign that the rate of cancer growth is accelerating. Hormone-resistant cancer should be fought like a fire that has the potential to grow exponentially, consuming everything in its path. Using this firefighter analogy, the goal should be to *extinguish*, not to *control*. The cancer should be attacked with maximal therapy at its earliest and weakest stage. It is easier to extinguish a fire burning in a wastebasket than one that has reached the curtains or is burning in the attic. *Low-Royal* is an opportunity to deliver multiple treatment punches before the cancer becomes further entrenched.

FIND THE METASTASIS!

Considering all that has been discussed above, every available means should be employed to locate the cancer. Putting a Band-Aid on the situation by suppressing PSA with Casodex is counterproductive. Generally, any new treatment should be withheld until energetic efforts are made to determine the site of the metastasis.* No expense should be spared to obtain the best available scans. F^{18} PET bone scans are available in most areas and are much more likely to find metastases than traditional technetium scans. Other types of scans should also be considered:

1. C^{11} Acetate PET is available at Phoenix Molecular Imaging, in Arizona.

2. C^{11} Choline PET is available at the Mayo Clinic, in Rochester, Minnesota.

3. Axumin PET is becoming commercially available in many locations.

---

* Men with metastases who start therapy prior to scanning can "mask" the metastatic sites. Effective therapy has the potential to shrink the metastatic sites and make them invisible on scanning, leading to the false perception that metastases are absent.

4. Gallium[68] PSMA PET is available commercially in Europe and on a research basis at several universities in the United States.

5. Combidex MRI is available at Radboud University, in Nijmegen, The Netherlands.

WHAT IF A METASTASIS SIMPLY CANNOT BE DETECTED?

Sometimes, men with low PSA levels have no detectable metastases despite searching with the best possible scans, a circumstance that forces hard choices. The question arises, "Should treatment be delayed until the PSA rises higher so that the metastases can be detected and targeted with radiation?" Waiting, as previously emphasized, is certainly undesirable. But what is the alternative? This is controversial. I think it is logical to consider four cycles of Taxotere combined with a second-line hormonal agent such as Xtandi or Zytiga. Although radiation will only "blindly" target the pelvic nodes, treating the pelvic node area in the absence of a positive scan may still be reasonable, since this is the most frequent site of early cancer spread. Using radiation, Taxotere, and Xtandi or Zytiga in this fashion for *Low-Royal* has not been proven to prolong survival. However, we should consider that experts can give the radiation with minimal toxicity, and missing a chance for a cure by delaying effective therapy while waiting for a scan to become positive seems less desirable.

Some experts, especially the academicians whose bread and butter is the publication of clinical trials, will certainly balk at the suggestion of using Taxotere for *Low-Royal*, citing concern about the absence of trials. There are, however, studies proving that early Taxotere is beneficial for *High-Azure*,[7] *Basic-Indigo*,[8] *High-Indigo*,[7] *Basic-Royal*[7] and *High-Royal*.[9] Early Taxotere also improves survival in breast cancer, lung cancer, and head and neck cancer, just to name a few. Considering Taxotere's amazing pedigree, it's not much of a stretch to conclude that men with *Low-Royal* will also benefit.

Another argument *against* using Taxotere for *Low-Royal* is based on the following idea: Perhaps the survival rates for *Low-Royal* are already good enough without Taxotere. Modern immunotherapy, secondary hormonal therapies, and *delayed* Taxotere are all known to be quite effective. Perhaps survival for *Low-Royal* is already so protracted it will be impossible to improve longevity further. The problem with this argument is that it ignores the benefits of achieving a complete *remission*. Early Taxotere gives longer remissions,[10] and some of these men may even be cured that is, achieve a *permanent* remission! Remission, permanent or otherwise, equals better quality of life.

Dynamic change is in the air for how *Low-Royal* is managed. The fact that *Low-Royal* is potentially life threatening is agreed upon by most, so experts are open to using more aggressive therapy at an earlier stage. However, new treatments are being discovered so rapidly, they outstrip our ability to measure their long-term impact. Studies to determine a survival advantage in earlier-stage disease take years to perform. *Low-Royal* men do not have that luxury of time. At least we know that aggressive treatment can cause long remissions, perhaps enabling some patients to go off hormonal therapy and achieve a better quality of life.

References

1. B Tombal and others. Modern detection of prostate cancer's bone metastasis: Is the bone scan era over? *Advances in Urology* 893193, 2012.

2. EY Yu and others. Detection of previously unidentified metastatic disease as a leading cause of screening failure in a phase III trial of zibotentan versus placebo in patients with nonmetastatic, castration resistant prostate cancer. *Journal of Urology* 188.1: 103, 2012.

3. DF Penson and others. Enzalutamide versus bicalutamide in castration-resistant prostate cancer: The STRIVE trial. *Journal of Clinical Oncology* 34.18: 2098, 2016.

4. PF Schellhammer and others. Lower baseline prostate-specific antigen is associated with a greater overall survival benefit from sipuleucel-t in the immunotherapy for prostate adenocarcinoma treatment (IMPACT) trial. *Urology* 81.6: 1297, 2013.

5. F Saad and others. Efficacy outcomes by baseline prostate-specific antigen quartile in the AFFIRM trial. *European Urology* 67.2: 223, 2015.

6. CJ Ryan and others. Relationship of baseline PSA and degree of PSA decline to radiographic progression-free survival (rPFS) in patients with chemotherapy-naive metastatic castration-resistant prostate cancer (mCRPC): Results from COU-AA-302. *Journal of Clinical Oncology* 31.15 suppl: abstr 5010, 2013.

7. ND James and others. Addition of docetaxel, zoledronic acid, or both to first-line long-term hormone therapy in prostate cancer (STAMPEDE): Survival results from an adaptive, multiarm, multistage, platform randomised controlled trial. *Lancet* 387.10024: 1163, 2015.

8. M Nakabayashi and others. Long-term follow-up of a Phase II trial of chemotherapy plus hormone therapy for biochemical relapse after definitive local therapy for prostate cancer. *Urology* 81.3: 611, 2013.

9. CJ Sweeney and others. Chemohormonal therapy in metastatic hormone-sensitive prostate cancer. *New England Journal of Medicine* 373.8: 737, 2015.

10. G Gravis and others. Androgen-deprivation therapy alone or with docetaxel in non-castrate metastatic prostate cancer (GETUG-AFU 15): A randomised, open-label, phase 3 trial. *Lancet Oncology* 14.2: 149, 2013.

Chapter 39

OLIGOMETASTATIC PROSTATE CANCER: *BASIC-ROYAL*

Jeffrey Turner, MD

*At a time in human history when technology has
the potential to profoundly affect people and society,
I can't think of a more exciting place to be.*

FRANK MOSS

RAPID IMPROVEMENTS IN medical technology are forcing us
to rethink our traditional approach to metastatic prostate cancer.
These new developments are multiple: The scans are better, the therapies
are more effective and have fewer side effects, and our understanding
of how cancer spreads has been greatly enhanced. A brief historical
review is in order.

THEORIES ABOUT HOW CANCER METASTASIZES
In 1889, Dr. Stephen Paget did autopsy studies in 735 women who
had died from breast cancer and concluded that the cancer metastases

occurred in a stepwise fashion, first near the tumor and subsequently in more distant parts of the body. His observations suggested that early treatment of metastases could possibly eradicate and cure the disease.

Paget's theory was quickly superseded in 1894, when Dr. William Halsted presented an alternative theory. He proposed that cancer spread locally to the adjacent lymph nodes *and* systemically throughout the rest of the body *at the same time*. He concluded that the detection of *any* metastasis signaled the presence of numerous undetected widespread *microscopic* metastases (micromets) in other parts of the body. Any attempt, therefore, to eradicate early-stage metastases would be futile, since the many occult (undetected) micrometastases would eventually appear, erasing any benefit from the previously administered therapy. Dr. Halsted's was the accepted viewpoint for almost 100 years.

More recently, over the last 15 years or so, an amalgamation of these two different theories has been adopted. Modern theory concedes that men with early metastases *may* have additional undetected *microscopic* metastases in other areas of the body. Attempts to cure such patients by treating the visible metastases will indeed be doomed to fail, since the untreated microscopic cancers will eventually grow larger, leading to cancer recurrence.

However, recent studies show that aggressive treatment, directed at all the visible metastases, can lead to durable remissions in some cases. Durable remissions have been seen in prostate cancer patients, as well as with other types of cancer such as melanoma, lung, kidney, and colon cancers.[1] These favorable outcomes confirm that a *subgroup* of patients with metastatic disease is free from additional micromets, or, if they are present, micromets are susceptible to eradication with systemic therapy. It is also becoming apparent that durable remissions are achieved more commonly if metastasis-focused treatment is combined with *systemic* chemo-hormonal treatment, which is active against the undetected micrometastases. This situation, the possibility that some cases of early-stage metastatic disease are curable, is termed "oligometastases." Some men achieve long-term remissions after treatment, which proves that treating oligometastases can be beneficial.

TREATMENTS FOR OLIGOMETASTATIC DISEASE

The basic component of therapy for this form of prostate cancer is either radiation or surgery. Radiation may be administered two ways: by intensity-modulated radiation (IMRT), or by stereotactic body radiation (SBRT). IMRT seems safer for treating a *region* of lymph nodes, whereas SBRT is better for bone metastases and perhaps for the treatment of an isolated lymph node. IMRT is given in small doses over a six- to eight-week period. SBRT is administered in only a few doses and completed in two weeks or less. Chapters 19 and 22 provide detailed reviews of IMRT and SBRT.

One benefit of radiation is the "Abscopal effect." Studies show that radiation incites a T-cell priming effect in the draining lymphatics. This T-cell effect may enable the immune cells to attack micrometastases in areas of the body outside the radiation field. This type of immune system activation by radiation is also discussed further in Chapter 42.

All the clinical trials cited below are in *hormone-sensitive* prostate cancer. As such, many of the studies add testosterone inactivating pharmaceuticals (TIP) to the radiation or surgery to improve the anticancer effect. TIP accomplishes two things: First, it enhances the killing effect of radiation. Second, TIP in some cases may be able to eradicate micrometastases that are in an area of the body outside the radiation treatment field. With the same rationale, consideration may be given to using Taxotere chemotherapy to enhance the anticancer effect against any undetected micrometastases.

STUDIES USING RADIATION TO TREAT OLIGOMETASTASES

In 2013, 50 patients were studied who had a limited number of metastases determined by state-of-the-art scanning with F^{18} and C^{11} acetate PET scans (Chapter 6).[2] The median PSA for the whole group was 6.7. Most of the men had regional node metastases *(Indigo),* though a minority had distant nodal or bone metastases. The cancer sites were treated with radiation along with TIP, which was continued for one year. Half of the patients also received *prophylactic* radiation to the surrounding pelvic lymph nodes (even in areas that did not light up on the scans). Three years after completing therapy, *one-half* of the men remained in remission. The men with fewer metastatic sites had the highest likelihood of remaining in remission.

Five additional studies evaluating a total of 126 men with prostate cancer were summarized in another article published in the *European Journal of Urology*.[3] Bone or lymph node disease was detected with Choline PET scans, and median PSA levels ranged between 1.7 and 5.6. Some patients were administered prophylactic pelvic node radiation with or without TIP. The median observation period after treatment ranged from six to 31 months. In two of these five studies, more than half of the men were relapse-free three years after radiation.[5,7] In two other studies, though, the median time to recurrence was more disappointing: 12 and 24 months, respectively. However, these less favorable results may be explained by the fact that only 25 percent of the men received prophylactic node radiation,[6] and none received TIP (the third study). In the fourth study,[4] the use of TIP and prophylactic node radiation, if any, was not reported. In the fifth study, 50 men were evaluated with either node or bone metastases. Median baseline PSA was 3.8. They received TIP for an average of only one month and had no prophylactic pelvic radiation. Nineteen months after radiation, half of the men had relapsed.[8]

These studies strongly suggest that treating oligometastases with radiation can result in extended remissions in about half of the men who undergo treatment, especially if the metastatic disease is in the lymph nodes. Better results are associated with the use of TIP and expansion of the radiation field to cover the surrounding "normal" lymph nodes.

SURGERY FOR OLIGOMETASTASES

From 2009 to 2013, the Mayo Clinic reported on 52 surgically treated men with rising PSA levels who underwent salvage surgery to remove cancerous lymph nodes.[9] Malignant nodes were detected by C^{11} Choline PET scanning. Median PSA was 2.2 at the time of the lymph node dissection. The median number of nodes removed was 21.5; the median number of nodes containing cancer was 3.5. Twenty months after salvage surgery, 46 percent of the men (24) remained in remission, 34 percent

(18) had started hormonal therapy, and 19 percent (10) had also received additional therapies.

Two other studies looking at surgery for malignant lymph nodes reported reasonably good results by adding varying amounts of TIP and prophylactic radiation to the surgery. Dr. Jilg[10] reported on 47 men with a median PSA of 11 prior to salvage surgery. The treatment of the 47 men was not uniform. Half of the men received prophylactic nodal radiation, and two-thirds received an unspecified duration of TIP. Two years after the surgery, about half of the 47 men were still in remission. Dr. Nazareno Suardi also reported on 59 men treated with surgery with a median PSA of 2.0. Again, treatment of the whole group was not uniform. One-third of the men were administered prophylactic radiation, and 40 percent were given two years of TIP. After five years, about half of the 59 men were still in remission.[11] A final study evaluating salvage surgery without the addition of any radiation or TIP reported less optimistic findings. Dr. Derya Tilki, from Germany, retrospectively evaluated 58 patients. Thirteen of them had their PSA drop to less than 0.2. However, the PSA began to increase in 12 of the 13 men over the ensuing 39 months of observation.[12]

These preliminary studies suggest that surgery alone is probably a less effective way to treat men who have cancer recurrences in their lymph nodes and no one is recommending surgery for bone metastases. The surgical studies that add treatment with radiation and TIP to the surgery seem to lead to a better outcome. Therefore, it's logical to ask, "Might these radiation- and TIP-treated men have done just as well without the surgery?" Despite my reservations about surgery, a rather optimistic review of the treatment for oligometastatic prostate cancer (with the major focus on surgery) was recently published.[13] This review suggests that local therapies, including prostatectomy and radiotherapy, can be performed safely in patients with oligometastatic prostate cancer.

Another excellent review[14] of treatment for oligometastatic prostate cancer suggests that metastases-directed therapies such as SBRT carry a very low risk for toxicity and that "emerging genomic data have suggested distinct biological differences between limited metastatic lesions and widely disseminated disease." This suggests that in the future we may develop the ability to genetically identify in advance what men are most likely to remain in a durable remission by using an aggressive, metastasis-directed treatment approach to eradicate all known disease sites.

USING TAXOTERE FOR OLIGOMETASTATIC, HORMONE-RESISTANT DISEASE

Our understanding of how to treat oligometastatic prostate cancer is rapidly evolving. The studies cited above indicate that an aggressive combination approach using radiation and TIP seems to give the best results. In addition, recent studies indicate that adding Taxotere may be beneficial. A large clinical trial involving almost 3,000 patients showed a 10 percent improvement in five-year survival rates for men with lymph node positive prostate cancer who were treated with Taxotere.[15] Since many of the men in this trial were *Basic-Royal,* this important new clinical study indicates that earlier use of Taxotere can lead to better outcomes.

Practically speaking, how should all these treatments be combined? Taxotere and pelvic radiation should be given *sequentially.* Excess side effects may occur if they are given at the same time. The largest study of pelvic radiation (in newly diagnosed men) reported better results by starting TIP two months before starting radiation.[16] This TIP-before-radiation policy has become standard. In the case of Taxotere, since Taxotere circulates and treats micrometastases throughout the whole body, it should probably be sequenced *ahead* of radiation. With all these considerations in mind, a possible treatment protocol for *Basic-Royal* might be as follows:

1. Lupron started (or continued) for 12 months
2. Taxotere started immediately (with Lupron): a total of four treatments, each administered three weeks apart
3. Radiation to all disease sites and possibly to the surrounding lymph-node chain, starting a month after the last dose of Taxotere

4. Xtandi or Zytiga for six to 12 months, if coverage by insurance can be obtained

5. Numerous precautions for side effects (Chapters 30 and 35)

With improved scanning technology that enables us to detect recurrent disease at a much earlier stage than was previously possible, the immediate, aggressive administration of multiple therapies improves the outlook for men with oligometastatic disease. Hopefully, the application of these measures will induce longer remissions and successfully bridge patients into an ever more exciting future era of scientific breakthroughs.

References

1. RR Weichselbaum and others. Oligometastases revisited. *Nature Reviews Clinical Oncology* 8.6: 378, 2011.

2. U Schick and others. Androgen deprivation and high dose radiotherapy for oligometastatic prostate cancer patients with less than five regional and/or distant metastases. *Acta Oncologica* 52.8: 1622, 2013.

3. P Ost and others. Metastasis-directed therapy of regional and distant recurrences after curative treatment of prostate cancer: A systematic review of the literature. *European Journal of Urology* 67.5: 852, 2015.

4. F Casamassima and others. Efficacy of eradicative radiotherapy for limited nodal metastases detected with choline PET scan in prostate cancer patients. *Tumori* 97.1: 49, 2011.

5. F Würschmidt and others. [^{18}F]fluoroethylcholine-PET/CT imaging for radiation treatment planning of recurrent and primary prostate cancer with dose escalation to PET/CT-positive lymph nodes. *Radiation Oncology* 6.1: 44, 2011.

6. KA Ahmed and others. Stereotactic body radiation therapy in the treatment of oligometastatic prostate cancer. *Frontiers in Oncology* 2: 215, 2012.

7. BA Jereczek-Fossa and others. Robotic image-guided stereotactic radiotherapy, for isolated recurrent primary, lymph node or metastatic prostate cancer. *International Journal of Radiation Oncology, Biology, Physics* 82.2: 889, 2012.

8. K Decaestecker and others. Repeated stereotactic body radiotherapy for oligometastatic prostate cancer recurrence. *Radiation Oncology* 9.1: 135, 2014.

9. RJ Karnes and others. Salvage lymph node dissection for prostate cancer nodal recurrence detected by ^{11}C-choline positron emission tomography/computerized tomography. *Journal of Urology* 193.1: 111, 2015.

10. CA Jilg and others. Salvage lymph node dissection with adjuvant radiotherapy for nodal recurrence of prostate cancer. *Journal of Urology* 188.6: 2190, 2012.

11. N Suardi and others. Long-term outcomes of salvage lymph node dissection for clinically recurrent prostate cancer: Results of a single-institution series with a minimum follow-up of 5 years. *European Urology* 67.2: 299, 2015.

12. D Tilki. Salvage lymph node dissection for nodal recurrence of prostate cancer after radical prostatectomy. *Journal of Urology* 193.2: 484, 2015.

13. JM Clement and CJ Sweeney. Evolving treatment of oligometastatic hormone-sensitive prostate cancer. *Journal of Oncology Practice* 13.1: 9, 2017.

14. JJ Tosoian and others. Oligometastatic prostate cancer: definitions, clinical outcomes, and treatment considerations. *Nature Reviews Urology* 14.1: 15, 2017.

15. ND James and others. Addition of docetaxel, zoledronic acid, or both to first-line long-term hormone therapy in prostate cancer (STAMPEDE): Survival results from an adaptive, multiarm, multistage, platform randomised controlled trial. *Lancet* 387.10024: 1163, 2016.

16. M Roach and others. Phase III trial comparing whole-pelvic versus prostate-only radiotherapy and neoadjuvant versus adjuvant combined androgen suppression: Radiation Therapy Oncology Group 9413. *Journal of Clinical Oncology* 21.10: 1904, 2003.

Chapter 40
TREATMENTS FOR *HIGH-ROYAL*

Richard Lam, MD

Attitude is a little thing that makes a big difference.
WINSTON CHURCHILL

METASTASES ORIGINATE FROM THE prostate and spread outside the gland to another part of the body, most commonly the lymph nodes and bones, and less often to the liver or lungs. Metastatic disease is usually a silent process without any symptoms. In the 1980s, before PSA was discovered, prostate cancer was typically diagnosed *after* metastases had already occurred. Back then, men came to the doctor seeking an explanation for bone pain or urinary blockage.

When cancer is widespread, removing or radiating the prostate becomes a lower priority; instead, a "whole-body" treatment plan is necessary. At this point in time, extensive metastatic cancer is generally thought to be incurable. However, certain exceptions may exist. I can recall at least three patients who were diagnosed with bone metastases more than 20 years ago, who were treated with Lupron and who continue to thrive, maintaining a steady low PSA level under 0.1 to this day.

HORMONAL THERAPY

The backbone of treatment for metastatic prostate cancer is hormonal therapy with testosterone inactivating pharmaceuticals (TIP), also known as androgen deprivation therapy or ADT (Chapters 23 and 27). Deprived of testosterone, prostate cancer cells are unable to replicate. They eventually die. Unfortunately for *Royal*, TIP usually loses effectiveness after a variable number of years.

Several factors predict a longer duration of cancer control with TIP: 1) a more limited extent of metastatic disease, 2) a lower Gleason grade, and 3) lower PSA levels. For example, a man with a Gleason score of 3+4=7, a PSA level of 10, and only six spots of metastatic disease will usually respond longer than a man with a Gleason score of 4+5=9, a PSA of 200, and 30 metastatic lesions.

THE PSA NADIR

The most important predictor of how long TIP will remain effective is determined by the *degree of PSA decline* after starting TIP, the so-called PSA nadir. The nadir is the PSA level when it arrives at its lowest point and thereafter stops dropping. A nadir of less than 0.1 is ideal. The outlook for a long response is most favorable when the PSA drops to less than 0.1.[1] When the nadir is above 0.1, hormone resistance and progressive disease is likely to develop much more quickly.

TREATMENTS FOR *ROYAL*

Patients in the *Royal* Stage of Blue usually require continuous treatment. The type of treatment selected is based on a patient's age, fitness, and the treatments that have been previously administered. Doctors try to strike a balance between a treatment's potency and its potential side effects. They discuss the pros and cons with their patients before deciding how to proceed. The various treatments for *Royal* are divided into six categories. As noted above, most patients stay on TIP indefinitely.

It is possible, if the PSA drops to less than 0.1, that some patients may be able to temporarily stop TIP, a practice called "intermittent therapy." However, intermittent therapy is not nearly as popular for *Royal* as it is for *Indigo*.

If the PSA begins to rise while taking TIP, or, alternatively, if there is a high PSA nadir, additional therapy will be necessary. The general categories of treatments commonly used for TIP-resistant disease are listed below. These can be used sequentially or in combination, depending on the circumstances surrounding the individual patient.

    I.   Immune-based therapy

    II. Secondary hormone approaches

    III. Chemotherapy

    IV. Bone-targeting agents

    V. Off-label agents FDA-approved for treating other types of cancer

    VI. Investigational drugs in clinical trials (Chapter 44)

I. IMMUNOTHERAPY

Prostate cancer has the distinction of being one of the first malignancies to have effective immunotherapy, a medicine called sipuleucel-t (Provenge). FDA-approval came in 2010 after a prospective, randomized trial demonstrated improved survival of slightly more than four months, compared with placebo. Provenge achieved this in men with relatively advanced disease, with PSA levels averaging over 50.[2] Further experience using Provenge reveals that there is an even greater survival benefit in men who begin treatment at an earlier stage with lower PSA levels. For example, with a PSA under 22, the median improvement in survival is 13 months.[3,4*]

---

* The prostate cancer world is changing so quickly! In 2013, when this study was published, "early-stage" was defined as a PSA less than 22! Now, due to PET scans, men can be treated with PSA levels as low as 1 or 2.

PROVENGE SHOULD BE THE FIRST TREATMENT

Provenge's convenience and lack of toxicity make it a logical first step in men who have become resistant to Lupron. Provenge only requires three visits to a specialized leukapheresisis center every two weeks. Leukapheresis is a three-hour process similar to dialysis. It filters out white blood cells (dendritic cells) from the bloodstream. These immune cells are saved and transported to a center in Seal Beach, California, for special processing. The dendritic cells are incubated and "trained" to recognize prostate cancer. The "primed" dendritic cells are then reinfused back into the patient three days later at the doctor's office. Dendritic cells activate the killer T cells that attack the cancer cells directly (Chapter 42). A total of three leukapheresis visits and three reinfusion visits are required, so the process is complete in four weeks. In general, side effects are mild, though occasionally patients will have transient fever, fatigue, nausea, headache, and flulike symptoms.

Convenience is not the only argument for putting Provenge first. The immune system *remembers* what it is taught and keeps working for the remainder of the patient's life. Therefore, if treatment is started when the disease is at an earlier stage, the *duration* of Provenge's effects on the immune system will be more prolonged and presumably more beneficial. For example, a very preliminary study using Provenge to treat *Indigo* saw three out of 48 men go into an extended remission.[5]

PROVENGE IS UNIQUE AND SOMETIMES MISUNDERSTOOD

Immunotherapy is a completely new realm of therapeutic technology. Unlike other types of therapy for *Royal*, PSA levels don't usually decline. Critics claim this is a sign that Provenge is ineffective. Criticism like this is ironic, considering that the FDA refuses to use PSA changes as an indicator of a drug's efficacy. Instead, the FDA demands proof of *extended survival* in prospective, placebo-controlled trials. Two such trials confirm that Provenge prolongs survival. Even so, some may wonder, "How can life be extended without PSA dropping?" One plausible explanation is that immune enhancement *impedes* the growth of new cancer cells without causing immediate mortality of the existing cells.*

It is quite remarkable that Provenge can extend life without causing serious side effects. Medicines that can extend survival in advanced cancer are rare and should be highly esteemed. Consider that several intriguing therapies—atrasentan,[6] zibotentan,[7] and denosumab—[8,9] all failed to show a survival advantage, even when they were tested in multimillion-dollar, multiyear, randomized trials against a much milder, earlier-stage type of prostate cancer (*Low-Royal*). Provenge improves survival, even in men with PSA levels above 50! As noted above, a greater survival benefit can be anticipated if Provenge is started before the disease becomes so advanced. There is also the possibility that Provenge's impact can be further increased by combining it with other types of immune treatment, an approach that is discussed in Chapter 42.

II. SECONDARY HORMONE THERAPY

For clarity in our discussion about TIP, let me define Lupron and other similar drugs like Firmagon, Trelstar, Eligard, and Zoladex as "primary" hormone therapy. These agents stop the *testicular production* of testosterone. Additional agents, ones that may be added or substituted when Lupron becomes ineffective, are termed "secondary" hormonal agents. One of the oldest secondary hormone medications is called bicalutamide (Casodex), which was approved in 1995 for use along with luteinizing hormone-releasing hormone analogues (such as Lupron) against metastatic prostate cancer. Nilutamide, an agent like Casodex but perhaps slightly more potent, was approved in 1997. Both Casodex and Nilutamide bind the androgen receptor, blocking the activity of testosterone, thus inhibiting cancer cell growth. Historically, when the combination of Casodex and Lupron (or Nilutamide) would become ineffective, the next secondary hormonal agent in line has been ketoconazole.

---

* This theory might be partially supported by a study performed by Dr. Eric Small at UCSF. When men with rising PSA levels were given Provenge plus Avastin, a drug that inhibits new blood vessel growth, a slower rate of PSA rise after treatment was observed.[10]

Doctors used to contend that the initiation of another secondary hormonal therapy should be delayed until the results of stopping Casodex were ascertained. In other words, they should wait to see if an "anti-androgen withdrawal response" occurred before proceeding with additional treatment. It is true that 10 to 15 percent of men who have a rising PSA on Casodex will experience a transient PSA decline lasting an average of three months when the Casodex is discontinued (the Lupron or Zoladex is continued but the Casodex is stopped). The "Casodex withdrawal maneuver" is rarely mentioned anymore. The responses are too infrequent and too brief to justify a delay in the initiation of another, more effective treatment.

KETOCONAZOLE

Ketoconazole was originally approved by the FDA for use as an antifungal antibiotic. It was later discovered to block *testosterone synthesis* (inside the cancer cell) when used in high doses. Ketoconazole has now been superseded by better agents (see below). However, at one time ketoconazole played an important therapeutic role, and certain treatment principles hold true for its modern replacements, Xtandi and Zytiga. The fact that ketoconazole is active in prostate cancer is undisputed. One study involving 79 men showed a 75 percent or greater PSA decline in 44 percent of the men.[11] After ketoconazole is started, the PSA should be checked every two to four weeks to determine whether it is effective. A rising PSA after 30 days does not invariably mean it won't work. Responses are sometimes delayed for 60 to 90 days. Ketoconazole has fallen out of favor because it is less potent than Xtandi or Zytiga. It also causes a wide variety of side effects, and has many interactions with other drugs.

ZYTIGA AND XTANDI

For a seasoned prostate cancer road warrior like myself, 2011 marked the start of the "Golden Age" of new prostate cancer therapeutics. This was when abiraterone (Zytiga) was first approved by the FDA. Zytiga was a giant leap forward both in terms of its anticancer effectiveness as well as its tolerability. It works by inhibiting CYP17, an enzyme essential for testosterone synthesis (the cancer cells rely upon CYP17 to manufacture their own testosterone internally). Self-production of testosterone is a characteristic of cancer cells that have developed resistance to the primary forms of hormonal therapy.

The approval of Zytiga resulted from two landmark studies. In the first, Zytiga was matched head to head with a placebo in TIP-resistant men who had already tried Taxotere. Zytiga was so effective, the study was closed early for ethical reasons.[12] In addition to extending life, this trial showed that Zytiga decreased PSA, decreased pain, and improved quality of life. Subsequently, Zytiga was tested in patients *before* Taxotere. The anticancer benefits of Zytiga were even more substantial.[13]

Unlike ketoconazole, Zytiga is well tolerated. If side effects develop, they are almost always quickly reversed, assuming the medication is stopped in a timely fashion. The most common issues are high blood pressure, low potassium, leg swelling, fatigue, and liver inflammation. During the first few months of starting treatment, regular lab testing is required to detect liver abnormalities or low potassium levels. Prednisone is given to sustain normal potassium levels in the blood. Rarely, prednisone increases blood sugar, so diabetics must monitor their glucose closely.

In 2012, the FDA approved enzalutamide (Xtandi), a different type of secondary hormonal agent. In a clinical trial evaluating Xtandi after Taxotere, Xtandi was proven to prolong survival.[14] Xtandi also delayed the onset of pain, bone cancer progression, and PSA progression, and showed an improvement in quality of life. The most common side effects were hot flashes and fatigue. There was also a slight risk of seizure (0.9 percent). In 2014, a second clinical trial using Xtandi prior to Taxotere showed that Xtandi delayed the need for chemotherapy by 17 months and improved survival, among other benefits. In this study, there was no increase in the incidence of seizures.[15]

Now we have two very effective hormonal agents to treat men resistant to Lupron. In making comparisons between Zytiga and Xtandi, there doesn't seem to be a major advantage of one over the other. So, is there a correct sequence? All I can suggest is to compare the pros and cons. With Zytiga, the requirement for an additional drug (prednisone) is a disadvantage. Zytiga also requires blood monitoring to check for potassium or liver problems, whereas Xtandi does not. On the other hand, Xtandi is associated with a small risk of seizures and causes fatigue more frequently. The sequence of Zytiga or Xtandi, therefore, depends on the needs for each individual's specific situation.

III. CHEMOTHERAPY

Taxotere was FDA-approved in 2004. Two prospective, randomized trials proved that it prolongs life.[16,17] These days Xtandi and Zytiga are used before Taxotere, as they have fewer side effects. However, if Xtandi and Zytiga stop working, Taxotere or Cabazitaxel (Jevtana) is often considered the next step.[10] Taxotere and Jevtana are quite similar, though Jevtana seems to have less side effects.[18] In general, most of the information provided here about Taxotere is also true for Jevtana.

TWO DIFFERENT ROLES FOR TAXOTERE

Taxotere has two basic roles to play. Historically, Taxotere has been reserved for men with progressive metastatic disease after Lupron, and now, more recently, for men who develop resistance to Xtandi and Zytiga. In this role Taxotere can be used as a single agent or combined with other agents such as Carboplatin[19] or Avastin,[20] agents that further enhance Taxotere's anticancer effects (see below).

Now, however, studies show that Taxotere can also be useful at an earlier stage, *before the onset of Lupron resistance.* Two studies have evaluated Taxotere in this role. The first study, CHAARTED, was published in 2015. It demonstrated that four months of Taxotere, added to TIP, *improved survival by 18 months* in men with metastatic, hormone-sensitive disease.[21] The second trial, called STAMPEDE, evaluated almost 3,000 newly diagnosed, hormone-sensitive men with extensive local disease or metastatic disease. STAMPEDE showed a significant survival advantage as well.[22] In addition, STAMPEDE also showed that in potentially curable patients, the cure rates are improved by 10 percent five years after treatment. The results of these two trials have turned the academic world on its ear. The early administration of Taxotere has, almost overnight, become the new standard of care for men with metastatic, hormone-sensitive disease.

The CHAARTED study has stimulated some discussion about the early use of Taxotere in men with oligometastases. Insufficient time has accrued to prove that there is a survival advantage for early Taxotere in *Basic-Royal*. Some experts have voiced a concern that these men will live such a long time with TIP alone that early Taxotere might be overkill. The problem is that the experts are forgetting that TIP plus Taxotere induces longer remissions[23] and thus a *better quality of life*. Some men may even be cured and able to go off TIP. A quality-of-life analysis from the CHAARTED study that was presented at the Genitourinary Cancers—American Society of Clinical Oncology meeting in 2016 supports this premise.[24] It was summarized by Dr. Robert Dreicer in *JAMA Oncology*:[25]

> "… patients treated with docetaxel plus ADT (TIP) had a decrement in overall quality of life while on treatment, but quality of life returned to baseline at 12 months *and was significantly better than in patients treated with ADT alone.*"

Survival is very important, but so is quality of life. Men who achieve remissions live better. This topic of optimizing treatment with early combination therapy is discussed further in the following chapter.

IV. BONE-TARGETED RADIATION

In 2013 the FDA approved Xofigo, a type of "smart radiation" that targets bone metastases. Bone-targeted radiation has been around for decades, but the older products (strontium[90] and samarium[53]) were ineffective and toxic. Xofigo uses *alpha-emitting* Radium[223]. Radium[223] is far more effective and much less toxic than the older radionucleotides. Xofigo showed a survival advantage when compared with "best clinical care" (Casodex, ketoconazole, and spot radiation) in a randomized prospective trial called ALSYMPCA.[26] The treatment itself consists of a simple one-minute injection given once a month for a total of six months.

Potential side effects are occasional nausea, vomiting, diarrhea, or low blood counts. Xofigo's effect on PSA is unusual. Although Xofigo extends survival, PSA levels may continue to rise. This "disconnect" between PSA and survival can be disconcerting to doctors and patients alike. Experts hypothesize that Xofigo *slows the rate* of cancer cell growth rather than causing precipitous cell death. This is not to say that notable declines in PSA with Xofigo don't occur. One of my patients dropped his PSA from 50 to 0. Another dropped his PSA from 150 down to 8. Xofigo has been a very welcome addition to our anticancer armamentarium.

BONE-TARGETED AGENTS—XGEVA AND ZOMETA

Two medications, Xgeva and Zometa, are commonly used to strengthen bone and arrest cancer growth in men with metastatic prostate cancer. Neither of these agents impacts survival, but Xgeva delays cancer growth in the bones.[27] Xgeva and Zometa work by inhibiting osteo*clasts*, the cells that induce bone breakdown. When the osteo*clasts* are inhibited, the bone matrix continues to expand due to the ongoing activity of the osteo*blasts*, resulting in a net increase in the amount of calcium deposited in the bone, which helps to reverse osteoporosis. Both agents reduce bone fractures, a common problem in men on TIP. Therapy is usually initiated with one of these agents at the first sign of bone metastases. Both Xgeva and Zometa can potentially lower calcium levels in the blood. As such, they should be stopped during the administration of Provenge (which also has the potential to lower calcium levels in the blood).

Zometa comes from a class of drugs called bisphosphonates. Other drugs in this class are Fosamax, Boniva, and Actonel, all of which are oral agents. Since Zometa is intravenous, bypassing the stomach, the potential for stomach irritation is avoided. Also, 100 percent of the drug gets into the system, compared with the 1 to 2 percent rate from the oral agents that must be absorbed from the GI tract. The most common side effect from Zometa is a brief, flulike muscle soreness lasting a day or so after the first infusion. Typically, these symptoms do not recur on subsequent infusions.

THE DANGER OF OSTEONECROSIS

Side effects from both Xgeva and Zometa tend to be mild except for a serious condition called osteonecrosis, which occurs in about 5 percent of men. Osteonecrosis consists of a breakdown of gum tissue due to underlying bone changes. The gum tissue recedes, leaving exposed bone that is susceptible to recurrent infections. This can be very painful and only reverses slowly after treatment is stopped. The risk of developing osteonecrosis is much higher when a tooth extraction occurs. The risk is also increased when treatment is continued for a longer period. To reduce the risk of osteonecrosis, some doctors have taken to administering Xgeva or Zometa on a less-frequent basis, quarterly rather than monthly.

V. "OFF-LABEL" CHEMOTHERAPEUTIC AGENTS

The various cancer treatments listed previously are often used in sequence: Provenge first, followed by Zytiga or Xtandi. Subsequently, Xofigo or Taxotere are used. The question will arise, "What will be the next step if all these agents stop working?" There are no definitive studies addressing this question, but clinical experience suggests that certain agents that are FDA-approved for other cancers can be considered. A list of such agents is provided in the following table:

Medication	Mechanism	FDA-Approved
Carboplatin	Chemotherapy	Lung Cancer
Xeloda	Chemotherapy	Breast Cancer
Ixempra	Chemotherapy	Breast Cancer
Avastin	Blocks New Blood Vessels	Colon Cancer
Lynparza	Stops DNA Repair	Ovarian Cancer

Carboplatin and Xeloda are most effective when used in combination with Taxotere, Jevtana, or Ixempra. In this combination role, even modest doses seem to improve response rates without adding much in the way of additional side effects. Nevertheless, Carboplatin can lower blood counts, induce nausea, and occasionally cause neuropathy, which is numbness of the feet and hands. Xeloda can also lower blood counts and occasionally causes temporary mouth sores or diarrhea. Preliminary trials of Taxotere in combination with each of an additional 30 different cancer agents have been published. None have suggested a notable improvement over Taxotere alone.[28]

We have generally used Ixempra as a single agent or occasionally in combination with Xeloda. The side effects of Ixempra are like those of Taxotere and Jevtana. Avastin, an angiogenesis inhibitor that is approved for colon cancer, has been tested in prostate cancer patients as an adjunct to Taxotere. (Cancer cells develop new blood vessels to grow, thus the reason for an angiogenesis inhibitor.) The largest study of Avastin did show a delay in cancer progression, although survival was not improved. However, two smaller phase II studies in men with very advanced, heavily pretreated disease reported that a three-drug combination of Taxotere, Avastin, *plus Thalidomide or Revlimid* (angiogenesis inhibitors) showed surprisingly high response rates and durable remissions.[29,30] The side effects, however, were notable, consisting of blood clots and severe numbness in the hands and feet.

Lynparza is FDA-approved for the treatment of ovarian cancer. A report in the *New England Journal of Medicine* indicates that men resistant to secondary hormonal agents and chemotherapy can have close to 90 percent response rates to Lynparza *if their cancers have a genetic mutation called BRCA.*[31] In general, it appears that BRCA or related mutations are present in about one-third of men with prostate cancer who have become resistant to secondary hormones and chemotherapy. This discovery is so new that the exact sequence of who should be tested for the mutation and who should be treated with Lynparza is still unknown. Even so, the discovery of this genetic type of prostate cancer, one that can specifically be targeted with an effective agent, is very exciting.

Before closing out this chapter, one relatively rare variation of metastatic prostate cancer, called neuroendocrine cancer or *small cell* prostate cancer, should be mentioned. Neuroendocrine prostate cancer may grow quickly and become advanced, even when the PSA level is not particularly high. Specialized blood tests, however, such as Chromogranin-A (CGA) and neuron-specific enolase (NSE) may be elevated and can be useful for tracking the disease's status. The organs to which small cell prostate cancer can spread are more unpredictable, compared with the usual pattern of lymph node and bone metastases associated with regular types of prostate cancer. TIP may be less effective with small cell prostate cancer, so chemotherapy, particularly with carboplatin, is often employed at an earlier stage.

Advanced prostate cancer is very dynamic, with a potential impact on various organs and bodily functions. As such, whenever PSA is tested, which may be as frequently as every three weeks in men receiving Taxotere, other blood tests—such as a CBC (anemia, blood clotting, and immune function), hepatic panel (liver function), and a basic metabolic panel (kidney function and electrolytes)—are also routinely checked. Blood tests may also detect treatment-related side effects or organ malfunction due to progressive cancer. Appendix III discusses these ancillary blood tests in more detail.

CONCLUSION

Five new agents have been approved to treat metastatic prostate cancer since 2010. Optimism for the treatment of metastatic disease is growing. How these new agents work runs a wide gamut, from immunotherapy to hormone therapy to chemotherapy to radiopharmaceuticals. Additional new mechanisms of cancer cell growth and resistance are being discovered, so more options will surely become available. With continued research, the goal is to convert *Royal*, from a life threatening condition, into one that can be managed as chronically and stabilized indefinitely.

References

1. M Hussain and others. Absolute prostate-specific antigen value after androgen deprivation is a strong independent predictor of survival in new metastatic prostate cancer: Data from Southwest Oncology Group Trial 9346 (INT-0162). *Journal of Clinical Oncology* 24.24: 3984, 2006.

2. PW Kantoff and others. Sipuleucel-T immunotherapy for castration-resistant prostate cancer. *New England Journal of Medicine* 363.5: 411, 2010.

3. PF Schellhammer and others. Lower baseline prostate-specific antigen is associated with a greater overall survival benefit from sipuleucel-T in the immunotherapy for prostate adenocarcinoma treatment (**IMPACT**) trial. *Urology* 81.6: 1297, 2013.

4. PF Schellhammer and others. Lower baseline PSA predicts greater benefit from sipuleucel-T. *Clinical Advances in Hematology and Oncology* 11.6: 377, 2013.

5. E Antonarakis and others. Sequencing of sipuleucel-T and androgen deprivation therapy in men with hormone-sensitive biochemically-recurrent prostate cancer: A phase II randomized trial. *Clinical Cancer Research* epub: 2016.

6. JB Nelson and others. Phase 3, randomized, controlled trial of atrasentan in patients with nonmetastatic, hormone-refractory prostate cancer. *Cancer* 113.9:2478, 2008.

7. K Miller and others. Phase III, randomized, placebo-controlled study of once-daily oral zibotentan (**ZD4054**) in patients with non-metastatic castration-resistant prostate cancer. *Prostate Cancer and Prostatic Diseases* 16.2:187, 2013.

8. MR Smith and others. Denosumab and bone-metastasis-free survival in men with castration-resistant prostate cancer: Results of a phase 3, randomised, placebo-controlled trial. *Lancet* 379.9810: 39, 2012.

9. MR Smith and others. Denosumab and bone metastasis-free survival in men with nonmetastatic castration-resistant prostate cancer: Exploratory analyses by baseline prostate-specific antigen doubling time. *Journal of Clinical Oncology* 31.30: 3800, 2013.

10. BI Rini and others. Combination immunotherapy with prostatic acid phosphatase pulsed antigen-presenting cells (Provenge) plus bevacizumab in patients with serologic progression of prostate cancer after definitive local therapy. *Cancer* 107.1: 67, 2006.

11. M Scholz and others. Long-term outcome for men with androgen independent prostate cancer treated with ketoconazole and hydrocortisone. *Journal of Urology* 173.6: 1947, 2005.

12. JS de Bono and others. Abiraterone and increased survival in metastatic prostate cancer. *New England Journal of Medicine* 364.21: 1995, 2011.

13. CJ Ryan and others. Abiraterone in metastatic prostate cancer without previous chemotherapy. *New England Journal of Medicine* 368.2: 138, 2013.

14. HI Scher and others. Increased survival with enzalutamide in prostate cancer after chemotherapy. *New England Journal of Medicine* 367.13: 1187, 2012.

15. TM Beer and others. Enzalutamide in metastatic prostate cancer before chemotherapy. *New England Journal of Medicine* 371.5: 424, 2014.

16. DP Petrylak and others. Docetaxel and estramustine compared with mitoxantrone and prednisone for advanced refractory prostate cancer. *New England Journal of Medicine* 351.15: 1513, 2004.

17. IF Tannock and others. Docetaxel plus prednisone or mitoxantrone plus prednisone for advanced prostate cancer. *New England Journal of Medicine* 351.15: 1502, 2004.

18. JS de Bono and others. Prednisone plus cabazitaxel or mitoxantrone for metastatic castration-resistant prostate cancer progressing after docetaxel treatment: A randomized open-label trial. *Lancet* 376.9747: 1147, 2010.

19. AO Sartor and others. Cabazitaxel vs docetaxel in chemotherapy-naive (CN) patients with metastatic castration-resistant prostate cancer (mCRPC): A three-arm phase III study (**FIRSTANA**). *Journal of Clinical Oncology* 34.15 suppl: abstr 5006, 2016.

20. PG Corn and others. A multi-institutional randomized phase II study (NCT01505868) of cabazitaxel plus or minus carboplatin in men with metastatic castration-resistant prostate cancer. *Journal of Clinical Oncology* 33.15 suppl: abstr 5010, 2015.

21. CJ Sweeney and others. Chemohormonal therapy in metastatic hormone sensitive prostate cancer. *New England Journal of Medicine* 373.8: 737, 2015.

22. ND James and others. Addition of docetaxel, zoledronic acid, or both to first-line long-term hormone therapy in prostate cancer (**STAMPEDE**): Survival results from an adaptive, multiarm, multistage, platform randomised controlled trial. *Lancet* 387.10024: 1163, 2016.

23. G Gravis and others. Androgen-deprivation therapy alone or with docetaxel in non-castrate metastatic prostate cancer (**GETUG-AFU** 15): A randomized, open-label, phase 3 trial. *Lancet Oncology* 14.2: 149, 2013.

24. LJ Patrick-Miller and others. Quality of life (QOL) analysis from E3805, chemohormonal androgen ablation randomized trial (**CHAARTED**) in prostate cancer (PrCa). *Journal of Clinical Oncology* 34.2 suppl: abstr 286, 2016.

25. R Dreicer. Highlights in genitourinary (prostate) cancer. *JAMA Oncology* 2.10: 1257, 2016.

26. C Parker and others. Alpha emitter radium-223 and survival in metastatic prostate cancer. *New England Journal of Medicine* 369.3: 213, 2013.

27. MR Smith and others. Denosumab in men receiving androgen-deprivation therapy for prostate cancer. *New England Journal of Medicine* 361.8: 745, 2009.

28. MD Galsky and others. Docetaxel-based combination therapy for castration-resistant prostate cancer. *Annals of Oncology* 21.11: 2135, 2010.

29. Y Ning and others. Phase II trial of bevacizumab, thalidomide, docetaxel, and prednisone in patients with metastatic castration-resistant prostate cancer. *Journal of Clinical Oncology* 28.12: 2070, 2010.

30. B Adesunloye and others. Phase II trial of bevacizumab and lenalidomide with docetaxel and prednisone in patients with metastatic castration-resistant prostate cancer. *Journal of Clinical Oncology* 30.5 suppl: abstr 207, 2012.

31. J Mateo and others. DNA-repair defects and olaparib in metastatic prostate cancer. *New England Journal of Medicine* 373.18: 1697, 2015.

Chapter 41

UNORTHODOX THERAPIES
FOR *ROYAL*

Mark Scholz, MD

*The most important thing in science is not so much to obtain
new facts as to discover new ways of thinking about them.*
WILLIAM BRAGG

A MEDICAL ONCOLOGIST SHOULD BE a fighter. Cancer is formidable, and the number of available weapons may be limited. And even if the options are running out, a good fighter should not give up easily. He keeps searching for creative solutions, ones that may even be outside the mainstream. This book has preached that the first step toward a successful outcome is the accurate characterization of the cancer's status by assigning the correct Stage of Blue and subtype. However, there are additional factors besides the Stage of Blue. This chapter covers three: *dialing down* treatment intensity in patients who are more frail or aged, *dialing up* treatment intensity by combining therapies, and drawing on treatments outside the standard prostate cancer armamentarium.

USING MILDER THERAPY IN OLDER MEN

Men who are more advanced in age may be unable to tolerate standard treatment due to a reduced capacity to tolerate the side effects. One common maneuver for reducing side effects from hormonal therapy is to substitute Casodex for Lupron. Casodex is about two-thirds as effective as Lupron but with one-third the side effects. In higher doses (three pills per day), Casodex is almost as effective as Lupron. Casodex blocks the androgen receptor *without eradicating testosterone*. This tempers the hormonal effects. For example, about half the men on Casodex maintain their sex drive (libido), whereas almost all men on Lupron lose their libido. One downside of Casodex, compared with Lupron, is an increased risk of breast enlargement. This, however, can be prevented by various means (Chapter 30).

Head-to-head trials comparing 50-mg-a-day of Casodex (the standard dose) with Lupron or surgical castration in advanced metastatic disease show that survival is better with Lupron.[1,2] However, when using three Casodex pills a day, the survival seems to be about the same, whereas energy levels and sex drive are better maintained.[3] Another study comparing Zoladex (a drug like Lupron) *plus* Flutamide (a drug like Casodex) with three Casodex pills a day also showed that survival was equivalent.[4] All these studies, when taken as a whole, indicate that Casodex by itself (in high dosage) is almost as effective as Lupron. The 50-mg-a-day dose of Casodex is less potent, and this is the commonly used dose in the US. Therefore, using Casodex monotherapy to treat younger men is questionable. For frail, elderly men, it is a welcome alternative.

OLDER MEN CAN TOLERATE TAXOTERE

With chemotherapy, there is a similar concern. Fatigue from chemotherapy can ruin an older man's quality of life. In younger men, fatigue usually lasts less than a week after each treatment. The problem is that older men don't bounce back as quickly, and the fatigue may become progressive with each successive cycle of treatment. One thing to consider, if the cancer is progressing and other commonly used treatments are ineffective, is that the side effects of Taxotere can be substantially reduced by using smaller weekly doses rather than the standard three-week protocol.

Back in 2001, we evaluated 20 elderly men (average age 78) receiving small weekly doses of Taxotere.[5] The oldest man in the study was 87. Treatment was well tolerated, and 17 of the 20 completed the prescribed course of therapy. Three of the men stopped early because of excess fatigue. To this day, we continue to utilize weekly Taxotere in men who would be unable to tolerate a larger dose given every three weeks, which is the way Taxotere is normally given. Advanced age, therefore, does not necessarily preclude Taxotere.

SEQUENTIAL TREATMENT VERSUS COMBINATION THERAPY

Longstanding tradition for *Royal* dictates that treatments are used one at a time. However, going back to an analogy used in a previous chapter, fighting uncontrolled cancer is an all-out battle and should be fought like a fire that has the potential to burn out of control. Using single agents may be suboptimal. Of course, enthusiasm for using multiple agents must be tempered by financial considerations, concerns about the cumulative toxicity, and a lack of trials proving the superiority of a combination approach.

The one-at-a-time policy originates from university research. The FDA requires that drugs be tested one at a time so that the study findings can be interpreted with clarity. However, the one-at-a-time policy has undergone a serious shakeup since the publication of CHAARTED[6] (Chapter 40), which proves that the earlier initiation of Taxotere *in combination* with TIP nets a whopping 17-month improvement in survival in men with metastatic prostate cancer. This study, along with the STAMPEDE study, which reached a similar conclusion, is forcing a global rethinking of the traditional sequential approach. Aside from these important studies showing better results with combination therapy, we should also recall that multiagent therapy is considered standard for many different cancers, as well as for serious infections such as pneumonia and AIDS. And now, there are more new agents for prostate cancer, creating the possibility of many new treatment combinations. Preliminary trials have been completed showing that the agents listed below can be administered together with reasonable safety:

- Taxotere combined with Zytiga or Xtandi[7,8]
- Provenge followed immediately by Zytiga or Xtandi (rather than waiting for the PSA to rise)[9]
- Xofigo combined with Zytiga[10]
- Zytiga combined with Xtandi[11]

This list is by no means exhaustive. Other combinations can also be considered. The point is that the historical taboo against combination therapy is over. Of course, the risks and benefits of using combination therapy need to be discussed, though there are ways to mitigate the risk. For example, treatments can be started at a lower dosage. If no side effects occur, the dosage can then be slowly escalated in accordance with the patient's ability to tolerate the combination. While combination therapy is unorthodox and, in some cases, risky, so is the threat from progressive cancer. Adopting an aggressive, outside-the-box treatment strategy may be justifiable if it improves the chance for achieving a good anticancer response.

In Chapter 40, Dr. Lam introduced four FDA-approved categories of treatment: immunotherapy, secondary hormonal therapies, chemotherapy, and various types of radiation. *Not all of these agents can be safely combined.* For example, it seems like a bad idea to use chemotherapy and immunotherapy together. Chemotherapy is known to cyclically *inhibit* the immune system, whereas the anticancer benefits of immunotherapy rely on immune system enhancement. As illogical as the combination sounds, one company actually tried combining Taxotere with GVAX, a type of immunotherapy that is discussed in the next chapter. The combination, as it turned out, was worse than the Taxotere alone. The trial failed and the company went bankrupt.[12]

Combinations of radiation, hormone therapy, and chemotherapy are beginning to be better understood. We now know that hormone therapy and chemotherapy are compatible, but in the past this was uncertain. At one time, both prostate cancer experts and breast cancer experts theorized that hormone therapy might *reduce* the effectiveness of chemotherapy. Studies subsequently proved this wrong. There was also a time of similar uncertainty about using hormone therapy and radiation together. We now know that hormone therapy *enhances* the anticancer effects of radiation.

Discussions about combination therapy also raise the question about optimal timing for the different therapies. Dr. Mack Roach, from UC San Francisco, designed a 1,500 patient study in which men were split into two groups. In group one, hormonal therapy and radiation were started the same day. In group two, hormonal therapy was first administered alone for two months, after which the radiation was started. The latter group did better. The best theoretical explanation I have heard to interpret these results is that since the hormonal therapy is known to cause an initial infiltration of immune cells into the dying tumor, immediate radiation kills the *infiltrating immune cells*. On the other hand, if the radiation is delayed two months, the immune cells have time to absorb the tumor antigens from the dying cancer cells and escape "ground zero" to do their immune magic in other parts of the body.

Another issue I frequently run across when doing second opinion consultations arises in discussions about the timing for secondary hormones (Xtandi or Zytiga) after Provenge. Many doctors postpone starting secondary hormonal therapy until *after* the patient has overt disease progression. Apart from the obvious disadvantage of delaying therapy, it is common knowledge that instances of PSA declining after Provenge are rare. Every oncologist knows that further therapy will be necessary at some point. Since the side effects of secondary hormone therapy are easily managed, postponing life-prolonging therapy with Zytiga or Xtandi makes no sense.

The ongoing discussions about combinations, sequencing, and timing are almost endless. Let's close this topic with a quick discussion about the timing of chemotherapy with radiation. Presently, there are no studies showing that lymph node radiation and chemotherapy can be safely given simultaneously. So typically, if both are planned, they are sequenced. But which one should come first? Since radiation has a more-established track record than chemotherapy, most doctors are comfortable with doing radiation first. But I prefer Taxotere first. The rationale for giving Taxotere before radiation is to get after the more dangerous micrometastases as quickly as possible.

SIR-SPHERES TO TREAT LIVER METASTASES

Another "outside-the-box" treatment to discuss is related to liver metastases, which are much more dangerous than metastatic cancer in the bones or lymph nodes. Liver metastases can quickly disrupt essential metabolic functions essential to sustain life leading to a rapid demise. Liver metastases are first suspected when a hepatic blood test becomes abnormal (Appendix II). Further investigation with a CT scan or MRI confirms the diagnosis. Alternatively, liver metastases may be picked up on a routine staging body scan prior to any changes in the blood. Once they are detected, however, liver metastases demands immediate attention. Men can live for years with bone and lymph node metastases. If left untreated, liver metastases can be fatal within months.

Stopping the liver metastases is the highest priority, even to the exclusion of concerns about how the disease is faring in other parts of the body. If not used previously, hormonal therapy with Lupron, Zytiga, and Xtandi—or chemotherapy with Taxotere, Jevtana, and Carboplatin—is the standard. However, there is a tendency for these treatments to lose effectiveness over time. Fortunately, much research has been done on the treatment of liver metastases in patients with colon cancer (the liver is the most common site where colon cancer spreads). One intriguing type of treatment that has been developed is an injection of SIR-Spheres, radioactive microspheres into the blood supply of the liver. SIR-Spheres have been shown to have notable efficacy against liver metastases with a very tolerable side-effect profile.

Prostate cancer cells and colon cancer cells have similar susceptibility to radiation. As such, it is logical to consider that SIR-Spheres might have an equally good restraining effect on prostate cancer, similar to that of colon cancer. In our clinic, we administered SIR-Spheres to several of our patients with liver metastases from prostate cancer. The results have been encouraging, with a notable improvement of survival, compared with our previous experience with standard therapy. Our finding were presented at the Interventional Radiology Symposium in Hollywood, Florida, in February 2016.[13]

Another new treatment for men with advanced cancer also uses injected radiation, like SIR-Spheres and Xofigo. It is based on technology that was briefly alluded to in Chapter 6, Gallium[68] PSMA PET scans. These scans target a unique surface feature on the cancer cells, called "prostate specific membrane antigen" (PSMA). What is intriguing is that PSMA can also be targeted with a *high-energy* radioactive molecule called Lutetium,[177] which is powerful enough to kill the cancer. Two small studies from Germany have reported favorable results using PSMA linked to Lutetium[177] in men with very advanced disease. Dr. Matthias Heck reported on 22 patients whom he treated. Patients were injected every eight weeks up to a total of four cycles. Their average PSA before treatment was 349. The most common side effects were dry mouth, anemia, and low platelet counts. A 30 percent or more decline in PSA after treatment occurred in 56 percent of the men.[14] In another study, Dr. Richard Baum reported on 56 patients.[15] Eighty percent of the patients had at least some degree of PSA decline. A couple of men reported dry mouths, but no anemia or lowering of blood counts was observed. Progression-free survival was 13 months. These studies look very hopeful, considering that these disease responses were accomplished in men with very advanced prostate cancer.

SUMMARY OF UNORTHODOX TREATMENTS

Factors that affect treatment selection, apart from Stage of Blue, are a patient's age, health status and disease that has spread to the liver. In frail, elderly men it is reasonable to consider reducing treatment intensity rather than withholding treatment altogether. At the other end of the spectrum, when considering treatment for young men with metastatic disease, it is reasonable to look at boosting treatment intensity by using multiple therapies in combination. "Borrowing" treatments used for other cancer types is another way to expand the number of therapeutic options.

References

1. G Chodak and others. Single-agent therapy with bicalutamide: A comparison with medical or surgical castration in the treatment of advanced prostate cancer. *Urology* 46.6: 849, 1995.

2. GT Bales and others. A controlled trial of bicalutamide versus castration in patients with advanced prostate cancer. *Urology* 47.1 suppl: 38, 1996.

3. P Iverson and others. Bicalutamide monotherapy compared with castration in patients with nonmetastatic locally advanced prostate cancer: 6.3 years followup. *Journal of Urology* 164.5: 1579, 2000.

4. F Boccardo and others. Bicalutamide monotherapy versus flutamide plus goserelin in prostate cancer patients: Results of an Italian prostate cancer project study. *Journal of Clinical Oncology* 17.7: 2027, 1999.

5. M Scholz and others. Low-dose single-agent weekly docetaxel (Taxotere) is effective and well tolerated in elderly men with prostate cancer. *American Society of Clinical Oncology Annual Meeting, abstr 2441*, 2001.

6. CJ Sweeney and others. Chemohormonal therapy in metastatic hormone-sensitive prostate cancer. *New England Journal of Medicine* 373.8: 737, 2015.

7. ST Tagawa and others. Phase 1b study of abiraterone acetate plus prednisone and docetaxel in patients with metastatic castration-resistant prostate cancer. *European Urology* 70.5: 718, 2016.

8. MJ Morris and others. Phase Ib study of enzalutamide in combination with docetaxel in men with metastatic castration-resistant prostate cancer. *Clinical Cancer Research* 22.15: 3774, 2016.

9. EJ Small and others. A randomized phase II trial of sipuleucel-T with concurrent versus sequential abiraterone acetate plus prednisone in metastatic castration-resistant prostate cancer. *Clinical Cancer Research* 21.17: 3862, 2015.

10. ND Shore and others. Open-label phase II study evaluating the efficacy of concurrent administration of radium Ra 223 dichloride and abiraterone acetate in men with castration-resistant prostate cancer with symptomatic bone metastases. *Journal of Clinical Oncology* 34.2 suppl: 177, 2016.

11. E Efstathiou and others. Enzalutamide in combination with abiraterone acetate in bone metastatic castration resistant prostate cancer. *Journal of Clinical Oncology* 32:5 suppl: abstr 5000, 2014.

12. EJ Small and others. A phase III trial of GVAX immunotherapy for prostate cancer in combination with docetaxel versus docetaxel plus prednisone in symptomatic, castration-resistant prostate cancer (CRPC). *Genitourinary Cancers Symposium Annual Meeting* abstr 7, 2009.

13. M Scholz and others. SIR-Spheres (SS) for prostate cancer (PC) metastatic to liver. *Genitourinary Cancers Symposium Annual Meeting* 2016.

14. MM Heck and others. Systemic radioligand therapy with ^{177}Lu labeled prostate specific membrane antigen ligand for imaging and therapy in patients with metastatic castration resistant prostate cancer. *Journal of Urology* 196.2: 382, 2016.

15. RP Baum and others. Lutetium-177 PSMA radioligand therapy of metastatic castration-resistant prostate cancer. *Journal of Nuclear Medicine* 57: 1, 2016.

Chapter 42

IMMUNOTHERAPY FOR PROSTATE CANCER

Charles Drake, MD

Cancer is not just a dividing cell. It's a complex disease:
It invades, it metastasizes, it evades the immune system.

Siddhartha Mukherjee

IMMUNE THERAPY IS SET TO BECOMe the biggest anticancer revolution ever seen. Over the last 30 years, many attempts to stimulate the immune system have failed. But things are quickly changing. In November 2015, the *New England Journal of Medicine* reported that Opdivo, a type of immune treatment, prolongs life in *lung cancer* patients, and does it substantially better than Taxotere, while only causing 20 percent of the side effects.[1] Lung cancer is a much harder disease to treat than prostate cancer. Immune therapy is rapidly making inroads in the toughest cancer arenas.

This chapter will discuss a variety of immune therapies available, or ones that are likely to soon become available, to treat prostate cancer:

Provenge, Leukine, Yervoy, Keytruda, Opdivo, PROSTVAC, GVAX, and the "Abscopal effect," which is an immune enhancing effect of radiation (see below). At the end of this chapter, we will briefly discuss how researchers are beginning to test these various therapies in combination.

For the purposes of our short discussion, three different types of immune cells need to be introduced: 1) The cells that *slow down* immune-system function are called the TRegs; 2) The soldier cells of the immune system that *directly attack* the cancer are called the killer-T cells; and 3) the cells that *detect* cancer and direct the killer-T cells to home in on cancer are called the dendritic cells.

PROVENGE

Provenge was FDA-approved for prostate cancer after a landmark study showed a 22 percent reduced risk of death compared with placebo.[1] Provenge is an immunotherapy that works by the mechanism of upregulated dendritic cell activity. Dendritic cells that have been removed from the patient's blood are mixed with PAP—a molecule present in prostate cancer cells—and Leukine (see below), a commercially available hormone that stimulates dendritic cell activity. After this process is complete, the activated dendritic cells are reinfused into the patient and help direct the immune system to attack the prostate cancer. Provenge was discussed in more detail in Chapter 40. Using Provenge in combination with other types of immunotherapy is discussed later in this chapter.

LEUKINE

As noted in the previous paragraph, Leukine is one of the components used in the formulation of Provenge. Leukine was FDA-approved back in the 1990s to counteract the immunosuppressive effects of chemotherapy. Subsequently, Leukine has been looked at as a type of prostate cancer therapy. One study reported a durable suppression of PSA lasting over five years in seven out of 29 men undergoing treatment for rising PSA levels after surgery (*Indigo*).[2] These days Leukine is rarely used as a standalone therapy, perhaps due to inconvenience, as it requires a daily injection. In addition, for prostate cancer, Leukine is "off label" and therefore less likely to be covered by insurance. Nevertheless, we cannot overlook Leukine. As you will see, it is a popular component used in various immunotherapy combinations.

IMMUNE CHECKPOINT INHIBITION: YERVOY, OPDIVO, AND KEYTRUDA

The discovery of "checkpoint inhibitors," a term I will explain momentarily, represents a monumental breakthrough. Historically, attempts at immune enhancement were thwarted by the intrinsic safeguards "built in" to the immune system. These safeguards are called "checkpoints." The safeguards exist to prevent serious immune *overactivity*, problems such as lupus, rheumatoid arthritis, or multiple sclerosis. Researchers have discovered that cancer cells exploit these immune checkpoints to their own advantage by fooling the immune system into inactivity, reducing its ability to fight against the cancer. Suboptimal immune activity, therefore, is not usually the result of *weakness* in the immune system as one might think. Rather, low immune activity comes from overamplified regulatory activity, which is often instigated by the cancer cells themselves.

Three FDA-approved medications that *reduce* overregulation of the immune system are Yervoy, Opdivo, and Keytruda. These medications have the capacity to *suppress* T-REG activity, which leads to *up-regulated* killer T-cell activity. While none of these medications have been FDA-approved for prostate cancer, Yervoy, which is manufactured by Bristol Myers, has been tested extensively in a large phase III trial.[3] Despite notable activity (when used in combination with radiation—see below) its potency fell slightly short of the level of activity demanded by the FDA. The problem may have been the way the trial was designed. Many men in the study had very advanced prostate cancer. Reanalysis of the study after completion showed a significant survival benefit for the men with earlier-stage disease. However, Yervoy failed to garner commercial approval because *after-the-fact* analysis is unacceptable by FDA standards. Unfortunately, when Yervoy was retested in another large phase III trial[4] in men with earlier-stage prostate cancer, treatment with radiation *was deleted from the protocol!* Also, only a median of four Yervoy treatments was given. Due to these factors, the long-term survival in these early-stage patients was probably more influenced by the other life-prolonging therapies given after the relatively brief course of Yervoy was stopped. The bottom line: There was no improvement in survival for the Yervoy-treated patients. In a much smaller pilot trial, a checkpoint inhibitor manufactured by Merck called Keytruda showed three rather dramatic remissions out of 10 men who were studied.[5] Opdivo, a third type of checkpoint inhibitor that is also manufactured by Bristol Myers, has yet to be tested for prostate cancer but is very active against other cancers like lung cancer, kidney cancer, and melanoma.

CANCER VACCINES

Another method to stimulate the immune system to fight cancer is to vaccinate patients with a genetically modified virus that has a PSA gene incorporated into the viral DNA. When the virus is injected into the patient, it generates a strong immune reaction against both the virus and the PSA. The problem with viral vaccines is that the immune reaction is so strong, it's not safe to give the same treatment over and over. One possible way to circumvent this problem is to *change the strain of virus* with each of the subsequent vaccinations, a method that is used in PROSTVAC.

PROSTVAC

The most fully developed viral vaccine is called PROSTVAC. PROSTVAC mixes PSA with a strain of virus called vaccinia and some additional components to rev up the immune system. Follow-up injections of PROSTVAC employ a different virus, called fowlpox. A randomized trial comparing PROSTVAC with a placebo showed an eight-month improvement in survival, and the data was updated in 2016.[6,7] This technology is now being studied in a much larger 1,200-patient trial. Unfortunately, preliminary reports at the time this book went to press, indicate that PROSTVAC failed to prolong survival.

GVAX

GVAX is an injection under the skin with genetically modified prostate cancer cells mixed with Leukine.[8,9] The prostate cancer cells are grown in the laboratory in Petri dishes. The cancer cells are inactivated with radiation prior to being injected into the skin of the patient. Unfortunately, clinical development of GVAX has been retarded due to an initial trial that was poorly conceived:[10] The testing was performed in very advanced prostate cancer patients. Even worse, the study was performed in *combination* with chemotherapy, which *suppresses* the immune system. As might be expected, adding GVAX to Taxotere showed no meaningful anticancer benefit. Another trial, however, one that compared GVAX *head to head* with Taxotere, showed equivalent survival to the men treated with Taxotere.[11] The intellectual property rights to the GVAX platform have been transferred to another company. Hopefully, clinical development will proceed and eventually lead to FDA approval.

THE EFFECT OF RADIATION ON THE IMMUNE SYSTEM: THE ABSCOPAL EFFECT

The word "radiation" usually communicates the fear of immune *suppression*. However, when used judiciously, radiation *stimulates* the immune system through the Abscopal effect.[12] The Abscopal effect works as follows: A beam of radiation focused on a tumor in the body damages the tumor cells. When cellular damage occurs, the immune system detects it. Immune cells naturally home in on damaged cells that are dying, if for no other reason than to remove the cellular debris. The radiation, therefore, leads the immune cells into direct contact with the cancer cells. The immune cells are then able to identify *tumor-specific molecules* emitted from the dying cancer cells. Thus, the immune cells, sort of like bloodhounds, "get the scent" of the cancer. With that scent obtained, the immune cells can circulate through the blood and attack tumors in other parts of the body. It seems that SBRT (Chapter 22), which delivers the largest radiation dose, induces a greater Abscopal effect than IMRT (Chapter 19), which relies on smaller doses of radiation given over a longer period. IMRT can cause the Abscopal effect but seems to do so less vigorously than SBRT.

Of course, the radiation also kills cancer cells directly. It accomplishes this by damaging the cancer's DNA. Performing spot treatment with high-dose radiation is relatively easy to do with modern technology. Doctors can safely administer radiation without causing serious collateral damage to the normal cells of the body near the tumor. The good news is that when the Abscopal effect is activated, cancerous tumors in *nonradiated areas of the body* can be killed by the newly activated immune cells.

COMBINATIONS WITH YERVOY

Yervoy has been a very popular drug to use in combination with other types of immunotherapy. At Prostate Oncology Specialists, a small pilot trial using Provenge in combination with a 10 percent dose of Yervoy showed encouraging results.[13] Seven men with hormone-resistant, metastatic disease underwent Provenge and Yervoy. Three years after treatment, only one of these advanced-stage patients has developed progressive disease and died of prostate cancer. The other six, at the time of this writing, have PSA levels under 8 and none have required chemotherapy.[14] Dr. Eric Small evaluated 24 patients with *High-Royal* who were given escalating doses of a combination of Yervoy plus Leukine.[15] Three out of the six men who were treated at the maximum level had a 50 percent or greater decline in PSA. Dr. Ravi Madan evaluated *High-Royal* patients with the combination of Yervoy and PROSTVAC. Out of 24 patients, 58 percent had a PSA decline, and in six patients the decline was more than 50 percent.[16] When Yervoy was tested with GVAX, more than 50 percent of the men had a PSA decline.[17]

CONCLUSION

The survival improvements documented using Provenge place immune treatment at the forefront of the future development of anticancer therapy for prostate cancer. The reason for the notable success of immune therapy for prostate cancer is not entirely clear. Some have speculated that prostate cancer's vulnerability to immune therapy is somehow related to its susceptibility to testosterone reduction.[18,19] Whatever the reason, in looking to the future, the notion of developing standard protocols that use vaccines, checkpoint inhibitors, and spot radiation in combination is very exciting.

References

1. H Borghaei and others. Nivolumab versus docetaxel in advanced nonsquamous non–small-cell lung cancer. *New England Journal of Medicine* 373.17: 1627, 2015.

2. BI Rini and others. Clinical and immunological characteristics of patients with serologic progression of prostate cancer achieving long-term disease control with granulocyte-macrophage colony-stimulating factor. *Journal of Urology* 175.6: 2087, 2006.

3. ED Kwon and others. Ipilimumab versus placebo after radiotherapy in patients with metastatic castration-resistant prostate cancer that had progressed after docetaxel chemotherapy (CA184-043): A multicentre, randomised, double-blind, phase 3 trial. *Lancet Oncology* 15.7: 700, 2014.

4. TM Beer and others. Randomized, double-blind, phase III trial of ipilimumab versus placebo in asymptomatic or minimally symptomatic patients with metastatic chemotherapy-naïve castration-resistant prostate cancer. *Journal of Clinical Oncology* 35.1: 40, 2017.

5. JN Graff and others. Early evidence of anti-PD-1 activity in enzalutamide-resistant prostate cancer. *Oncotarget* 73.3: 52810, 2016.

6. PW Kantoff and others. Overall survival analysis of a phase II randomized controlled trial of a Poxviral-based PSA-targeted immunotherapy in metastatic castration-resistant prostate cancer. *Journal of Clinical Oncology* 28.7: 1099, 2010.

7. PW Kantoff and others. Revised overall survival analysis of a phase II, randomized, double-blind, controlled study of PROSTVAC in men with metastatic castration-resistant prostate cancer. *Journal of Clinical Oncology* 34:122, 2016.

8. WJ Urba and others. Treatment of biochemical recurrence of prostate cancer with granulocyte-macrophage colony-stimulating factor secreting, allogeneic, cellular immunotherapy. *Journal of Urology* 180.5: 2011, 2008.

9. G Dranoff and others. Vaccination with irradiated tumor cells engineered to secrete murine granulocyte-macrophage colony-stimulating factor stimulates potent, specific, and long-lasting anti-tumor immunity. *Proceedings of the National Academy of Science* 90.8: 3539, 1993.

10. E Small and others. A phase III trial of GVAX immunotherapy for prostate cancer in combination with docetaxel vs. docetaxel plus prednisone in symptomatic, castration-resistant prostate cancer (CRPC). *Genitourinary Cancers Symposium Annual Meeting* abstr 7, 2009.

11. C Higano and others. A phase III trial for GVAX immunotherapy for prostate cancer versus docetaxel plus prednisone in asymptomatic castration-resistant prostate cancer (CRPC). *Genitourinary Cancers Symposium Annual Meeting* abstr LBA 150, 2009.

12. FG Herrera and others. Radiotherapy combination opportunities leveraging immunity for the next oncology practice. *CA: A Cancer Journal Clinics* 67.1: 65, 2017.

13. M Scholz. Sipuleucel-T in combination with mini-dose ipilimumab for metastatic, castrate-resistant prostate cancer. *Journal of Clinical Oncology* 33.15 suppl: abstr e22104, 2015.

14. S Yep and others. Phase I clinical trial of sipuleucel-T combined with escalating doses of ipilimumab in progressive mCRPC. *Poster: Prostate Cancer Foundation Scientific Retreat,* 2016.

15. L Fong and others. Potentiating endogenous antitumor immunity to prostate cancer through combination immunotherapy with CTLA4 blockade and GM-CSF. *Cancer Research* 69.2: 609, 2009.

16. RA Madan and others. Ipilimumab and a poxviral vaccine targeting prostate specific antigen in metastatic castration-resistant prostate cancer: A phase I dose-escalation trial *Lancet Oncology* 13.5: 501, 2012.

17. W Gerritsen and others. Expanded phase I combination trial of GVAX immunotherapy for prostate cancer and ipilimumab in patients with metastatic hormone-refractory prostate cancer (mHPRC). *Journal of Clinical Oncology* 26.15 suppl: abstr 5146, 2008.

18. JB Aragon-Ching and others. Impact of androgen-deprivation therapy on the immune system: Implications for combination therapy of prostate cancer. *Frontiers of Bioscience* 12: 4957, 2007.

19. ES Antonarakis and others. Sequencing of sipuleucel-T and androgen deprivation therapy in men with hormone-sensitive biochemically-recurrent prostate cancer: A phase II randomized trial. *Clinical Cancer Research* clincanres-1780, 2016.

Chapter 43

GENETICALLY TARGETED THERAPY

Mark Scholz, MD

There is one thing that gives radiance to everything.
It is the idea of something around the corner.

G.K. CHESTERTON

SOMEDAY ALL TREATMENT SELECTION will be guided by the unique genetic characteristics of each individual cancer. A relatively recent example of this was published in the November 2015 issue of the *New England Journal of Medicine*. Lynparza, an FDA-approved medicine for ovarian cancer, was administered to 50 men with very advanced prostate cancer. Lynparza resulted in a 90 percent response rate in a subgroup of 15 of the 50 men who had a specific genetic mutation in the BRCA gene or other closely related genes. Everyone is hopeful that in the future, genetically determined treatment will become the rule rather than the exception.

Five new life-extending treatments—Provenge, Zytiga, Xtandi, Xofigo, and Jevtana—have become available in the last seven years. Despite these hopeful developments, 28,000 men succumb to prostate cancer each year. In most cases, mortality follows the development of treatment resistance. When resistance occurs, the next step will often be *off-label* treatments, medicines that are FDA-approved for other types of cancer, such as kidney cancer or lung cancer. The problem is the vast number of options. If you are going to take a shot in the dark, how do you pick the gun that is most likely to be effective?

Now that research is progressing, the identification of a genetic abnormality may point to a specific therapy. Hundreds of cancer medications are available, but how can we know which one to use? Men with very advanced prostate cancer have a limited survival window. They don't have enough time to try all these alternatives by trial and error. While a genetically based treatment-selection approach is still in its baby stages, the upside is potentially huge.

A REMARKABLE TURNAROUND STORY

The successful selection of an effective agent can have a huge upside. Let me relate the story of a patient of mine named Bill. He was diagnosed in late 2010. Initially, things looked good. His PSA was only 4.2 with a Gleason score of 3+4=7. He underwent surgery, and soon things started to become more serious. After the surgery, his Gleason score was upgraded to 4+5=9. His PSA never dropped to zero. He had radiation, but the PSA remained low for only a brief period. He then started Lupron, but resistance developed within a year. Over the next three years, Bill was treated with all the medicines listed above: Provenge, Zytiga, Xtandi, and Taxotere. By the summer of 2014, his cancer was spreading extensively throughout his bone marrow. Xofigo had been started in February 2014. Unfortunately, he developed progressive bone marrow failure, a common development in men with uncontrolled prostate cancer. He became so anemic, he could only be kept alive with monthly blood transfusions. When the Xofigo was stopped in August, his PSA had risen to over 120. Bill's chances for living another six months were bleak.

AN OFF-LABEL MEDICATION THAT WORKED

Fortuitously, right before Bill was referred to our office, he had started a medication called Mekinist, a pill that is FDA-approved for metastatic melanoma. Since off-label use is not covered by insurance, Bill purchased it himself, at a cost of $10,000 per month. His investment quickly paid dividends. By December 2014 his PSA had dropped to 18, his bone marrow had started functioning again and he no longer needed further blood transfusions. Bill's health improved. He returned to his job full time and took trips with his family to Europe over the next two years. The Mekinist was well tolerated without any notable side effects. Unfortunately, resistance eventually developed and the cancer began to progress. Further intensive efforts to find another magical off-label treatment were unsuccessful, and he succumbed to the disease in early 2016.

The decision to give Mekinist to Bill was an amazingly lucky pick. After showing such a great cancer response, his insurance company even started paying for it. A turnaround of such a late-stage cancer is truly remarkable—a testament to the new types of groundbreaking products being developed in the pharmaceutical industry. With each additional treatment that becomes commercially available, the odds for more patients to get last-minute turnarounds are improving.

TARGETING TREATMENT FOR PROSTATE CANCER BY GENETIC TESTING

The problem is that there are over 100 different types of cancer, and the number of new cancer agents is increasing. How do you know what agent to pick? We have tried giving Mekinist to a few additional patients without any major benefit. This is not surprising, considering that there are scores of different genetic types of prostate cancer. Even prior to the era of genetic testing, we had known that a wide variation exists in how patients respond to different agents. The hope of genetic testing of tumor cells is that we may be able to determine in advance what treatment will be most beneficial.

FINDING THE BAD GENES

The idea is to pick a treatment that is known to counteract the bad effects of a specific mutated gene, once it is identified. Uncontrolled cancer cell growth is due to misbehaving genes. A mutated gene, for example, can be stuck in the "on" position, thus promoting uncontrolled growth of the cell. Abnormal genes can now be identified with a laboratory process called "gene sequencing." Genetic analysis of tumor tissue shows that in patients with advanced disease, about four genes, on average, are mutated. But the number of detectable bad genes ranges from as low as zero or one up to 10 or more.

ISSUES STILL TO BE WORKED OUT

As exciting as this sort of "smart selection" sounds, there are still several challenges to overcome. Gene sequencing can consistently identify malfunctioning genes by name, but we don't always know the gene's actual function. Nor do we necessarily have a medicine that can fix it. Even when an active medication exists and is proven to help the specific mutated gene that has been identified, there is no guarantee it will work in prostate cancer. For example, Mekinist is thought to be effective in counteracting the misbehavior of a gene called GNAS in patients with melanoma. However, as of yet, we don't have data showing that Mekinist will be effective for prostate cancer patients with GNAS.

BIOPSY IS NOT EASY

We attempted to obtain cancer cells from Bill's bone for genetic testing by doing a biopsy. Unfortunately, no viable tumor cells could be obtained. In our experience, biopsy to obtain tumor cells from the bone for genetic testing in prostate cancer patients only yields diagnostic information about half the time. Bone biopsy is cumbersome and uncomfortable, but until recently, bone biopsy was the only way to access the genetic material in tumor cells.

Fortunately, the ability to analyze DNA released *into the blood* from cancer cells may now replace the need for bone biopsy. One assay, performed by Guardant Health, tests for 70 of the most common mutations seen in various cancers, including prostate cancer. Studies indicate that mutations diagnosed this way match the abnormalities detected by bone biopsy.[1,2] The testing of cell-free DNA in the blood appears to be a welcome alternative to obtaining tumor DNA from bone biopsy, and in some cases it may be able to identify in advance what patients are likely to obtain a good response to Taxotere.[3]

Genetically derived information for the selection of off-label cancer treatments may lead to four possible outcomes:

1. No therapy exists for the abnormal cancer gene that has been detected.

2. FDA-approved treatment for prostate cancer is available to treat this specific gene abnormality.

3. FDA-approved treatment exists for this specific gene abnormality, but it is only available for another type of cancer (lung, kidney, melanoma, etc.).

4. New agents presently in the process of undergoing clinical trials are available for this specific genetic abnormality, either in prostate cancer or another type of cancer.

In practical terms, the first two outcomes are not going to be much help to patients. Specifically, in regard to outcome number 2, most patients who undergo genetic testing for prostate cancer have already exhausted the FDA-approved options for prostate cancer. But outcome numbers 3 and 4, however, may point to a therapy that would otherwise be lost in the background of the numerous off-label treatments that might be considered.

It's unfortunate that despite our best efforts, Bill's gene profile could never be obtained. Nevertheless, Mekinist had a stupendous impact on his longevity and quality of life. At this point we don't know if his excellent response occurred due to his having a malfunction of the GNAS gene, another gene, or a specific combination of genes. However, now with easier access through blood testing, we will be able to detect specific gene abnormalities and select off-label treatments more intelligently.

References

1. D Robinson and others. Integrative clinical genomics of advanced prostate cancer. *Cell* 161.5: 1215, 2015.

2. RB Lanman and others. Analytical and clinical validation of a digital sequencing panel for quantitative, highly accurate evaluation of cell-free circulating tumor DNA. *PLoS One* 10.10: e0140712, 2015.

3. T Gourdin and others. Genomic profiling of metastatic prostate cancer through analysis of circulating tumor DNA. *Journal of Clinical Oncology* 34.2 suppl: abstr 17, 2016.

Chapter 44

CANCER RESEARCH: STRIVING TO LIVE LONGER AND BETTER

Luke Nordquist, MD

The consequence was, that the most sudden and visible good effects were perceived from the use of oranges and lemons; one of those who had taken them being at the end of 6 days fit for duty.

JAMES LIND

A HISTORY OF CLINICAL TRIALS

Dr. James Lind, a Scottish physician and pioneer of naval hygiene in the British Royal Navy, was credited with carrying out the first clinical research in 1747. At that time, scurvy, caused by a deficiency in Vitamin C, was a major cause of death of sailors at sea. Back then the concept of vitamins was unknown. Dr. Lind was not the first to suggest citrus fruits as a potential treatment for scurvy, but he was the first to conduct an experiment to test this theory. He divided 12 sailors affected with scurvy into six groups of two. Each group of two sailors was given a different treatment: a quart of cider daily, 25 drops of sulfuric acid, six spoonfuls of vinegar, half a pint of seawater, barley water, or oranges and lemons. Despite running out of the oranges and lemons early, the two sailors assigned citrus fruit recovered from their disease. This may not represent the most well-conducted study, but it does represent the birth of clinical trials.

CLINICAL TRIALS TODAY

In 1971 the National Cancer Act was signed into law by President Richard M. Nixon, declaring war on cancer. At that time, there were an estimated three million cancer survivors in the US. Today there are over 12 million cancer survivors, thanks to improvements in treatments discovered through clinical trials. In 2000, there were just over 5,000 clinical trials registered for all diseases, including cancer. Today there are over 200,000 clinical trials in all 50 states and abroad.

Clinical trials can be credited with curing testicular cancers, many types of lymphomas, and childhood leukemia, to name a few. However, even when cancers aren't curable, new treatments have changed many otherwise fatal cancers into chronic diseases. And even though we congratulate ourselves on these accomplishments, we also realize that there is still too much suffering and death from cancer and much more that needs to be done.

THE TAKE-HOME MESSAGE FROM THIS CHAPTER

As I write this chapter, my intention is not to list the most exciting new research drugs for prostate cancer. Clinical trial options change too quickly, and this chapter would rapidly be out of date. My cancer center, like many others, may have several new clinical trials added each month. Instead, the purpose of this chapter is to describe the clinical trials *process*, how vital it is to the development of new cancer treatments, and what a cancer patient should consider in regard to his treatment options.

WHY DO WE NEED CLINICAL TRIALS?

I don't think anyone would argue with the statement: "We need more treatments for cancer—and faster!" Therefore, until every cancer is cured, we will need more trials. However, truth be told, there isn't necessarily a shortage of new treatments to be investigated. In fact, there is an abundance of potential investigational treatments in the research pipeline. A major hurdle is a shortage of patient participation. Sadly, only three percent of cancer patients ever participate in a clinical trial. Just imagine how many more studies could be completed if even 10 to 15 percent of cancer patients participated. That would lead to a more efficient pipeline of potentially lifesaving treatments.

Before we dive into why the percentage of clinical trial participants is so low and what can be done about it, let's step back and look at some of the components of a clinical trial and how a new treatment progresses from an idea, to an investigational treatment in patients, to, finally, an FDA-approved treatment.

WHAT ARE CLINICAL TRIALS?

The first step is for a researcher to come up with a new treatment idea, called a "hypothesis." A hypothesis is a proposal about how a new cancer treatment might work in a particular cancer. The new treatment may be a drug, a type of therapy, or even a combination of drugs. Clinical trials, research trials, and studies all refer to the path or process that investigates the effectiveness of a new treatment.

Once a treatment hypothesis is formulated into an actual drug (pill, injection, or intravenous treatment), it moves into the "preclinical" phase. Preclinical work is done in laboratories prior to experimenting in humans. This includes Petri dishes, mice, etc. Promising preclinical studies then lead to "clinical research" trials. Clinical research means human testing. All human testing requires approval by an independent outside entity called an Institutional Review Board (IRB), which has the task of ensuring that the study is ethical and that all safety measures have been considered for the participants. The company that is developing the investigational treatment and paying for the costs of performing the research is called the "sponsor." The physicians who administer the treatments to patients are referred to as the "investigators." There are three main phases of clinical trials that an investigational treatment goes through to receive FDA approval: phase I, phase II and phase III studies.

- **Phase I:** These trials explore initial investigational treatments in humans. These trials are small, often only enrolling around 20 to 80 patients, and are commonly conducted at a single cancer center. All patients will receive the investigational treatment in a phase I trial. The focus of these studies is to determine a safe and effective dose of the treatment.

- **Phase II:** These trials are a little larger, with up to a few hundred patients enrolled. They are often conducted at several cancer centers. The goal of a phase II trial is to further evaluate the safety and establish the effectiveness of the drug in a specific cancer. Most phase II study participants will receive the investigational treatment, but occasionally there are randomized phase II trials. Randomized trials compare the investigational treatment to another treatment or to a placebo.

- **Phase III:** These trials are very large and may enroll up to several thousand patients. They are conducted at multiple cancer centers, often globally. The goal of a phase III trial is to confirm the safety and efficacy of the drug in comparison to the current, most effective "gold standard" of therapy. Patients on phase III clinical trials are often randomized to a treatment that could be the investigational treatment, a standard-of-care treatment, or a combination of both the investigational and the standard treatments.

- **Note:** There is also a **phase IV** clinical trial, which investigates additional safety issues, potential benefits, and optimal use *after* the drug has been FDA-approved and is on the market.

THE PATIENT PROCESS IN A CLINICAL TRIAL

The clinical-trial-enrollment process starts when a patient signs an "informed consent agreement," which is a document explaining the study purpose, how it will be performed, and the possible side effects and potential benefits of the treatment. After the consent has been signed, research staff will have the patient complete a screening process, which might involve drawing blood for lab tests, imaging with Xrays or CT scans, EKGs, and a more comprehensive medical history. Screening ensures that a patient meets all of the study's predetermined inclusion criteria.

After a patient has passed the screening process, he is assigned to treatment. There might be only one treatment arm in which the patient is guaranteed to receive the treatment, or there might be multiple treatment arms and the patient will be assigned to one of the options. Typically, a clinical trial that is comparing two or more different treatments will be randomized, which means that neither the patient nor the physician chooses the treatment. Instead, a computer allocates the treatment, ensuring balance between treatment arms.

Once a patient is enrolled in a study, everyone involved (the patient, the physician, and the research team) follows the very structured and defined research protocol until the study ends or the patient is taken off the study. It is important to also note that patients can remove themselves from a study at any point for any reason.

HOW DO WE DETERMINE IF A STUDY IS SUCCESSFUL?

A study is designed from the beginning to test a specific premise, called the "endpoint." These endpoints include, but are not limited to, safety, feasibility, response rate, the improvement in overall survival, quality of life, and time to progression of the cancer. If an investigational agent successfully meets the predetermined endpoints, such as an improvement in survival, the clinical trial will typically move on to the next phase of development and, potentially, to FDA approval.

In order for a cancer drug to receive FDA approval, it needs to have been proven safe and to prolong life or improve quality of life. A survival benefit—making someone live longer—is the most common requirement for an FDA approval. There is no prespecified length of survival improvement required for FDA approval. For example, in 2005, a drug called erlotinib (Tarceva) was FDA-approved for advanced pancreatic cancer after it demonstrated only a 12-day improvement in survival. Twelve days! Does that mean that erlotinib will only prolong survival by less than two weeks in all patients? The answer is no.

Let me explain how such a small increment of increased life could justify FDA approval. A sponsoring pharmaceutical company is a business and is managed in a fashion that limits spending. It can cost the company upward of *$1 million a day* to conduct a clinical trial. With that in mind, if you were the CEO of a pharmaceutical company with a promising new drug, would you study cancer survival in early-stage disease, when men would be expected to live many years? Of course not; the expense would be too prohibitive. Instead, studies include patients who are near the end of their lives. Most studies designed to achieve FDA approval of a new drug are conducted in late-stage patients. Therefore, the average survival improvements, even with effective therapy, are relatively short. The amount of benefit in earlier-stage disease should be much greater. Taxotere is a good example. In studies for very advanced disease, there was only a *two-month* survival benefit. However, in *earlier-stage* disease, the benefit was *17 months*. One good question to ask is, "How advanced were the patients who participated in the study?"

HOW ARE CLINICAL TRIALS FUNDED?

Cancer research can be divided into publicly and privately funded research. Publicly funded research primarily refers to taxpayer funds allocated by Congress to the National Institute of Health, National Cancer Institute, Department of Defense, etc. This form of research is commonly accomplished through grants and often carried out by academic centers or large cooperative groups. Unfortunately, because of cuts in government spending, this form of research has been under great strain. In fact, the current government spending for cooperative group studies only supports about 13,000 cancer patients a year, which represents only 0.8 percent of all newly diagnosed cancer patients in the US.

Privately funded research, on the other hand, is typically accomplished through pharmaceutical companies, called "sponsors." Privately funded research has really opened the doors to community cancer centers getting involved with research. Community cancer centers offer the sponsors efficiencies that can't always be accomplished at academic centers or with cooperative groups, saving the sponsors significant dollars in the drug development process.

WHY DON'T MORE PATIENTS PARTICIPATE IN CLINICAL TRIALS?

The first reason is the medical community. Most physicians don't participate in clinical trials. It requires a significant time commitment with extensive paperwork. Extra time must be allocated for patient education. Extra staff is needed, and this leads to an increase in overhead. Another problem is that patients are anxious about placebos. But most cancer clinical trials don't use placebos. It's only ethical to have a placebo when there is no other effective treatment available. Thirdly, there may be cost concerns. However, clinical trials can be a possible *solution* to the cost problem. Non-FDA-approved drugs must be provided for free by the sponsor. Lastly, no one wants to be a "guinea pig" for an unproven type of therapy. But no treatment is totally free from a risk of side effects. Newly discovered treatments often have *fewer* side effects than those of older ones.

HOW DO PATIENTS FIND A CLINICAL TRIAL?

If a patient is interested in participating in a clinical trial, I would recommend he start with his treating physician, who is most familiar with his case. However, if he doesn't receive satisfactory options, he should seek information elsewhere. A second opinion from an expert in his type of cancer is a logical next step. In addition, there are valuable websites (i.e., clinicaltrials.gov) that provide listings of clinical trials. In April 2017, a search for "prostate cancer" indicated 3,800 active trials.

WHAT'S THE FUTURE FOR CANCER TREATMENTS?

We have made great strides in our treatments for cancer. The primary focus of early cancer treatment was broad-spectrum cellular poisons such as chemotherapy. These agents still play an important role but are plagued by significant side effects. The focus is shifting to "targeted therapies." Although still not curing cancer, targeted treatments have proven to be more effective, with fewer side effects. Chapters 42 and 43 describe how we are moving toward "precision medicine" and immune therapies. Individual patients can have the mutations in their cancer identified, so that personalized treatment can be prescribed. The most precise treatment of all involves the immune system. Major strides have led to the unraveling of the mysteries of the immune system, enabling us to harness it to attack cancer cells.

THE FINAL WORD

I think it is important for patients to realize that clinical trials should not be reserved only for the time when all other treatments have failed. They should be viewed as an added tool in one's bag of treatment options. Medical advances are occurring so quickly that new medicines may only be available in a clinical trial. A new agent may allow a patient to reserve the "standard" treatment as a backup option. In addition, clinical trials may save money by providing access to expensive medications free of charge. Lastly, clinical trials advance medical science. Clinical trial participants are pioneers and part of the growing treatment team of professionals and experts who want to stop cancer from being the number two cause of death in the US. We all need to offer our thanks to every cancer patient who has taken the important step of participating in a clinical trial.

Chapter 45

PAIN MANAGEMENT

Mark Scholz, MD

Not knowing what to do is the worst kind of suffering.
PAULO COELHO

FORTUNATELY, EVEN THOUGH prostate cancer commonly spreads to the bone, the metastases are frequently not associated with pain. However, when pain occurs, good pain control is essential. Art and skill are required for effective pain management. When I suspect that a patient is hurting, I analyze the situation using a five-step process:

I. Query the patient to see if he acknowledges the pain.

II. Pursue an accurate diagnosis. Is the pain cancer-related?

III. If the pain is caused by cancer, select a new treatment for the cancer.

IV. Initiate a stepwise escalation of analgesics and other supportive medications.

V.   Consider radiation, nerve blocks and other means if Steps I to IV don't work.

I. ACKNOWLEDGE THE PAIN

Pain comes with a strong psychological and emotional component. It sends a loud signal: something is endangering our most valuable possession—our health. Pain, therefore, is often associated with fear, which further magnifies the pain. Many men have told me they fear pain and suffering more than death itself. Fear may lead to *denial* as a psychological defense mechanism. This has been confirmed through surveys, one in particular sponsored by Bayer. Men may choose to ignore their pain rather than talk about it with their doctors.

In the Bayer survey, 410 men with advanced prostate cancer were queried. *Two-thirds* of the men were handling their pain by ignoring it! When questioned further, one-third explained that, to them, acknowledging pain made them more fearful, raising anxiety about the possibility that their cancer is progressing. One-fourth of the men found it difficult to talk about their pain, because it made them feel weak. Doctors and family members need to be aware that men commonly use denial to fight pain. Denial can be effective as a short-term bridge for pain control. But using denial to fight pain in the long-term is psychologically draining, leaving men very fatigued. Since pain can almost always be remedied, and denial blocks access to a real solution, doctors and caregivers need to be alert and query men closely about how they feel.

II. DEVELOP AN ACCURATE DIAGNOSIS

Once pain is acknowledged, the next step is to determine whether it is coming from cancer or from some other condition, such as arthritis. Determining the cause of the pain is a diagnostic process. Diagnosis starts by determining the pain's location, duration, intensity, temporality (i.e., when it started and how long it has been going on), and nature (e.g., sharp, dull, burning, etc.). Cancer pain is characteristically located in the bone (not joints). The pain tends to be continuous and progressive. Bone pain from metastatic cancer can be confirmed by checking the patient's most recent bone scan to see if the pain's location matches a spot detected on the scan. If no spot is present, another cause besides cancer should be considered.

III. START A NEW TREATMENT FOR THE CANCER

Uncontrolled cancer pain indicates that the existing anticancer treatment is ineffective. The best treatment for cancer pain is effective anticancer medication. While waiting for a new anticancer medicine to kick in and relieve the pain, short-term pain medicines should be used. Reliance on long-term pain medications, rather than treating the cause of the pain with an effective cancer therapy, results in unnecessary side effects from the pain medications, such as drowsiness, loss of appetite, constipation, and mental confusion. The best quality of life and the best longevity come by controlling the cancer with effective therapy. Usually, the earliest sign of effective therapy is pain reduction, which occurs before the PSA declines or the scans improve.

IV. USE MEDICATIONS IN A STEPWISE MANNER

Pain medications are selected based on their potency. Milder analgesics like Advil, Motrin, Aleve, and Celebrex are usually initiated first. Their effectiveness is enhanced when used on a regular basis and with an adequate dosage. Overall, they are well tolerated. However, stomach upset with heartburn and even stomach ulcers can occur. Antacids like Prilosec and Pepcid may help counteract this problem.

Narcotic pain medications are divided into two classes—short- and long-acting. Generally, milder, shorter-acting narcotics like Vicoden and Norco are tried first. If pain control is inadequate, a stronger, short-acting narcotic like Dilaudid is tried. Once adequate pain control is achieved with the short-acting narcotics, a long-acting narcotic such as MS-Contin or slow-release Oxycontin may be substituted to maintain blood levels around the clock. Since narcotic pain medications can cause drowsiness, compensatory stimulants may be helpful. Laxatives are usually required to maintain normal bowel function, because narcotic pain medications frequently cause constipation.

A remarkable degree of short-term pain relief can often be obtained with cortisone medications such as prednisone or Decadron. Their analgesic effect may last for days, weeks, sometimes even months. The long-term use of cortisone, especially at high doses, may become problematic, because it can suppress the immune system, raise blood sugar levels, accelerate osteoporosis, and even cause stomach ulcers. Despite these problems, cortisone can work short-term wonders as a stop-gap measure for managing uncontrolled pain.

As noted above, there is a psychological component to pain, which is magnified by fear. Sometimes antianxiety medications like Ativan or Xanax reduce the fear level and help control pain. Antidepressants like Celexa, Zoloft, Paxil, and Wellbuturin may have a similar benefit. Combinations of all the approaches described above are often helpful. Successful pain management involves a high level of continuous communication between the doctor and the patient, because a "trial-and-error" approach, starting with milder analgesics and building up to more potent agents, is the correct process for finding optimal therapy.

V. USE RADIATION AND/OR NERVE BLOCKS

Pain may be localized in one specific area of the body or generalized in many spots throughout the body. An *injectable* type of radiation, called Xofigo (Chapter 40), is a good treatment if there are multiple painful areas. If the pain is in one area, a beam of radiation aimed directly at the painful area is very effective and usually free of side effects. The problem is that excess beam radiation can *permanently* suppress bone marrow function if too large an area of the body is treated. Excessive beam radiation is therefore to be avoided. Bone marrow is the source of very important functions, such as immune system activity, the normal clotting of blood, and the production of red blood cells.

Neuroleptic pain is due to a cancerous tumor growing and pushing against or pinching a nerve. Neuroleptic pain can be very severe and difficult to control with medications. The pain is very sharp and intense. It may radiate from one area of the body (the back, for example) down the leg or the arm. Pain may be absent in one body position and excruciating in another position. Sometimes neuroleptic pain can be controlled with a nerve block. Doctors who specialize in pain management are trained in how to inject Novocain into the area where the nerve is compressed to block the nerve and relieve the pain. In certain situations, off-label use of medications that are FDA-approved to treat seizures, such as gabapentin, can be effective against nerve pain.

PRACTICAL ASPECTS OF NARCOTIC PAIN MEDICATIONS

The accurate monitoring of a response to pain is critical. If something is not working, the medication dose needs to be increased or another agent needs to be substituted or added. Overdosage with long-acting pain medications can be dangerous, as they can suppress breathing. Therefore, the dose of long-acting pain medications needs to be escalated slowly—every two to three days. In the meantime, while waiting for the long-acting narcotics to kick in, the dosage of the short-acting narcotics can be increased more aggressively. With good communication and proper medical management, pain can almost always be effectively controlled.

As can be seen from this chapter, proper pain management relies on a diagnostic and therapeutic sequence that accurately determines the source of the pain and utilizes medications in a stepwise, escalating fashion. However, the field of pain management is vast. If the basic measures are unsuccessful, consultation with a pain specialist is the logical next step.

Having completed this section related to the *Royal* Stage of Blue, you can now jump to the section midway through the next chapter to the subhead "Non-Prostate Health Issues."

SECTION VII

LIFESTYLE AND GENERAL HEALTH ISSUES

Chapter 46

HEALTH ISSUES FOR MEN WITH PROSTATE CANCER

Jeffrey Turner, MD

Any intelligent fool can make things bigger and more complex. It takes a touch of genius—and a lot of courage—to move in the opposite direction.

E. F. SCHUMACHER

MILLIONS OF MEN ARE ALIVE and in remission after having undergone surgery or radiation for prostate cancer. These men all require ongoing cancer surveillance. Depending on their original Stage of Blue, they are all at some degree of risk for the cancer coming back. The risk of relapsing within the first five years after treatment can be as low as 5 percent for *Sky* or close to 50 percent or more for *High-Azure*, depending on how it was treated. Regular testing with PSA is the mainstay. The general policy after treatment is to do PSA tests quarterly for the first two years, biannually for the next three years and annually thereafter. For radiation patients, a yearly digital rectal examination is recommended. Routine imaging studies are rarely needed, unless the PSA increases.

Interpreting PSA after surgery is straightforward and should always incorporate an *ultrasensitive* PSA assay. Within six weeks after surgery, the PSA should be undetectable and remain so indefinitely. Any sequential rise in PSA typically signals a cancer relapse. However, occasionally after the operation, a very low level of PSA may be detected for *noncancerous* reasons because sometimes the surgeon fails to remove the prostate gland in its entirety. *But, if the cancerous portion of the prostate* has been fully removed, sequential testing will show that the PSA remains stable at a very low level. *There will be no pattern of rise over time.* Other than this one exception, any rise (confirmed by repeat testing) signals a cancer recurrence.

Interpreting PSA levels after radiation takes much more skill. Men who were initially treated with some form of radiation still have a prostate gland. As we all know, the prostate makes PSA. Therefore, PSA after radiation will not be undetectable. PSA after radiation is only abnormal when it rises above a certain threshold. As a starting point for general discussion, let's set the "normal" PSA level after radiation at 1.0 or less. There are, however, factors besides recurrent cancer that can cause the PSA to rise above 1.0—prostatitis or benign prostatic hypertrophy, for example. Since this issue of interpreting PSA after radiation is complex, Chapter 33 and 36 address how to determine if a rise in PSA is due to cancer or some other cause.

TESTOSTERONE RECOVERY

In patients who received TIP, testosterone levels are checked along with PSA to confirm its recovery after TIP is stopped. *PSA cannot be accurately interpreted if the testosterone level remains low.* Delayed testosterone recovery after TIP occurs commonly in men who are older, in men who had a more extended duration of TIP, and in men who began with a low testosterone prior to starting TIP.[1] For example, nine months of TIP may result in a three- to six-month delay in testosterone recovery. One study of long-term TIP (two years) reported that an *additional* two years were required before most had recovered.[2]

TESTOSTERONE REPLACEMENT THERAPY AND POTENTIAL SIDE EFFECTS

Some men, particularly the more elderly, will be left with chronically suppressed testosterone after TIP. Symptoms include muscle loss, weight gain, decreased libido, fatigue, and poor memory. The question arises, "Is it advisable to administer testosterone after curative therapy?" Several studies suggest that giving testosterone is safe. To date, 11 placebo-controlled, randomized trials and 29 non-placebo-controlled trials have been conducted that address this question. None of the studies show an increased risk of prostate cancer, cancer progression, or relapse.

Patients taking testosterone need to monitor their PSA closely, just like any other prostate cancer patient. A recent analysis of 292 patients treated with testosterone after prostate cancer treatment concluded that, if there is any increased risk of cancer recurrence, it is less than 1 percent. However, an increased risk of stroke and heart attack was noted. Therefore, another blood test, called the CBC (complete blood count), must be checked for abnormally high red blood cells (RBC). *Excessively high RBCs predispose to a heart attack or stroke.* The specific component within the CBC that measures RBC is called the "hematocrit" (HCT). If the HCT rises above 50 percent, the risk of stroke rises. An elevated HCT can be reduced by lowering the dosage of testosterone. Alternatively, a unit of blood can be "donated" on a periodic basis. (Donations from cancer patients will not be accepted by the Red Cross, but any oncology office can remove a unit of blood in a process called phlebotomy.) Typically, men will need a unit removed every few months, after which the HCT will stabilize at an acceptable level.

RISK OF SECONDARY MALIGNANCY FROM RADIATION

Patients treated with radiation may have a very small risk of secondary bladder or rectal cancer. The occurrence of secondary cancer can only be established by the following criteria: 1) it occurs five or more years after the radiation, 2) it occurs within the prior field of radiation, and 3) it is a different type of cancer than the initially treated one. The risk of secondary malignancy, in a worst-case scenario, is about 1 in 300. However, many studies have reported that the risk is far lower, and possibly negligible. The risk is probably higher with older radiation techniques such as 3D conformal radiation. Patients who have had seed implants probably have the lowest risk.

Surveillance for secondary tumors relies on checking the urine or stool for blood. The problem is that radiation itself makes men more prone to bleeding, unrelated to harboring cancer. So, blood may garner less attention than it should. Some experts have recommended an annual bladder cystoscopy.[3] This, however, can be very traumatic to the urethra, which is already been compromised by the previous radiation. Less invasive surveillance strategies are cytologic testing of the urine for atypical or malignant cells or doing a urine test called NMP-22. At Prostate Oncology Specialists, we recommend bladder wall imaging with ultrasound starting about 10 years after radiation.

NON-PROSTATE CANCER HEALTH ISSUES

Men are notoriously reluctant to visit a doctor. However, after a previous brush with cancer they become more amenable. The requirement for post-treatment prostate cancer surveillance presents a convenient opportunity to screen for non-prostate-cancer-related issues such as heart disease, hypertension, colon cancer, and other maladies. In this chapter, I'll share a couple of examples. A more detailed *Men's Health Brochure* is posted online at www.prostateoncology.com.

HEART DISEASE

The number one cause of mortality is heart disease. "Hardening of the arteries," or atherosclerosis, results from cholesterol infiltrating the arterial wall, causing inflammation and scarring. Over time, this scarring leads to calcification. Calcification combined with fat causes plaque. If plaque breaks free and blocks the artery, a heart attack or stroke occurs. Screening for impending arterial blockage requires a stress test or a coronary calcium score. Men with high cholesterol levels or high blood pressure, or men who are overweight, smoke, or have a family history of heart disease, are at the greatest risk. Aspirin and statin drugs can reduce the risk of heart attack while also providing anticancer benefit (Chapter 29).

IMMUNIZATIONS/VACCINES

It is advisable to receive an annual flu vaccine. Also, everyone should be aware that an antiviral flu *antibiotic* called Tamiflu is quite effective if it is started near the onset of easily recognized flu symptoms: sore throat, body aches, and fever. These symptoms usually come on suddenly. If one member of the family gets the flu, the other members can be treated with Tamiflu "prophylactically" to prevent them from contracting the disease.

Prevnar-13 and Pneumovax are once-in-a-lifetime vaccines recommended for patients over the age of 65 to reduce the risk of pneumonia. Zostavax to prevent shingles is also recommended for patients over the age of 60 who previously had chickenpox. Perhaps more importantly, this vaccination reduces the risk of a dreadful complication of shingles, called "post-herpetic neuralgia," which is associated with *lifelong intense burning, shooting, or stabbing nerve pain.*

LUNG CANCER

The US Preventive Services Task Force now recommends annual CT scans of the chest (low-radiation protocol) for current smokers or ex-smokers who quit within the past 15 years. Regular scanning is needed because by the time that cancer-related symptoms such as cough and chest pain occur, the disease is almost always incurable. Lung cancer is almost universally fatal if not diagnosed early. CT scans can detect small lung cancers at a curable stage, when the tumor can still be surgically removed or radiated.

COLON CANCER

Colon cancer, like most cancers, is easily cured when detected early. Patients over the age of 50 (or earlier, with a family history) should obtain regular screening colonoscopies. Alternatively, a less-invasive stool test is now available, called Cologuard.

OSTEOPOROSIS

Osteoporosis occurs more frequently in men who have low testosterone, especially those who have been treated with TIP. Bone fractures have dire consequences, including loss of height, pain, and shortened survival. Conditions besides TIP that predispose to osteoporosis are cigarette smoking, excess alcohol intake, and hormonal imbalances. Performing a bone density scan at age 70, or earlier in men who are at increased risk, should be considered. Treatment for osteoporosis include 250 mg of calcium daily at bedtime, 2,000 units of vitamin D3 daily, and pharmaceuticals such as Boniva/Fosamax or Prolia. Exercise is very important. Chapter 48 outlines a weight-training routine. Chapter 30 reviews the subject of male osteoporosis in greater detail.

ANNUAL PHYSICAL

Every man age 40 and older should have an annual physical, including a skin exam and an eye exam. Common blood tests like CBC, hepatic panel, basic metabolic panel, and lipid panel—as well as hormonal and vitamin screening that includes B12, thyroid, vitamin D, and testosterone—should be performed. The rationale and interpretation of these tests is discussed in Appendix III. The old saying bears repeating: "An ounce of prevention is worth a pound of cure." Considering that men will be required to go to the doctor's office anyway to track their prostate situation, why not make sure that some of the common and preventable maladies like high blood pressure and high cholesterol are not missed along the way?

WHAT ABOUT OTHER MEN IN THE FAMILY?

Prostate cancer can run in families. As our patients become more sophisticated about their health, their minds naturally run to concerns about their fathers, sons, and brothers. What can someone do about an elevated PSA without overreacting? Rushing into a urologist's office and undergoing a 12-core random biopsy is foolish. Rereading Chapters 4 and 5 will be helpful. Additionally, *Invasion of the Prostate Snatchers*, explains what is going on in the prostate cancer world in much greater depth. PSA screening should be withheld until patients are comfortable that they understand the big picture. Well-intentioned PSA screening leads to unanticipated harm in people who are ill-informed.

Good health is our greatest asset. For the most part, our bodies function quietly and efficiently without complaint. But many problems (such as prostate cancer) don't cause symptoms until the condition is advanced. Waiting until "something hurts" is the old-fashioned way to do medical care. New technology is changing the game. Live longer by diagnosing problems early, before they get out of control.

References

1. B Dai and others. Kinetics of testosterone recovery in clinically localized prostate patients treated with radical prostatectomy and subsequent short-term androgen deprivation therapy. *Asian Journal of Andrology* 15.4: 466, 2013.

2. M Khera and others. Androgen replacement therapy after prostate cancer treatment. *Current Urology Reports* 11.6: 393, 2010.

3. F Suriano and others. Bladder cancer after radiotherapy for prostate cancer. *Reviews in Urology* 15.3: 108, 2013.

Chapter 47

WHOLE NUTRITION FOR PROSTATE HEALTH AND RECOVERY

Verne Varona

On-street interviewer:
"Can you name the four basic food groups?"

Woman's answer:
"Frozen, instant, canned, and chocolate."

AS STRANGE AS THIS MIGHT SOUND, many people do not know what foods make up the basic food groups, or the real meaning of a balanced diet. From educators to physicians, we are constantly told to eat "a balanced diet." But what does this really mean? Contrary to a common theory, a balanced diet is not a cookie in each hand ... Ideally, the bulk of human food intake should be from *whole food* sources, with only a small percentage coming from food *products*.

Whole Foods – Whole foods are unprocessed, unadulterated, and natural foods. This category of staple foods was consumed for thousands of years by traditional cultures throughout the world.

Food Products – Food products are processed, refined, boxed, bottled, canned, packaged, and powdered. They consist of *former* whole foods that human hands have changed in some way. While brown rice might be considered a whole grain, brown rice flour/bread/crackers/muffins are *grain products*. The label might boast, "Natural Whole Grain Bread," but don't be deceived. They were *originally* whole grains, but they are "whole" no longer.

NUTRITION 101—WHOLE FOODS VS. FOOD PRODUCTS

When you select whole, natural foods, you provide your body with essential nutrients that are often absent from the common foods that make up the Standard American Diet (SAD). You avoid many harmful additives and other undesirable substances that make up modern processed foods. Over 14,000 human-made chemicals are added to our food supply. The corporate justification for these chemicals is to extend the shelf life of the food, increase visual marketability, and appeal to an ever-increasing desire for added sweet flavors.

Today we eat the same macronutrients, but they come from different food sources:

Macronutrients	Traditional Source	Modern Source
Carbohydrate	Whole grains, grain products, vegetables	Grain products (bread, pasta) vegetables, fruits, refined sugars
Fats	Vegetable oils, nuts, *minimal* animal products	Meat, dairy, oils, nuts
Proteins	Beans, bean products, *minimal* animal products	Animal products, dairy

The first difference between these two approaches is the amount of *meat*. In the Traditional Model, there is a reduced quantity of animal protein compared to the Modern Diet. The second difference relates to a sharp increase in the amount of simple carbohydrates (sugars). There are two kinds of sugar: complex and simple. Complex carbohydrates are often called the "bland" stuff, while simple carbohydrates are known by their immediate sweet taste. Put a piece of chocolate on your tongue and contrast that with a teaspoon of cooked rice: sweet versus bland—unmistakable. From decades of examining client dietary records, I've learned that most people are eating a diet that lacks *complex* carbohydrates (the primary fuel source for our brain and physical energy). This leads to sugar cravings.

Complex carbohydrates from whole grains, beans, and vegetables are composed of long chains of sugar molecules, called "polysaccharides." In the digestion process (which begins in the mouth), these long chains are broken down into smaller sugar units. Thus, the carbohydrate is absorbed into the bloodstream *gradually*. All carbohydrate *eventually* becomes sugar; the critical difference is the *speed* at which it does so. Complex sugar (from whole grains, beans, vegetables, and fruit sources) gives *enduring* energy, whereas simple sugar offers quick but fleeting energy. Think of complex carbohydrates as a hardwood log burning in a fireplace with a consistent flame. Conversely, the burning of simple sugar is like a newspaper tossed into a fireplace; it immediately flames big and bright but quickly extinguishes into cool ash.

Blood sugar highs and lows create hormonal and chemical stress that predisposes to inflammation and mood swings.

Blood Sugar Wave with Refined Sugar Consumption

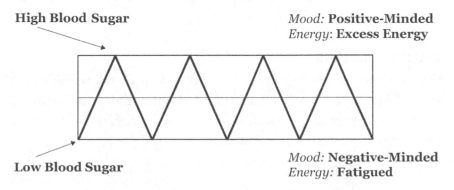

High Blood Sugar

Mood: **Positive-Minded**
Energy: **Excess Energy**

Low Blood Sugar

Mood: **Negative-Minded**
Energy: **Fatigued**

"Longevity Blood Sugar Wave" with Complex-Carbohydrate Foods

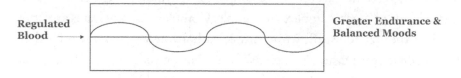

Regulated Blood ———▶   Greater Endurance & Balanced Moods

The "longevity blood sugar wave" results from a *whole foods* diet. Making your blood sugar bounce all over the place can sometimes be fun and stimulating, but as a steady diet, it becomes destructive. The negative consequences of erratic blood sugar are a compromised immune system, inflammation, strong cravings for sugar or salt, and fatigue. And for cancer patients, maintaining a consistently lower blood sugar lowers insulin and discourages cancer growth.

THE MODERN DIET—QUANTITY AND QUALITY

Apart from the concern about excessive swings in blood sugar, the modern diet is high in animal protein, fats, and refined chemicalized food. Excesses of these specific foods, as was discussed above, leads to *inflammation*.[1] Inflammation plays an integral role in the process of atherosclerosis—hardening and narrowing of the arterial pathways. Excessive consumption of saturated fats (found mainly in animal products) and partially hydrogenated vegetable oils (also known as trans-fats) also stimulates the process of atherosclerosis. The argument over animal protein is not a black-and-white, to-have-or-have-not issue. It's about volume and frequency. We simply eat excessive amounts of animal protein, and do it far too frequently.

QUALITY CONCERNS

Most commercial foods are poor in quality, with chemicals added for preservation, taste, and color. Some of these food additives are: artificial sweeteners (Aspartame, Acesulfame-K, Saccharin, Sucralose, etc.); food dyes; mycoproteins (meat substitutes); partially hydrogenated oils (trans-fat); refined sugars; high-fructose corn syrup; processed meat additives such as sodium nitrates; bovine growth hormones; pesticides; herbicides; and numerous preservatives designed to increase shelf life.

Of concern are the *processed meats,* such as bacon, sausage, hot dogs, sandwich meat, packaged ham, pepperoni, salami, and virtually all red meat used in frozen prepared meals. Typically, they are manufactured with a carcinogenic ingredient known as sodium nitrite.[2] (In addition, meat companies traditionally use nitrates as a color fixer to make meats appear a bright red color, creating the illusion of freshness.)

Research has shown that sodium nitrite consumption results in the formation of nitrosamines in the human body, leading to a dramatic increase in cancer risk for those who consume them. A University of Hawaii study in 2005 found that processed meats increase the risk of pancreatic cancer by 67 percent.[3] Another study revealed that every 50 grams of processed meat consumed daily increases the risk of colorectal cancer by 21 percent.[4]

WHAT THE DESIGN OF YOUR BODY REVEALS

Most drivers know that their standard car engine is designed for unleaded gas. What happens if they use leaded? For a brief while they might get away with it, but they risk destroying the oxygen sensors, which decreases fuel mileage, and ruin the catalytic converters, which convert pollutant gasses into less harmful ones. This is analogous to the dietary fuel that nourishes our blood and cells. Our body is simply not designed for the modern diet, with its excess of very concentrated foods. We are designed to consume a predominantly plant-based, whole foods diet occasionally enhanced with *small* quantities of animal protein—*if* desired.

While some historians and anthropologists claim that humans are *historically omnivorous,* our physical structure (teeth, jaws, and digestive system) are far better suited to a plant-based diet. The physical characteristics of carnivores and humans differ and make clear nature's preferences for our healthful eating. Here are some differences that illustrate this point:

Animals that Consume Meat	Plant-Based Human Physiology
Carnivores have sharply pointed teeth for tearing but no flat molars for grinding.	The human mouth contains few sharp teeth (but we have four flat molars for grinding).
Carnivores have naturally strong stomach acids that help break apart and digest animal proteins.	Humans have stomach acids that are at least 10 times weaker than those of a meat eater.
Carnivores have salivary secretions that are acidic with no alkaline enzymes to predigest complex carbohydrates.	Humans have alkaline enzymes in saliva that predigest complex carbohydrates.
Meat eaters have no lateral movement in their jaws.	Human jaws have a unique ability to use lateral movements in chewing.

HOW MUCH PROTEIN DO WE REALLY NEED?

Contrary to what most people believe, an adult's established protein requirement is not very high. Per a 2009 study published in *The American Journal of Clinical Nutrition*, 0.8 grams of protein per kilogram (2.2 lbs.) of body weight per day is the average requirement for adults. This translates into about 54 grams of protein daily for a 150-pound adult. A 7-ounce steak can deliver 54 grams of protein, but this source adds an undesirable mixture of saturated fat, hormones, and steroids. By consuming a variety of quality vegetable proteins, such as whole grains, beans, and bean products, one can easily meet this protein requirement without the negative additional factors. A plant-based dietary plan is a healthier choice than getting excessive amounts of protein from animal sources, such as red meat, poultry, and eggs. A 2009 study published in *The Physician and Sportsmedicine Journal*[5] reported that daily aerobic exercise, along with a low-fat, high-fiber diet consisting of whole grains, fruits, and vegetables, reduces insulin levels. Overweight men, particularly those who carry extra midsection weight, run higher insulin levels, a potential stimulus to cancer cell growth.

STARTING POINT: A FLEXIBLE TEMPLATE

Next is a sample food plan for healthy eating. The three categories of staple, secondary, and pleasure foods (for those in good health) are like diets in many traditional cultures. Staple foods such as grains and beans, as well as vegetables and foods from these groups, should make up the bulk of your diet. The percentages below are approximate and not fixed, but are starting points for experimenting and determining how your body best reacts to various combinations of food groups.

Supplemental foods are animal proteins, oils, seeds and nuts, fruits, and beverages. The Animal Protein portion of this category is optional. If you exclude or minimize this category, you should increase your consumption within the Beans category. Finally, the Pleasure Foods category is the smallest. Leaving a very small percentage of your diet for treats is fine. From time to time, we find ourselves in social situations in which we can exercise more flexibility with food choices. This category is shown as WYW on the pie chart, which stands for "Whatever You Want!"

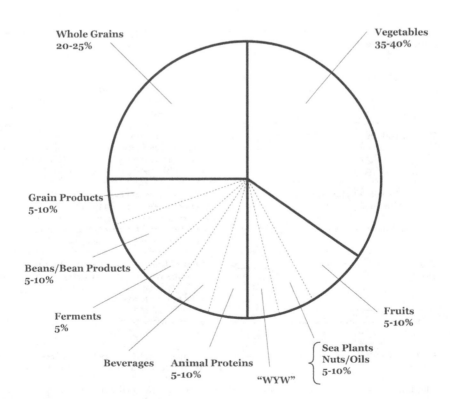

Whole Grains
20-25%

Vegetables
35-40%

Grain Products
5-10%

Beans/Bean Products
5-10%

Ferments
5%

Fruits
5-10%

Beverages   Animal Proteins
5-10%

"WYW"

Sea Plants
Nuts/Oils
5-10%

Example of a Good, Balanced Diet

EXAMPLES OF STAPLE FOODS

Whole Grains, 30%	Brown rice, oats, barley, millet, quinoa, buckwheat
Grain Products, 10%	Unrefined whole grain bread, pasta, crackers
Vegetables, 40%	Root, green leafy, and ground vegetables
Beans, Bean Products, 10%	Dried/canned beans and bean products (tempeh, tofu, miso)

EXAMPLES OF SUPPLEMENTAL FOODS

Animal Protein, 10%	Fish, poultry, wild game
Small Percentages	Seeds/vegetable oils, nuts, seasonal fruits, beverages

FOOD EXCHANGES

Standard Foods	Alternative Whole Food Choices
Red Meats →	Reduce volume & frequency of red meats -- Gravitate toward **white meats** -- Eat more vegetable protein sources (**beans, bean products**)
Dairy Products →	Reduce & or eliminate diary foods -- Increase **vegetable oils, nuts & seeds** -- Take more mineral source foods (**green vegetables** and **sea vegetables**)
White Breads, Enriched Breads, Pasta, Muffins, etc. →	**Whole grain cereals, whole grain bread & whole grain pasta.**
Canned & **Frozen Vegetables** →	**Minimized frozen vegetables, fresh vegetables,** organic, when possible
Refined Sugar & Sweetened Deserts →	**Fruits, limited juices, natural jams, cookies with natural sweeteners** such as **agave, barley malt, rice syrup, maple syrup, honey**
Soda Pop →	**Fruit spritzers** (fruit juice & carbonated water)
Coffee & Caffeinated Beverages →	Gradual **caffeine reduction → black tea → green tea → herbal & grain teas**
Alcohol →	Occasional **natural beer** and spirits, **non-alcoholic beer**

FOOD EXCHANGES

Before you radically leap into a global change of your diet from SAD to whole foods, you can make incremental healthy choices by exchanging some of your customary foods for healthier options. In the Food Exchange diagram on the previous page, the left side is composed of conventional choices, while the right side represents healthier alternatives. These food transitions can make a noticeable and prompt difference in your feeling of well-being and your ability to heal.

THE HEALING PATH

The healing path is composed of many roads that eventually lead to the same destination: a place where body, mind, and spirit are unified. The roads that we choose should fulfill the incomplete areas of our lives, the areas we need to pay more attention to, the areas of ourselves that need to be expressed more fully and that we need to nurture.

These areas of our lives may be named: *Purpose, Nutrition, Love, Honesty, Compassion, Humor, Spirit, Forgiveness, Faith, and Gratitude.* In the relatively young field of allopathic medicine, we've only recently recognized that healing efforts must be personalized for patients and offer some degree of control as well. Patients need to learn how to make informed choices instead of being pressured by "experts" into believing that there are no other options available. Choice is what makes us exceptional. Sometimes, our exceptionality can defy the statistical categories into which we are lumped, allowing us to overcome grim odds. Part of us needs to prepare for the worst, but a bigger part needs to expect a miracle.

BECOME YOUR OWN BEST ADVOCATE

Making healthier choices should be based on education, common sense, and self-experimentation. Today, corporations that dominate the American food and agricultural landscape have a strong influence over the FDA and USDA. Consumers are not offered real protection from dangerous chemicals indiscriminately added to foods, medicines, and personal care products. So, the question remains: How do you protect yourself? Here are some simple rules for transforming yourself from a passive consumer into an active advocate in your quest for good health. Learning to take an active stance is the first step. Here are some more:

1. **Read Label Ingredients.** By going online, you have access to an immediate education about chemicals, foreign ingredients, and symptoms.

2. **Get Organized!** While cooking and food preparation require "work," planning makes it all doable and easier. Plan wisely and in advance. Keep grocery lists; prepare foods in advance that you can freeze or refrigerate (such as whole grains, beans, and soups).

3. **Know Where to Eat.** Learn about the healthiest restaurant menu options in your neighborhood. Carry some herbal tea bags or condiments, so you can personalize restaurant meals. Custom order instead of ordering standard dishes from a menu. Ask questions about ingredients, portions, and freshness.

4. **Research!** Learn how to do online research. Refuse to accept negative medical predictions or timelines for death. You are exceptional and not a statistic. If you have a concern about a symptom and your healthcare professional tells you, "Just don't worry about it," explain that you need more—or find another physician who will be responsive to your concerns. They are part of *your* team!

5. **Communicate!** Express your concerns, fears, or opinions to your medical professional. Make sure you are heard and that you understand what you are told.

6. **Second Opinions.** Get one! Get a third, if you feel the need.

7. **Trust Your Intuition.** It may not always be accurate, but it's worth investigating. It's a quiet, calm voice that constantly speaks to you. Take time to listen.

The end result of becoming a stronger advocate for yourself is empowerment. When you take control and do the work you need to do, you will benefit. If you don't, who will?

Let food be thy medicine and medicine be thy food.
HIPPOCRATES

References

1. D Giugliano and others. The effects of diet on inflammation: Emphasis on the metabolic syndrome. *Journal of the American College of Cardiology* 48.4: 677, 2006.

2. Processed Meats Too Dangerous for Human Consumption—The Institute for Natural Healing. http://institutefornaturalhealing.com/2015/07/processed-meats-declared-too-dangerous-for-human-consumption.

3. U Nöthlings and others. Meat and fat intake as risk factors for pancreatic cancer: The multiethnic cohort study. *Journal of the National Cancer Institute* 97.19: 1458, 2005.

4. V Bouvard and others. Carcinogenicity of consumption of red and processed meat. *Lancet Oncology* 16.16: 1599, 2015.

5. M Aryal and others. Oxidative stress in benign prostate hyperplasia. *Nepal Medical College Journal* 9.4: 222, 2007.

Chapter 48
FITNESS AND LONGEVITY

Mark Scholz, MD

Get comfortable with being uncomfortable ... will is a skill.
JILLIAN MICHAELS

ONE MORNING I REACHED a fitness milestone. I could stand on one leg at a time without leaning on anything, and pull on my shoes and socks without falling over. This didn't happen overnight. I'd previously hired a personal trainer.

My goal in hiring a trainer wasn't to perform balancing acts. For years, I had lived with a guilty conscience about my lack of exercise—guilty because I am so familiar with the scientific studies related to fitness. Fitness affects health in many more ways than most people realize: *The risk of a sedentary lifestyle is about the same as a pack-a-day smoking habit.* To quote Anton, my trainer, "Sitting is the new smoking."

Strength training is imperative for optimal health. After age 60, men lose 1 percent of their muscle every year. Without countermeasures, decrepitude becomes inevitable. Loss of muscle and strength leads to

poor balance, unsteadiness, and falls. Hormonal treatments accelerate the loss of muscle. Weakness and frailty are the essence of what it
means to be "old." Despite these scary realities, no one is ever "too old"
to get on the fitness bandwagon. Exercise can make muscles grow and
strengthen at any age.

This is powerful information, but only if you act. For three years,
with good intentions, I bought gym memberships, purchased an exercise machine, and got a set of weights. But I only used the equipment
a few times. What was wrong? Most of you know. Exercise is painful.
I already have enough pain in my life with no desire for more. It feels
good to *avoid* exercise. Only when I scheduled regular appointments with
a trainer did I begin to sustain a regular exercise program. It's expensive,
but it works. The hardest part was getting started. Soon there was an
increased sense of well-being, more energy, a smaller waistline, more
dietary freedom, and better balance. Even my tennis game improved.

Selecting the right trainer is the first step. Trainers need to be discern-
ing and intelligent. A poorly conceived exercise program leads to injury.
That's why they are called *personal* trainers. In an optimal program, a
good trainer customizes the exercise program per each individual's needs.
Interview several trainers—you are looking for a congenial personality
(you will be spending significant time together). Once you get started,
there will be paybacks: a better golf game, improved sleep patterns, a
happier mood, and, of course, improved self-esteem. Fitness *is* achievable. Break out the checkbook and get help! No drug can match the
benefits of strength training.

For those of you who want to go it alone, a reasonable program
is provided below. It was designed by Clifford Felarca, a former nurse
practitioner in my office. Before starting, he recommends doing some
stretching and warm-up exercises, wearing loose, comfortable clothing,
and having some water handy. He also cautions to build up the exercise
intensity slowly. You can start *without any weights whatsoever.* Then,
slowly add weight as you gain strength.

Cliff recommends *daily* exercise. The muscles need 48 hours to
recover. Therefore, he recommends *alternating* every other day with the

"Push/Pull" exercise routine outlined below. Using this method, the whole body is exercised every 48 hours.

Weightlifting Protocol

"Push Day"	Do 3 sets of 12 repetitions
Pectorals	Raise your arms up in front of you while lying on your back. Lower back down until almost touching the ground.
Pectorals	(Advanced) Wall Press: Stand an arm's length from a wall and, at chest level, place your hands flat on the wall. Bend your arms slowly with a straight back. Straighten out and then return to the starting position.
Triceps	Extend your arm (or a weight if you have begun using weights) behind you while leaning forward over a chair or table.
Shoulders	Extend your arms straight out by the sides, parallel to the floor, and start to make circles with each outstretched arm. (You can add light weights to each arm.)
Deltoid	Extend your arms out to each side while standing (with or without a weight in each hand). Lower both arms back to your side with a controlled, smooth motion.
Abdomen	Torso twists (Do 3 sets of 25 repetitions.) Google: "torso twist" for details.
"Pull Day"	Do 3 sets of 12 repetitions
Biceps	Curl your arm (or the weight) up in front of you while standing.
Back muscles	Sitting, pull your shoulder blades together; hold for 5 to 7 seconds; relax and repeat.

Back muscles	While leaning forward with one hand supported by a chair or table, dangle a weight in the free arm and pull it straight up toward your chest. Then straighten your arm until it again is fully extended; repeat.
Legs	Deep knee bends: Stand normally. Use something next to you for balance, if necessary. Bend both legs squatting down about halfway to the floor, then straighten up; repeat. Keep your knees behind your toes.
Calves	Start flat-footed with your feet shoulder-width apart. Push up so you are standing on your toes, then release; repeat.
Abdomen	Sit-ups (Do 3 sets of 25 repetitions).

This program emphasizes resistance training over aerobics. *The goal is to build up the mass of the muscles.* The muscles are the batteries of our bodies. Increasing their size increases your energy. In addition, muscle tissue uses energy at a faster clip, *burning calories even when we are sedentary.*

Exercise is hard, so most people don't do it. Success comes by having a plan. It also helps to have a motivating passion and a vision for maximizing your longevity: Perhaps you want to extend your retirement years, live to see your grandchildren graduate, or keep yourself in robust health to support your spouse. Without a motivating purpose, the daily pains of life will wear us down. One of my very clever patients, Gary Driggs, wrote a booklet back in 2003 with a provocative title: *How Prostate Cancer Can Make You Live Longer.* Gary used a prostate cancer diagnosis as a wakeup call to improve his overall health practices. It sure has worked. Now, at 82, he is still going strong, preaching the same message.

Chapter 49

SUPPLEMENTS FOR PROSTATE CANCER

Mark Moyad, MD

Intellectuals solve problems, geniuses prevent them.
ALBERT EINSTEIN

WHEN IT COMES TO DIETARY supplements, the general rule
is that *less is more*. Megadoses are never better. In fact, studies of megadose supplements suggest a *worse* outcome or prognosis in
patients with cancer. Supplements in cancer are controversial, but less
so for preventing or treating the side effects of conventional treatment.
I have written several books about dietary supplements, including "The
Supplement Handbook" and the Promoting Wellness Series. This chapter only provides a short outline, but it will be helpful in your journey
against a disease I believe can be controlled, conquered, or wiped out
in my lifetime.

B-VITAMINS: B1, B2, B3, B6, B12, AND FOLIC ACID

Numerous clinical trials were started in the hope of finding that high doses of B vitamins could reduce the risk of cardiovascular disease and cancer. However, researchers have been surprised to learn that excess B vitamins may *promote* heart disease and *encourage* cancer growth. Many cancers, including prostate cancer, have *surface receptors* for B vitamins, especially folic acid. *In other words, researchers believe that tumors can use vitamins as nutrients to help them grow.* Vitamin B12 may be needed in some individuals if their blood tests show an insufficiency or deficiency. The most effective B12 preparations are designed to melt under your tongue (sublingual).

VITAMIN C

Ascorbic acid, or vitamin C, is very popular, but researchers have not found that it helps prevent or treat prostate cancer. There has been some interest in taking megadoses (thousands of milligrams) from pills or even intravenously from a doctor. Studies in patients with advanced cancer showed it could make some patients feel better, but it had no impact on improving their survival. It is possible that intravenous vitamin C may still play a role in reducing some cancer treatment side effects or improving quality of life, but this is preliminary and I am truly bothered by what some clinics charge for this service. Studies of vitamin C for colds showed the most benefit at a moderate dosage (about 500 mg per day).

VITAMIN D

Studies evaluating the treatment of prostate cancer with high-dose vitamin D have showed conflicting results. The deleterious effects of *low* vitamin D on general health, and specifically on prostate cancer, have been clearly established. Prostate cancer patients should have a blood test to measure their vitamin D. I generally recommend 1,000 IU daily if the level is found to be below normal. Be aware that blood levels require several months to adjust after there is a change in intake.

VITAMIN E

Most nonsmokers (or ex-smokers) need only 15 to 30 mg (or IU) of natural or synthetic vitamin E to normalize their blood levels. You can get this amount from a children's or adult multivitamin or from healthy foods, particularly nuts, seeds, and plant-based cooking oils. Larger amounts of individual vitamin E supplements were shown to have a *negative* impact on prostate cancer patients in a very large placebo-controlled prospective trial. Men with prostate cancer *should not* take an individual vitamin E supplement.

FISH OIL (OMEGA-3 FATTY ACIDS)

Several studies have suggested that taking fish oil pills containing the two primary fish oils, EPA and DHA (500 to 1,000 mg per day), may reduce the risk of sudden cardiac death and may reduce the risk of other cardiovascular events. In addition, fish oil may have antiarthritic and antidepressive properties, but more controversial is whether or not fish oil has anticancer properties. Personally, I would be surprised if they did, and some new research suggests it could encourage the growth of some prostate cancers. I like fish oil right now for those with difficult-to-treat depression or arthritis; interestingly, it is being studied in a major clinical trial to reduce the symptoms of chronic dry eye.

GINGER

At a dose of 500 to 1,000 mg per day, ginger may be effective for reducing symptoms of nausea during and after chemotherapy. My favorite brand was the one tested in the largest cancer clinical trial thus far to show some efficacy and safety, and that product is known as "Zindol DS" from Aphios (Google it, please).

KOREAN RED GINSENG (PANAX GINSENG), MACA, L-ARGININE, L-CITRULLINE

These options all have very good preliminary data to show they improve sexual health (erectile function/libido) in men, and MACA and Panax ginseng even has data to support that it potentially helps women. It appears that Panax ginseng may also help reduce fatigue in cancer patients, based on a recent small study from the MD Anderson Cancer Center. Real exciting stuff, especially since many of the prescription sexual health products are so darn expensive!

PANAX QUINQUEFOLIUS (ALSO KNOWN AS AMERICAN GINSENG)

This dietary supplement (1,000 to 2,000 mg per day) has helped some patients reduce their fatigue and improve energy levels during chemotherapy or other cancer treatments. Interestingly, physicians really have few other options to improve energy levels or reduce fatigue from cancer treatment, apart from weightlifting/resistance exercise and caffeine. So many drug trials have failed! However, American ginseng from the Ginseng Board of Wisconsin has now become arguably the SAFEST, CHEAPEST AND MOST EFFECTIVE OPTION FOR FATIGUE! I am so excited about this, I can't even stand it! And, many argue that supplements have no role in cancer? WHAT?! This is silly! Some supplements have a specific role in cancer (to help with fatigue or to help prevent nausea, for example), especially after receiving adequate research.

GLUCOSAMINE, PYCNOGENOL, OR SAM-E DIETARY SUPPLEMENTS

Taken for osteoarthritis, these have a very good safety record. Glucosamine is now available in liquid options, but there is no evidence suggestive of antiprostate cancer activity. SAM-e has garnered some impressive research as an antidepressant, especially when used for difficult-to-treat depression, per a recent Harvard study.

LYCOPENE

There have been only a few studies of men taking lycopene supplements for prostate cancer, and the results thus far are inconclusive and controversial. More studies are desperately needed, but in the meantime, I am not a big supporter of lycopene dietary supplements for prostate cancer. The foods that are high in lycopene are tomatoes, watermelon, guava, pink grapefruit, papaya, and apricots. This is what gets missed in all the lycopene hype: Some of the strongest research evaluated lycopene from food sources, not from pills. I just interpret the lycopene data as another reason to consume more veggies and fruit (especially veggies—asparagus, carrots, ... yes, they have lycopene, too)!

MULTIVITAMINS

One of the largest studies of men taking a single pill, a low-dose multivitamin once a day (actually Centrum Silver), seemed to show it prevented cancer and might reduce the risk of recurrence of some cancers. But another study showed that taking two or more multivitamin pills a day *increased the risk for advanced and fatal prostate cancer.* In other words, less is more when it comes to multivitamins. It is possible that higher doses of these pills may feed prostate tumors. I am particularly suspicious of multivitamins that contain a high concentration of antioxidants. Taking a children's multivitamin several times a week, not to exceed one multivitamin pill a day, makes more sense. Be especially careful of any multivitamin that asks you to take more than one pill a day. Please be most careful about folic acid and zinc in higher amounts, *because they have been associated with a higher risk of aggressive prostate cancer in human studies.*

QUERCETIN

This is a compound found in grapes, garlic, and other natural sources that has some anti-inflammatory properties. We have no idea if it helps to prevent or treat prostate cancer, but it has been used with some success in treating chronic nonbacterial prostatitis. Prostatitis causing pain and inflammation of the prostate is more common than previously realized and is frequently a cause of unexplained PSA elevations. One of the most clinically tested and under-utilized products in the world is Q-Urol. However, first check with your doctor to see if you qualify for it or another quercetin-based product. It is not uncommon to combine quercetin with prescription medication for chronic nonbacterial prostatitis.

RESVERATROL

This so-called antiaging compound is widely sold as a supplement, but I prefer red wine as my source of resveratrol. And, the ongoing evidence with resveratrol and prostate cancer is so controversial. For example, one lab study showed it could theoretically encourage the growth of some prostate cancers. Bottom line: Studies show no consistency in helping prostate cancer patients.

SAW PALMETTO AND OTHER BPH SUPPLEMENTS

Saw palmetto is one of the most popular herbal products around the world used to provide some relief for the symptoms of benign prostatic hyperplasia (BPH). In two major clinical trials (STEP and CAMUS), the most commonly used dosage (320 to 960 mg per day) was very safe but worked no better than a placebo. However, a placebo works well for some men with mild BPH (no kidding here). There is no strong human research that supports using saw palmetto to prevent or treat prostate cancer.

SELENIUM = STAY AWAY FROM INDIVIDUAL SUPPLEMENTS NOW!

In a large and definitive clinical trial, selenium dietary supplements did NOT work to prevent prostate cancer at a dosage of 200 mcg per day—and it may have increased the risk of aggressive prostate cancer! However, another clinical trial may have found a benefit in getting smaller amounts of selenium from healthy food sources and a vitamin-and-mineral-combination supplement (low-dose multivitamin). Bottom line: There is no reason to take *extra* selenium, and several clinical trials that have recently been completed suggest the same thing—individual selenium supplements could increase the risk of prostate cancer recurrence or encourage the growth of prostate cancer.

TEA AND TEA SUPPLEMENTS

Most forms of tea, including black, green, herbal, and oolong, are healthy and have few or no calories, so enjoy drinking them. However, please keep in mind that tea-based dietary supplements or pills (not the drink) have no solid proof from human studies that they do anything against prostate cancer. A large clinical trial of high-dose green tea supplements in patients with advanced cancer showed no real benefit. Additionally, there has been a recent concern about tea dietary supplements (especially green tea supplements) increasing the risk of liver damage. So, a quick review, from the comedy *Young Frankenstein:* "Drinking tea, good. Taking tea supplements, bad." (Or not so good.)

WHEY PROTEIN OR PROTEIN POWDER (CASEIN, SOY, BROWN RICE, PEA, HEMP)

This can be taken as a powdered drink supplement (never as a pill) for any man needing more high-quality protein for health or weight loss, and to support muscle health. I usually recommend vanilla, chocolate, strawberry, or plain whey protein isolate or a plant-based product like pea protein with no sugar or fancy extras (a clean product). It should contain about 25 grams of protein per 100 calories. It tastes great when mixed with water (my favorite, and the favorite of most patients—Jay Robb Protein powders)! There is no protein bar in the world that can compete with this product's numbers! In fact, I always like to say, "The only thing you should get from a bar is a beer!" Okay, there are a few healthy protein bars, but the best supplement sources of protein are these powders. The maximum overall protein intake is roughly half your weight in grams per day (food or supplements), so a 200-pound person should get a maximum of 100 grams per day of total protein to help maintain muscle mass. A 150-pound person should get a maximum of 75 grams.

ZINC FOR EYE-HEALTH

Zinc has been promoted as an eye-healthy, immune-healthy, and prostate-healthy dietary supplement. However, zinc supplements in high dosages, 80 to 100 mg per day or more, should be avoided. Recent human research has linked higher doses of zinc from dietary supplements to abnormal immune changes, a potential reduction in the impact of bone-building drugs, abnormal changes in cholesterol blood tests, increased risk of urinary tract infections, kidney stones, prostate enlargement, and an increased risk of aggressive prostate cancer.

MARIJUANA CURES EVERYTHING, DUDE?!

Over the past several years as I've traveled around the country, and even the world, I always knew that at least one person in the audience would ask THE QUESTION. And, if I gave a lecture in Colorado I would get THE QUESTION many, many times! The question is whether "Marijuana is beneficial or is a treatment for [*every possible disease that has impacted humankind since the beginning of time.*] So, excuse me for using the words "dude" or "man" a lot in this section, but we *are* talking about marijuana. I mean Cheech and Chong used "man" and "dude" all the time in their records and films. (For you young people, please Google "Cheech and Chong"—no it is not a breakfast cereal or a phone app).

One of the best reviews and meta-analysis of marijuana[1] (a.k.a. "cannabinoids," a class of active ingredients) for medicinal use concluded with the following after examining 79 clinical trials (with over 6,450 participants):

> "There was evidence to support the use of cannabinoids for the treatment of chronic pain and spasticity. There was also evidence suggesting that cannabinoids were associated with improvements in nausea and vomiting due to chemotherapy, weight gain in HIV infection, sleep disorders, and Tourette syndrome. Cannabinoids were associated with an increased risk of short-term adverse events."

The adverse events that were more common in these clinical trials were the following: dizziness, dry mouth, nausea, fatigue, sleepiness, sedation, euphoria, vomiting, disorientation, drowsiness, confusion, loss of balance, and hallucination. OUCH!!!

Next, an expert from HAAAARVARD (I love to say that) looked at 28 randomized trials[2] and stated the following:

"Use of marijuana for chronic pain, neuropathic pain, and spasticity due to multiple sclerosis is supported by high-quality evidence." YEAH!!

However, this author expressed some concerns about the side effects with marijuana use such as, "... addiction and worsening of psychiatric illnesses such as some anxiety disorders, mood disorders, psychotic disorders, and substance use disorders ..." OUCH!!!

And there was this:

> "Regular marijuana use can result in physical problems as well. It is associated with increased incidence of symptoms of chronic bronchitis and increased rates of respiratory tract infections and pneumonia. Preliminary research points to an association between marijuana use and myocardial infarction, stroke, and peripheral vascular disease." OUCH, OUCH!!!

And in one of the most recent respiratory reviews of marijuana,[3] the following concerns were expressed after looking at 48 articles:

> "The research indicates that there is a risk of lung cancer from inhalational marijuana as well as an association between inhalational marijuana and spontaneous pneumothorax, bullous emphysema, or COPD. A variety of symptoms has been reported by inhalational marijuana smokers, including wheezing, shortness of breath, altered pulmonary function tests, cough, phlegm production, bronchodilation, and other symptoms." OUCH x 3!

Look, I am excited about marijuana and some of its medically active ingredients (a.k.a. "cannabinoids") to help patients with a variety of conditions, including a reduction of cancer pain, nausea, and vomiting, and perhaps an improvement in appetite. And I think it is interesting to consider for kids and adults with seizures who do not respond to other options. HOWEVER, it is also overhyped ("fights cancer"???) and comes with various side effects, including the cost! Medical marijuana has now become a massive area of profit for many state governments and owners of those groovy medical marijuana facilities. So finding the real truth, apart from the hype and cash flow, is a challenge!

PLEASE TELL ME MORE, DUDE MAN!

Let's just review a few quick, one-liner facts about marijuana[1,2,3] (since people no longer have the attention spans to read long paragraphs without being distracted):

- Marijuana has many synonyms or its own vernacular: "pot," "weed," "grass," "ganja," "joint," "reefer," "dope," "Scholz" (okay I made that last one up).

- Before the Marijuana Tax Act of 1937, cannabis was used medicinally, and in 1970, it was officially classified as a Schedule 1 drug because of its potential for abuse, lack of safety, and other reasons. Other schedule 1 drugs include ecstasy, heroin, and LSD.

- Over half of the states in the US currently have laws legalizing marijuana in some form! Wow! Wow spelled backwards! Marijuana itself is not FDA-approved to treat any medical condition (ahhhhh the irony).

- Marijuana = Cannabis = from the Cannabis sativa plant. And, over 60-plus cannabinoids and 400 compounds have been found in marijuana. Cannabinoids are some of the active ingredients in marijuana that could treat some diseases.

- The most well-known cannabinoid is THC (tetrahydrocannabinol), which is the primary ingredient thought to cause the "high" or "buzz." (This is what I am told; I have no experience with it, except in college when someone FORCED me to smoke and inhale it, or else they would not let me leave the fraternity house.)

- Interestingly, two cannabinoid (THC-like) drugs known as dronabinol (THC in sesame seed oil) and nabilone (another THC copycat) were FDA-approved in 1985. They are both oral prescription drugs available in the USA! These drugs were approved for nausea and vomiting from cancer chemotherapy. It is also useful for appetite stimulation in medical situations, as well as some forms of cancer or HIV infection that could cause large, unhealthy amounts of weight loss ("wasting" or "cachexia"). Interestingly, there is even some evidence that dronabinol helps "dysgeusia." In other words, it improves the taste of food.

- Another cannabinoid that is getting a lot of interest is Cannabidiol (CBD), *which does not cause intoxication.* CBD is being tested now in countless medical situations—as a topical oil for cancer pain or other types of pain, such as arthritis, for example. In fact, I have known many patients in the past five years who've told me they get good relief when using topical CBD oil right on the actual site of their pain. One concern in future studies is the potential for drug interactions, because cannabidiol can block the enzymes that the liver normally uses to deactivate drugs in your system. Therefore, it could increase the concentration of some drugs to dangerous levels.[4]

DR. MOYAD'S HIP AND GROOVY SUMMARY

So, let's review: Personally, if you are healthy, I think the risks of marijuana outweigh the benefits, unless of course you win the lottery and just want to try it one time to celebrate the fact that you never again have to listen to your boss or some of your annoying coworkers. Marijuana has NOT been proven to be heart-healthy, and in fact it could be heart-*un*healthy. And the smoke does not make the lung tissue happy, even though you could feel temporarily happy.

I frequently hear, "Marijuana is natural." So should I get excited about it? Just because it is natural is not the reason I get excited about diddly squat (a.k.a. anything). I mean, poison ivy and arsenic are natural, folks, but I usually do not recommend those things—except to my big brother when he pushed my face in the snow when we were kids …

Do I think it's possible that marijuana or one of its compounds can fight cancer or encourage the growth of cancer? Yes! But at this point, we have no conclusive evidence one way or the other. It's dangerous to treat humans, unless studies *in humans* show that it works. In Europe, a laboratory study showed that a certain drug could impact a cannabinoid receptor in the brain. "Experts" were convinced that it would be a great weight-loss drug, and it was marketed briefly under the trade name of Acomplia (Google that bad boy). It was removed from the market because of serious side effects, such as anxiety, suicidal ideation, nausea, and, in some cases, the development of multiple sclerosis.[5] The bottom line is that for every laboratory cannabinol study that suggests it fights cancer, there are other studies that suggest the opposite, or that it has toxic effects on normal cells.[6,7] THC has been shown to *promote* tumor growth in some immunocompetent animals.[8] Look, if you are a mouse or a rat, we can cure you of almost anything today, but until we get more human studies, we have no idea if it fights or accelerates or does nothing to the growth of cancer.

FINAL THOUGHTS

Always talk to your doctor about whether you qualify for any pill or supplement based on both your medical history and the results of your latest medical tests. If you do qualify, talk to your doctor about the precise dose, frequency, and form or brand name of the supplement that was used in the best objective clinical studies that suggested a benefit. In other words, use the same approach as you would use for a prescription medication. Dietary supplements should be treated in the same manner.

References

1. PF Whiting and others. Cannabinoids for medical use: A systematic review and meta-analysis. *Journal of the American Medical Association* 313.24: 2456, 2015.

2. KP Hill. Medical marijuana for treatment of chronic pain and other medical and psychiatric problems: a clinical review. *Journal of the American Medical Association* 313.24: 2474, 2015.

3. MP Martinasek and others. A systematic review of the respiratory effects of inhalational marijuana. *Respiratory Care* 61.11: 1543, 2016.

4. K Detyniecki and others. Cannabidiol for epilepsy: Trying to see through the haze. *Lancet Neurology* 15.3: 235, 2016.

5. EB Russo. Cannabidiol claims and misconceptions. *Trends in Pharmacology Sciences* 38.3: 198, 2017.

6. P Bagavandoss and others. Inhibition of cervical cancer cell proliferation by cannabidiol. *Planta Medica* 81.S01: S1, 2016.

7. L Deng and others. Quantitative analyses of synergistic responses between cannabidiol and DNA-damaging agents on the proliferation and viability of glioblastoma and neural progenitor cells in culture. *Journal of Pharmacology and Experimental Therapeutics* 360.1: 215, 2017.

8. MP Davis. Cannabinoids for symptom management and cancer therapy: The evidence. *Journal of the National Comprehensive Cancer Network* 14.7: 915, 2016.

Chapter 50

THE KEY: KNOWING YOUR STAGE OF BLUE

Mark Scholz, MD

Caveat Emptor: Let the Buyer Beware.
ENGLISH COMMON LAW

THIS BOOK IS A RESOURCE for patients. A cancer diagnosis is shocking. It's easy to be bowled over by a powerful $10 billion-a-year prostate cancer business and rush into poor choices. Even sophisticated patients are no match for the carefully orchestrated sales pitches they will encounter. How can anyone be prepared? No one gives prostate cancer a second thought until a diagnosis occurs.

When the fateful day arrives, the common false assumption is that the doctors are there to help you. This is naive. *The prostate cancer world is a competitive business.* Medicare pays $28,000 for IMRT. Proton therapy costs more than $100,000 per patient. In Southern California, where I work, advertisements costing millions of dollars blanket the radio waves advertising robotic surgery and proton therapy. Prostate cancer is a big business, heavily influenced by powerful, underlying financial incentives.

The best protection is a good working knowledge of prostate cancer, especially knowledge about your Stage of Blue. Imagine visiting a car dealership unprepared. Failing to research the invoice price of a new car almost always means paying a higher price. Prostate cancer ignorance leads to suboptimal treatment, unnecessary side effects and lower cure rates. Accurate information improves your confidence when discussing frightening treatments with experienced doctors. You must know your Stage of Blue! Staging guides doctors and patients to the best therapy, protecting you from being assigned to the wrong treatment.

Accurate staging provides a broader perspective about a cancer's potential impact on future *survival*, called the cancer's *prognosis*. Perspective and context help keep all the factual details in order. Treatments are evaluated and compared *in the context of the disease's severity*. Men with more life-threatening disease may need more intense treatment (and should be willing to put up with greater side effects). Men with harmless types of disease should eschew treatment altogether. Given these important considerations, let's summarize the potential impact of each Stage of Blue on longevity:

> *Sky*—Even with no immediate treatment, shortened longevity is not a risk.
>
> *Teal*—Even with relatively mild treatment, shortened longevity is a small risk.
>
> *Azure*—Even with combination treatment, shortened longevity is a possibility.
>
> *Indigo*—Even with combo therapy, there is a substantial risk of shortened longevity.
>
> *Royal*—Even with maximal therapy, shortened longevity occurs in over half of men.

Knowing the prognosis enables men to learn whether their treatment should prioritize survival or quality of life. Since even the bad types of prostate cancer are associated with long survival, quality of life will always retain some degree of importance. With the milder cancers, maintaining quality of life is the main priority. As we have learned for *Sky*, treatment is much worse than the cancer.

The greatest danger, therefore, for men with early-stage disease (the *Sky* and *Teal* Stages) is overtreatment. With the other Stages, the risk is greater for *under*treatment. As recently as 15 years ago, treatments for advanced-stage disease were limited to Lupron, bone radiation and morphine. Back then, surgeons (urologists) were adequately equipped to manage advanced prostate cancer. Now things are very different. With so many new, life-prolonging therapies available, the old-fashioned policy of "letting nature take its course" is no longer acceptable.

So, to recap: This book exists to forewarn and forearm. The starting place is your Stage of Blue. We have presented 15 different subtypes of prostate cancer—five Stages of Blue, each with three subtypes (Appendix I and II). The best results come from knowing precisely what you are treating so that treatment is personalized for everyone's specific subtype of prostate cancer.

Medicine is both a science and an art. You should make every effort to select the best possible physician partner to help you navigate the treatment selection process. The amount of new information about prostate cancer is expanding rapidly. A physician who sees many prostate cancer patients in daily practice is probably best. Hopefully our book has been helpful. We want to wish you the very best good fortune in your endeavor toward achieving an optimal outcome.

ACKNOWLEDGMENTS

THIS MULTIYEAR PROJECT HAS BEEN SUPPORTED BY SOME RATHER SPECTACULAR PEOPLE:

Lindsay Amaral: One of the professional editors who reviewed the manuscript.

Micah Chancey: A gifted writer who can detect logical fallacy from across the room.

Barry Clark: A presence who unknowingly holds me accountable to a much higher standard.

Joel Copeland: Bestowed with the gift of simplification.

Michele DeFilippo: One of the professional editors who reviewed the manuscript.

John East: Rapidly gobbles verbiage and understands its implications better than anyone.

Judith Gurewich: Provided invaluable advice and kindly published my first book.

Abigail Harris: One of the professional editors who reviewed the manuscript.

Harry Hathaway, Esq: Generously reviewed and offered useful advice.

413

Larry Martin: Generously provided the cover design concept.

Alexandra Oakley: One of the professional editors who reviewed the manuscript.

Ronda Rawlins: One of the professional editors who reviewed the manuscript.

Robert Reback, Esq: Provided excellent legal advice.

John Sarian: My spiritual mentor. A constant, sensible voice in my life.

Alex Scholz: Everyone's angel, the Rock of Gibraltar who finds what others overlook.

Dennis Scholz: My amazing mom, bolstering me with unstinting confidence.

John Scholz, Esq: My brother, who offered his well-trained lawyerly eye.

Juliet Scholz: My wife, my best friend and one who can proofread with the finest.

Natalie Scholz: My brilliant daughter, blessed with wisdom way beyond her years.

Kaili Shewmaker: My right arm, left arm, right leg, left leg, brain, eyes (I'll stop there).

James Stein: Kindly proofed the manuscript.

Larry Urish: One of the professional editors who reviewed the manuscript.

Sabrina Yep: A jack of all trades who does everything extremely well, including editing.

APPENDIX I

THE FIVE STAGES OF BLUE

Sky *(Low-Risk)* is a relatively harmless condition. The biggest risk for *Sky* is overtreatment. Within *Sky*, the most favorable subtype of all (*Low-Sky*) is defined by all the usual *Sky* criteria of Gleason 3+3=6, PSA less than 10 and minimal or no palpable disease on DRE. In addition, to qualify as *Low-Sky*, the PSA density must be less than 0.15 (Chapter 2), there can be no more than two biopsy cores containing cancer and no single core can be more than 50 percent involved. Men in *Low-Sky* have the best chance for staying on surveillance long-term without requiring treatment. At the other end of the spectrum (within *Sky*) is *High-Sky* which is defined by all the usual *Sky* criteria but with one or more of the following: palpable disease, a PSA density over 0.15 or more than 50 percent of the biopsy cores containing cancer. These men are at somewhat greater risk for disease progression, (i.e., the eventual need to go off active surveillance and undergo treatment). *Basic-Sky* falls between the *Low* and *High* subtypes. As would be expected, the risk for men with *Basic-Sky* to require future treatment is intermediate between *Low* and *High*.

Teal *(Intermediate-Risk)* is a generally low-grade condition associated with excellent long-term survival, though unlike *Sky* most men undergo

415

treatment. In addition to all the usual *Teal* criteria of Gleason 7, PSA from 10-20 or palpable T2b disease (Chapter 1), men who qualify for *Low-Teal* must have *only one* of these elements. In addition, the Gleason score must be 3+4=7 not 4+3=7, the amount of Grade 4 per the pathology report must be under 20 percent. In addition, no more than two biopsy cores can contain cancer. Many men with *Low-Teal* can be managed like *Sky*, that is with active surveillance (Section II). The criteria for *Basic-Teal* (also known as *favorable Intermediate-Risk*) is like *Low-Teal* except for having three to six biopsy cores containing cancer. *High-Teal*, also known as *unfavorable Intermediate-Risk*, is defined by having two or more of the usual *Teal* criteria or more than six biopsy cores that contain cancer. Chapter 20 discusses the different treatment approaches to consider for *Basic-* and *High-Teal*.

Azure (High-Risk) also contains three subtypes. *Low-Azure is* Gleason 4+4=8 with all other criteria being favorable—two or less positive biopsy cores, no biopsy core more than 50 percent involved with cancer, a PSA less than 10 and minimal or no palpable disease (T1c or T2a). Men with *Low-Azure* can consider having treatment along the lines of what is used for *High-Teal*. *High-Azure* is defined by having at least one of the following: A PSA over 40, Gleason 9 or 10, more than 50 percent positive biopsy cores, or cancer that spreads overtly outside the prostate. *Basic-Azure* falls between the *Low* and *High* subtypes. *Basic-Azure* is managed aggressively with an extended duration of hormonal therapy, seeds and IMRT as is *High-Azure*, possibly with the addition of Zytiga or Taxotere.

Indigo (Relapsed Disease) occurs when surgery, radiation, or some form of focal therapy fail to cure the disease. Men who are *Low-Indigo* are judged to be at very low risk for harboring any lymph node metastases. To qualify as *Low-Indigo* the PSA must be under 0.5 after previous surgery, less than 5.0 after previous radiation or focal therapy and the PSA doubling time must be over 8 months. In addition, the original Stage of Blue prior to initial therapy with surgery, radiation or focal therapy must be *Sky*, *Low-* or *Basic-Teal*.

Men with *High-Indigo* have metastases, but only into the pelvic lymph nodes. The metastases are proven to exist by either surgery or with scans showing *unequivocal* pelvic node involvement. Scans and surgical pelvic lymph node staging in men with *Basic-Indigo* show no overt lymph node metastases. However, in men with *Basic-Indigo*, various factors suggest a *significant likelihood* that *microscopic* pelvic lymph node disease is present. Such factors include higher PSA levels, a fast PSA doubling time or a Stage of Blue prior to initial treatment with surgery or radiation that was higher than *Basic-Teal*. Appendix II provides the specific thresholds. The intensity of treatment selected for *Low-Indigo* may be relatively mild, since less aggressive therapy may be curative and further options can subsequently be implemented, if necessary. Aggressive combination therapy is often used for *Basic-* and *High-Indigo* for two reasons: To enhance longevity and to try and cure the disease so as to eliminate the need for lifelong hormonal therapy, with the goal of achieving better quality of life.

Royal (Hormonal-Resistance or Mets Outside the Pelvic Nodes) is what defines *Royal. Low-Royal* is "pure" hormone resistance without any proven metastases. Hormonal resistance is defined as a rising PSA with a testosterone level less than 50. *Basic-* or *High-Royal* means that metastases outside of the pelvic nodes are proven to exist. With *Basic-Royal* the total number of metastases is five or less. Men with *High-Royal* have more than five metastases. Clearly, the likelihood of detecting metastases is influenced by searching with the best available type of scan. PET scans, for example (Chapter 6), may convert men who were thought to be *"Low-Royal"* using an older type of scan technology to *Basic-* or *High-Royal*.

Treatment recommendations for *Royal* can vary widely because doctors are struggling to digest the explosion of new knowledge. Better treatments, improved scans and a deeper understanding of staging, genetics and immunotherapy have all conspired to complicate and increase the controversy about how to select optimal therapy. Overall, however, we can certainly be thankful for these breakthroughs and the additional discoveries that are coming in the near future.

APPENDIX II

FACTORS COMPRISING THE FIVE STAGES OF BLUE

Stage of Blue	Prior Local Rx	Gleason Score	PSA	# Biopsy Cores with Cancer	DRE Stage	MP-MRI or CDU Scans	CT & Bone Scan	Other
Sky						No SVI, Gross ECE, or increase in lesion size over time	No need	PSA Density
Low	No	3+3=6	<10	1 or 2	T1c			<0.15
Basic				3 to 6				
High				>6	T2a			>0.15
Teal		7			*Low-Teal* = a **"Small"** lesion		Clear	*Low-Teal:* The % of Gleason 4 in the biopsy cores must be <20%
Low	No	3+4=7	<10	1 or 2	T1c/T2a			
Basic			<10	3 to 6	T1c/T2a	No **SVI**, Invasion or Gross **ECE**		
High		4+3=7	10–20	>6	T1c/T2a T2b			

Rx = Treatment; **DRE Stage:** Clinical Stage Per Digital Rectal Exam (Chapter 1 Table.); **MP-MRI** = Multiparametic MRI; **CDU** = Color Doppler Ultrasound; **CT** = CAT scan; **ECE** = Extra-Capsular Extension; **"Small"** = < 12 mm; **SVI** = Seminal Vesicle Invasion; **N1** = Pelvic Lymph Node Metastases; **Mets** = Metastases; **PSADT** = PSA Doubling Time; **PET** = C[11] Acetate, C[11] Choline, Axumin or PSMA Ga[68]; **XRT** = Radiation; **Testo** = Testosterone; **BS** = Bone Scan

Stage of Blue	Prior Local Rx	Gleason Score	PSA	# Biopsy Cores with Cancer	DRE Stage	MP-MRI or CDU Scans	CT & Bone Scan	Other
Azure		8 to 10				*Low-Azure* = a **"Small"** lesion		*Low-Azure:* The % of cancer in the biopsy cores must be <50%
Low		4+4=8	<10	1 or 2	T1c/T2a			
Basic	No	4+4=8	10–40	3 to 6	T1c, T2a/T2b	*Basic-Azure* = No **SVI**, invasion or Gross **ECE**	Clear	
High		9 or 10	>40	>6	T3a/T3b T4/N1			
Indigo			PSA and **PSADT** after Surgery/Radiation				Bone, **CT & PET** scans	Prior Stage of Blue
Low	Yes	3+4 or Less	Surgery < 0.5 / Radiation < 5 **PSADT** >8 months			No **SVI/ECE**		Less than *High-Teal*
Basic		Any	Surgery > 0.5 / Radiation > 5 **PSADT** < 8 months			Positive **SVI**, Gross **ECE**	clear	*High-Teal, Azure*
High		Any	PSA < 100; any **PSADT**			**N**₁	BS (–)	Any
Royal			>100					Royal = Any rising PSA with a low testosterone and / or any **Mets** outside pelvic nodes
Low	Yes		<10			All scans clear		
Basic		Any	<20	Any	Any	<6 **Mets,** 1 or more outside of pelvic nodes		
High	Yes or No		Any			>5 **Mets** with at least 1 outside pelvic nodes		

Rx = Treatment; **DRE Stage:** Clinical Stage Per Digital Rectal Exam (Chapter 1 Table.); **MP-MRI** = Multiparametic MRI; **CDU** = Color Doppler Ultrasound; **CT** = CAT scan; **ECE** = Extra-Capsular Extension; **"Small"** = < 12 mm; **SVI** = Seminal Vesicle Invasion; **N1** = Pelvic Lymph Node Metastases; **Mets** = Metastases; **PSADT** = PSA Doubling Time; **PET** = C¹¹ Acetate, C¹¹ Choline, Axumin or PSMA Ga⁶⁸; **XRT** = Radiation; **Testo** = Testosterone; **BS** = Bone Scan

APPENDIX III

INTERPRETING LABORATORY BLOOD TESTS

ACH OF THE SIX BLOOD PANELS presented below is a grouping of semirelated tests. Some tests within a specific panel will have greater medical significance than others. For example, in the first panel, the *Metabolic Panel*, glucose, potassium, and creatinine tend to have much greater relevance for patient management than chloride, which often adds little new information. In any case, a brief description of each of these individual blood tests is provided, along with a short explanation about the most common clinical usage. Laboratory medicine is a vast field. These explanations are introductory, not encyclopedic.

The six blood panels are the *Basic Metabolic Panel* (BMP), which focuses on kidney function and electrolytes (blood levels of minerals); the *Hepatic Panel*, which focuses on liver function; the *Lipid Panel*, which includes good and bad cholesterol and triglycerides; the *Thyroid Panel* (self-explanatory); the *Androgen Profile*, which checks testosterone, free testosterone, and pituitary function (which controls testicular function); and the *Complete Blood Count* (CBC), which evaluates immune function via the white blood cell count (WBC) and its subtypes, the granulocytes, lymphocytes and monocytes, as well as the platelets, which participate in coagulation. CBC also includes measurement of the red cells, which transport oxygen. When the red-cell count is low, it is called anemia.

Basic Metabolic Panel (BMP)

Blood glucose (GLU) levels vary before and after meals. It is normal for patients to have "elevated" glucose for several hours after a meal. So, an out-of-normal-range glucose only signals diabetes if flood for the BMP is drawn when the patient is fasting. Patients with diabetes have blood sugar levels that remain persistently elevated, even when the patient is fasting. Since blood glucose can vary quickly in response to food intake, a more accurate measure is a test called "glycohemoglobin," which must be ordered separately since it is not included in the routine panels. *Low levels* of glucose occur in patients on macrobiotic diets and are desirable in prostate cancer patients, because less sugar is available to feed the growing tumor cells. Low levels of glucose in diabetic patients may be indicative of excess medication or insulin. Occasionally, low glucose may be reported if there is a delay in the lab's processing of the blood. If the tube of blood sits a while before being tested, the ongoing metabolic activity of red cells continues in the glass tube, consuming the glucose.

Blood Urea Nitrogen (BUN), elevations can result from dehydration. The more severe the dehydration, the more the BUN increases. BUN is very sensitive, and changes may occur in response to modest stimuli. A modest elevation of BUN does not necessarily signal a need for intervention. The elevation of BUN can also occur with kidney malfunction. When this is the case, there is almost always the simultaneous elevation of creatinine (see below). BUN can also be elevated by a high protein diet. Low BUN levels are of no consequence.

Creatinine (CREA) is a quick and accurate way to measure kidney function. Elevated creatinine indicates some degree of kidney impairment. Changes in creatinine with elevation above a historical baseline (compared to previous tests) needs to be explained. Deterioration of kidney function is potentially serious. Occasionally, severe dehydration elevates creatinine. Minor elevation of creatinine can be seen from aging and is usually not of significance if the minor elevation remains stable. Creatinine levels below the normal range are usually not consequential.

Sodium (Na) is the basic ingredient of standard table salt. The kidneys and adrenal glands regulate its concentration in the blood. Sodium plays an important role in water balance. Drinking too much water, heart failure, or kidney malfunction can cause abnormally low amounts of sodium in the blood. Levels of sodium outside the normal range represent a significant problem that needs evaluation and correction.

Potassium (K) blood levels outside the normal range are of critical significance and can be associated with heart arrhythmias. Low potassium can result from diuretics (water pills) if potassium hasn't been supplemented by taking potassium pills alongside diuretics. High blood levels of potassium can result from kidney disease or from taking too much potassium. Occasionally, the elevation of potassium occurs due to the blood being "traumatized" during phlebotomy (the act of drawing blood). When this is suspected, a repeat blood draw is indicated. Levels of potassium outside the normal range represent a significant problem that needs evaluation and correction. Abnormal chloride (CL) levels usually accompany abnormalities of sodium or potassium. Borderline low or high levels of chloride generally have no significance.

Calcium (Ca) in the blood is tightly regulated by parathyroid hormone and vitamin D. Calcium can be lowered by medications such as Zometa, Xgeva, Actonel, Fosamax, and Provenge. Low levels can also be observed in malnourished patients whose albumin levels are low (albumin is a component of the *Hepatic Panel*). The accuracy of the blood calcium test is enhanced by using a more accurate test, called "ionized calcium." Elevated calcium results from the excess intake of vitamin D or over-active parathyroid glands. A high calcium level can be dangerous and potentially cause sleepiness and heart arrhythmias. Low levels can cause muscle spasms, which typically occur in the hands.

Hepatic Panel (Liver Function Tests)

Transaminases (AST/ALT) are the most sensitive indicators of liver cell irritation or damage. AST and ALT (also known as SGOT and SGPT) can occasionally rise above the normal range due to viral infections or from excess alcohol. Larger degrees of elevation may indicate the toxic effect of medications, viral hepatitis, or the spread of cancer to the liver. AST/ALT elevation can also occur after a heart attack. Low levels of AST/ALT are of no significance,

Bilirubin (TBIL) is a breakdown product of old, used-up red cells. Elevations of bilirubin can occur with bile duct blockage and gallbladder problems. Elevated bilirubin can also occur if the rate of red-cell breakdown is accelerated. A benign syndrome, called Gilbert's disease, is a harmless common disease that causes the mild chronic elevation of bilirubin. (DBIL) is a subfraction of bilirubin. Relative changes of the two forms provide useful diagnostic information that helps to explain some of the different causes of bilirubin elevation.

Alkaline Phosphatase (ALP) is produced by bone and liver. Elevations of ALP can be due to problems originating from the liver, bone, or both. Since ALP can be elevated from bone metastases, tracking elevations and declines may be useful for determining a response to therapy (Chapter 37). Another blood test, called the "Fractionated ALP," can be ordered by your doctor to help determine if the source of elevation originates from liver or bone. Elevations of ALP, especially in conjunction with elevated bilirubin, indicate bile duct blockage. Low ALP levels are not of concern.

Total Protein (TP) is a simple measure of the amount of protein in the blood, including albumin. The non-albumin portion of the blood includes antibodies, which function as a portion of the immune system.

Elevated levels of TP can be seen in immune derangements in which antibodies are overproduced.

Albumin (ALB) acts as a storage reserve for protein. Low albumin levels are reflective of malnutrition, liver disease, or kidney disease. The elevation of albumin is usually of no consequence, though it can occur in the setting of dehydration.

Lipid Panel

Triglyceride (TRIG) is simply another name for fat. The triglyceride levels in the blood vary up and down after meals, somewhat after the fashion that glucose varies throughout the day. Thus, triglyceride levels drawn soon after a meal can be substantially elevated. An elevated *fasting* triglyceride level indicates a higher risk for coronary arteriosclerosis. However, triglyceride levels are not as accurate at predicting arteriosclerosis as cholesterol. In the old days, *total* cholesterol (CHOL) levels over 200 were thought to be indicative of an increased risk for arteriosclerosis. This is true. But LDL and HDL (see below) are much better indicators of arteriosclerosis risk than total cholesterol.

Low Density Lipoprotein (LDL), or, as it is more commonly known, "bad cholesterol," correlates with the risk for developing arteriosclerosis. This is the type of cholesterol that is more likely to stick to the walls of blood vessels and lead to clogging. The American Heart Association recommends that LDL cholesterol should be less than 100 to prevent the deposition of cholesterol on the arterial wall. This is a very conservative threshold. In men with previous coronary problems, cardiologists recommend lowering the LDL to 60. Modern statin drugs such as Lipitor dramatically lower LDL levels in the blood and can lead to a reversal of blood vessel clogging.

High Density Lipoprotein (HDL) cholesterol is called "good cholesterol." Higher levels of HDL protect *against* the development of arteriosclerosis by scavenging excess cholesterol from the walls of the blood vessels. HDL levels can be increased with exercise and, to a smaller degree, by statin medications. Studies show that the higher the level of HDL, the lower the risk for heart disease. Levels of HDL under 40 represent a concern.

Thyroid Panel

Thyroid Stimulating Hormone (TSH) is released into the bloodstream from the pituitary gland, at the base of the brain. TSH arrives at the thyroid gland and stimulates it to increase the production of thyroid hormone. Elevated TSH suggests that the production of the thyroid hormones (called T3 and T4) is inadequate. Low TSH indicates thyroid *overactivity* or that patients who are being treated with thyroid medication are on too much medication.

Androgen Profile

Free Androgen Index (FAI) is calculated by dividing the SHBG level (see below) into the level of testosterone. For example, if testosterone is 200 and the SHBG is 20, the FAI equals 10. An FAI level of 10 or higher indicates a normal amount of *free* testosterone in a young man. FAI levels normally decline with age. FAI is a better indicator of male hormone activity than the total testosterone level.

Sex Hormone Binding Globulin (SHBG) tightly binds testosterone and renders it inactive. Therefore, the *total* testosterone, much of which is bound to SHBG, is a rather poor indicator of the true testosterone activity.

Testosterone (TEST) is the predominate male hormone. It normally declines with age. The side effects of low testosterone are described in detail in Chapter 30. Testosterone drops to low levels (<50) with hormonal treatments such as Lupron. Normal levels range between 250 and 1,000.

Luteinizing Hormone (LH) and Follicle Stimulating Hormone (FSH) are hormones released from the pituitary gland that stimulate the testicles to produce testosterone. Medications such as Lupron and Zoladex block the testicular production of testosterone by fooling the pituitary into lowering its output of LH. When hormone blockade is stopped, LH and FSH levels increase and spur increased testosterone production by the testicles.

Complete Blood Count (CBC)

The CBC contains several blood tests of importance. Anemia is a relative reduction of red cells in the blood compared to normal levels. It results in a decrease in the oxygen-carrying capacity of the blood. Severe anemia can be felt as tiredness and shortness of breath. Anemia is measured by three factors in the CBC: hematocrit (HCT), hemoglobin (HGB), and red blood count (RBC). An HCT level less than 40 in men is abnormal. Symptoms of tiredness and shortness of breath do not usually occur, however, until the HCT declines to around 32, though there are occasional exceptions. A severely low HCT is treatable with medications or transfusion. The most common reason for mild to moderate anemia in prostate cancer patients is low testosterone from hormonal blockade.

The other important measures in the CBC take on greater significance in patients receiving chemotherapy. Chemotherapy can reduce the platelet count (PLT) and white blood count (WBC). Platelets help the blood clot normally. Severe lowering of the platelets from chemotherapy alone is uncommon. However, extensive infiltration of the bone by cancer or extensive amounts of previous radiation to the bone are both potential contributors to a low platelet count. The white blood cells comprise a significant portion of the immune system. The WBC is broken down into granulocytes (GRAN), lymphocytes (LYM), and monocytes (Mon). Elevated granulocytes is indicative of an underlying bacterial infection or treatment with an immune-stimulating drug, such as Neulasta, which is used to counteract the effects of chemotherapy. Viral infections can cause low lymphocyte counts and high monocyte counts. MCV, MCH, and MCHC are measures of red cell dimensions. Low MCV can be seen in iron deficiency. It also occurs in an inherited congenital anemia called "thalassemia." High MCV can be a sign of liver disease or B12 deficiency. The elevation of RDW, a measure of red cell size variability, can be an early sign of iron deficiency. Abnormalities of MCH and MCHC are rarely consequential.

Important Individual Blood Tests

Regular blood testing in patients with active cancer, and annual testing in otherwise healthy men, provides important information about a patient's status. In addition to the above panels, it is prudent to test for vitamin D and vitamin B12 levels. These are discussed in Chapter 49. Deficiencies of these may show up as fatigue, which may be overlooked in an active cancer patient who may already be fatigued due to the side effects of treatment.

APPENDIX IV
AUTHOR BIOGRAPHIES

Fabio Almeida, MD graduated at the top of his class and with honors from Chicago Medical School. He completed a residency and fellowship in nuclear medicine at the University of San Francisco, and is certified by the American Board of Nuclear Medicine and the Certification Board of Nuclear Cardiology. He was in academic practice at the University of California, San Francisco, and was in private practice until 2005. Dr. Almeida is one of the pioneers in the development and implementation of cross modality fusion for cancer imaging (SPECT, PET, CT and MRI). He also worked for the Centers for Disease Control and Prevention after 9/11 for several years as a physician and informatics specialist consultant. He currently serves as the medical director of Phoenix Molecular Imaging.

Duke Bahn, MD is the director of the Prostate Institute of America. Certified by the American Board of Radiology, he specializes in the early detection and staging of prostate cancer using color Doppler ultrasound with tissue harmonics. He is also a pioneer in using cryotherapy, as both a primary and salvage treatment for prostate cancer. His published data was the impetus for obtaining Medicare approval for cryotherapy as a viable treatment for prostate cancer. Dr. Bahn has held many academic and professional appointments, including clinical professor of urology at the Keck School of Medicine, University of Southern California.

John Blasko, MD is the former director of clinical research for the Seattle Prostate Institute and a clinical professor in the Department of Radiation Oncology at the University of Washington School of Medicine. A member of the board of directors of the American Brachytherapy Association, Dr. Blasko has published several hundred articles, abstracts, and book chapters about radioactive seeding. He received his medical degree from the University of Maryland School of Medicine and served his residency at the University of Washington School of Medicine.

Ralph Blum was a cultural anthropologist and author. He graduated Phi Beta Kappa from Harvard University with a degree in Russian Studies. He reported from the Soviet Union, a first for *The New Yorker*, consisting of a series on Russian cultural life. He wrote for various magazines, among them *Reader's Digest, Cosmopolitan,* and *Vogue.* Blum published three novels and five nonfiction books. He coauthored of *Invasion of the Prostate Snatchers*, an exposé about the use of overaggressive treatment for prostate cancer in the United States.

Stanley Brosman, MD is board-certified in urology. He is the former chief of urology at UCLA/Harbor General Hospital, a clinical professor of surgery/urology at UCLA, and associate director of urologic oncology at the John Wayne Cancer Institute. Dr. Brosman is past president of the urology section of the California Medical Society and past president of the Los Angeles Urologic Society. He is the author or coauthor of more than 80 peer-reviewed scientific articles and over 50 book chapters or monographs. He practices urology with a focus on prostate cancer in Santa Monica, California, at the Pacific Urology Institute.

Kelly Chiles, MD, is an assistant professor of urology specializing in all areas of male sexual and reproductive medicine, as well as an experienced urologic microsurgeon. Dr. Chiles received her bachelor's degree in microbiology from Pennsylvania State University and her master's degree in biotechnology from Johns Hopkins University. After completing medical school at Penn State, she went on to complete her internship and residency at the University of Connecticut. Dr. Chiles completed an intensive two-year fellowship in male sexual and reproductive medicine at Weill Cornell Medical College and Memorial Sloan Kettering Cancer Center prior to joining The GW Medical Faculty Associates.

D. Jeffrey Demanes, MD received his bachelor of arts degree from UC Berkeley and his medical degree from the David Geffen School of Medicine at UCLA. He completed residencies in internal medicine and radiation oncology at UCLA and his medical oncology fellowship at UC San Francisco. He is the past chairman and president of the American College of Radiation Oncology. Dr. Demanes specializes in brachytherapy, the surgical subspecialty of radiation oncology. He founded the California Endo Curietherapy Center (CET) in 1981 and has performed more than 10,000 surgical radiation implants. He is a professor emeritus in the department of radiation therapy at UCLA.

Jonathan Epstein, MD received his doctorate from Boston University. He completed his residency in anatomic pathology at Johns Hopkins Hospital and a fellowship in oncologic pathology at Memorial Sloan Kettering Cancer Center in New York. He then joined the staff at The Johns Hopkins Hospital as professor of pathology, urology, and oncology, where he was named the Reinhard Chair of Urological Pathology and Director of Surgical Pathology. He is the past president of the International Society of Urological Pathology. Dr. Epstein has 744 publications in peer-reviewed literature and has authored 50 book chapters with an H-factor of 118, an indication of the influential and far-reaching impact of his work. His most-frequently-cited first- or last-authored publication is "Pathological and Clinical Findings to Predict Tumor Extent of Nonpalpable (stage T1c) Prostate Cancer," published in *JAMA*. The study establishes the criteria for active surveillance.

Peter Grimm, DO was a radiation oncologist in Seattle, affiliated with Swedish Medical Center-Cherry Hill. He received his medical degree from Chicago College of Osteopathic Medicine and was adjunct assistant professor of radiation oncology at the UCLA Department of Radiation Oncology. Dr. Grimm practiced for 36 years as a seed implant expert. He received various awards, including an American Cancer Society Fellowship and the President's Award from the American Brachytherapy Society. He held at least six patents related to radioactive seed implantation and authored or coauthored more than 60 peer-review publications. Dr. Grimm also created a popular prostate cancer educational website that provides comparative outcomes for many types of treatment: pctrf.org.

Laurence Klotz, MD is the past chief of urology at Sunnybrook Health Sciences Centre and professor of surgery at the University of Toronto. He is also chairman of the World Uro-Oncology Federation and a past president of the Urological Research Society and the Canadian Urological Association. Dr. Klotz was the founding editor-in-chief of both the *Canadian Journal of Urology* and the *Canadian Urology Association Journal*, and is now editor emeritus of the *CUAJ*. He was the founder and is chairman of the Canadian Urology Research Consortium. Dr. Klotz obtained his medical degree from the University of Toronto and completed his residency at the University of Toronto's Gallie Program in Surgery. Dr. Klotz continued his postgraduate studies with a special fellowship in uro-oncology and tumor biology at Memorial Sloan Kettering Cancer Center in New York. Dr. Klotz is a widely published uro-oncologist with over 300 publications and four books. His main research interest is prostate cancer. He serves on the boards of many medical/scientific organizations and journals, including the SUO and Prostate Cancer Canada, and the journals *Prostate Cancer and Prostatic Diseases, Brazilian Journal of Urology, Italian Journal of Urology,* and *World Journal of Urology*. He was recently awarded the Queen's Jubilee Medal for meritorious public service.

Richard Lam, MD has been a board-certified internist and oncologist specializing in prostate cancer since 2001. He is director of clinical research at Prostate Oncology Specialists, Inc. Dr. Lam has written numerous articles based on his research. He received his undergraduate degree in biology, magna cum laude, at UCLA. He then went on to earn his medical degree at the David Geffen School of Medicine at UCLA before completing his residency training in the specialty of internal medicine at the UCLA Center of Health Sciences. He completed his oncology and hematology fellowship at Harbor-UCLA Medical Center.

Gary Leach, MD is former chief of the Department of Urology and director of the Urodynamics Laboratory at Kaiser Los Angeles Medical Center. He completed his medical training at Wayne State University, in Detroit, Michigan. Dr. Leach is the past president of the Los Angeles Urologic Society and past president of the Urodynamic Society, whose members specialize in the diagnosis and treatment of incontinence. He has written many scientific articles and has contributed to several definitive textbooks on incontinence. In addition, he serves as a member of the Multiple Sclerosis Society Advisory Board. Dr. Leach has written over 100 scientific articles related to urology.

Sean McBride, MD, is a board-certified radiation oncologist with an expertise in treating primary genitourinary (prostate, bladder, kidney, and testicular) and head and neck (oral cavity, base of tongue, tonsil, larynx, hypopharynx, sinus, nasopharynx, and thyroid) malignancies. Dr. McBride works with a dedicated team of medical oncologists, surgeons, and medical physicists to help deliver individualized care using sophisticated radiation therapy techniques, including image-guided, stereotactic radiosurgery (IGRT), intensity-modulated radiation therapy (IMRT), and brachytherapy.

Daniel Margolis, MD earned his bachelor's degree from UC Berkeley and his MD from USC, followed by an internship in internal medicine at VA West Los Angeles Medical Center. He completed his residency in diagnostic radiology at UCLA, and a prestigious fellowship funded by the National Cancer Institute at Stanford University. He was an associate clinical professor at the David Geffen School of Medicine at UCLA until 2016 and is now an associate professor of radiology and the director of prostate MRI at Weill Cornell Medical College. He has authored or coauthored over 60 peer-reviewed scientific articles.

Mark Moyad, MD, is arguably the world's leading medical expert on diet and dietary supplements. He is the Jenkins/Pokempner Director of Complementary and Alternative Medicine at the University of Michigan Medical Center-Department of Urology. He graduated from the University of South Florida College of Public Health and the Wayne State University School of Medicine. He is the primary author of over 150 published medical journal articles and the past editor-in-chief of the medical journal *Seminars in Preventive & Alternative Medicine,* and he has given over 5,000 lectures around the world to the public and healthcare professionals in virtually every medical specialty and major medical center. He is coauthor or author of 14 academic and consumer books, including *The Supplement Handbook: A Trusted Expert's Guide to What Works & What's Worthless for More Than 100 Conditions.* He has been a consultant for and/or interviewed by most of the major magazines, websites, and radio and television shows devoted to health in the US, and appears regularly on a variety of network news and feature programs.

John Mulhall, MD is director of both the Male Sexual and Reproductive Medicine Program and the Sexual Medicine Research Laboratory at Memorial Sloan Kettering Cancer Center. In addition, he is professor of urology in the Department of Urology at Weill Cornell Medical College. Professor Mulhall has had more than 250 papers published in peer-reviewed journals, and has published numerous books, such as *Contemporary Management of Urologic Emergencies* (1999*), Sexual Function in the Prostate Cancer Patient* (2009), and *Saving Your Sex Life: A Guide for Men with Prostate Cancer* (2008). He has contributed in excess of 30 book chapters and has also edited textbooks, such as *Cancer and Sexual Health*

(2011) and *Fertility Preservation in Male Cancer Patients* (2012). Professor Mulhall has been editor-in-chief of *Current Sexual Health Reports* (2003–2008) and an associate editor of reviews for *Urology* (2006–2010). He is currently editor-in-chief for the *Journal of Sexual Medicine*. Professor Mulhall is the recipient of numerous awards, including the Career Development Award from the VA (1998), the Robert P. Nelson Award from the Sexual Medicine Society of North America (2001), and the Young Investigator Award (2000) and the Jean Francois Ginestie Award (2002) from the International Society for Sexual Medicine. In 2005, he was honored with the Gold Cystoscope Award from the American Urological Association.

Luke Nordquist, MD is board certified in internal medicine and medical oncology. He completed his oncology fellowship at Memorial Sloan Kettering Cancer Center and his residency in internal medicine at the University of South Florida/H. Lee Moffitt Cancer Center. He also has a bachelor's degree in pharmacy from Creighton University. Dr. Nordquist was selected by the American Society of Clinical Oncology (ASCO) to sit on its Government Relations Committee, representing the interests of cancer physicians and patients on Capitol Hill. This influential committee is made up of 19 oncologists who are current ASCO leaders and several previous ASCO presidents. He is an expert panel member for the development of National Prostate Cancer Treatment Guidelines, and a selected CALGB member for the design of new research studies for prostate and urologic cancers across the nation.

Christopher Rose, MD, is a board-certified radiation oncologist. He received his bachelor's degree from Massachusetts Institute of Technology and his doctorate from Harvard Medical School. His residency in radiation oncology was at the Harvard Joint Center for Radiation Therapy. Dr. Rose was a visiting clinical scientist at the Institute for Cancer Research, Royal Marsden Hospital, University of London, in Great Britain. He was an assistant professor of radiation oncology at Harvard Medical School, and chairman of the board of directors and president of the

American Society of Therapeutic Radiology and Oncology (ASTRO). He is past president of the Council of Affiliated Regional Radiation Oncology Societies of the American College of Radiology, past president of the California Radiation Oncology Society, and counselor of the American College of Radiology. He is currently a member of the Medicare Coverage Advisory Commission and vice chair of the NCI-sponsored Quality Research in Radiation Oncology Study. Dr. Rose has published more than 50 peer-reviewed articles. He received the Donald Coffey Clinician Scientist Award from the PCF. He is the 2008 Gold Medalist of ASTRO. Dr. Rose currently serves as chief clinical officer of radiation oncology at McKesson Specialty Health.

Carl Rossi, MD is a radiation oncologist specializing in proton beam therapy, specifically for prostate cancer and lymphomas. He is also the current medical director for the Scripps Proton Therapy Center, which provides treatment to target tumors with high control and precision. In addition to treating a variety of cancers with radiation, the center also treats some noncancerous conditions. Dr. Rossi has a research focus on the quality of life and cure rate in prostate cancer and lymphoma treated with proton beam radiation.

Howard Sandler, MD graduated from the University of Connecticut summa cum laude, where he also received his MD and master's degree in physics. He is the Newman Family Professor of Radiation Oncology at Cedars-Sinai Medical Center and chair of Ronald H. Bloom Family Chair Cancer Therapeutics. He is the principal investigator for a national Radiation Therapy Oncology Group study examining radiotherapy and chemotherapy for prostate cancer. He is coauthor of more than 200 peer-reviewed scientific articles.

Mark Scholz, MD is the medical director of Prostate Oncology Specialists, Inc. He is also the executive director of the Prostate Cancer Research Institute. He received his medical degree from Creighton University, in Omaha, Nebraska. Dr. Scholz completed his internal medicine residency and medical oncology fellowship at the University of Southern California Medical Center. He is coauthor of *Invasion of the Prostate Snatchers*. He has authored over 20 scientific publications related to the treatment of prostate cancer.

Peter Scholz is the creative director of the Prostate Cancer Research Institute (PCRI). He received his BA in English literature from the University of California, Los Angeles. In addition to branding, design, and media production for the organization, his interests at PCRI are in simplifying, curating, and presenting prostate cancer information in ways that are understandable and accessible to patients.

Michael Steinberg, MD is Professor and Chair of the Department of Radiation Oncology at the David Geffen School of Medicine at UCLA. Dr. Steinberg currently serves as Director of Clinical Affairs for the Jonsson Comprehensive Cancer Center at UCLA. He served as the PI for a National Cancer Institute Cancer Disparity Research and as a manuscript author at the RAND Corporation. He is the founding Chair of the Health Policy Council of American Society for Radiation Oncology (ASTRO) and past President and Chairman of the Board of ASTRO. He previously served for the AMA CPT Editorial Panel and the Medicare Evidence and Coverage Advisory Committee. He is also Chair of the IT Steering Committee for UCLA Health Sciences. Dr. Steinberg is Chair of the Clinical Chairs in the David Geffen School of Medicine and currently serves on the Governing Group of the UCLA Health System. Dr. Steinberg graduated Occidental College Phi Beta Kappa, was elected to AOA at University of Southern California School of Medicine and did his radiation oncology residency and fellowship at UCLA.

Jeffrey Turner, MD is a board-certified internist and medical oncologist specializing full time in prostate cancer since 2009. Dr. Turner is an active member of the American Society of Clinical Oncology, American Society of Hematology, and American College of Physicians-Internal

Medicine. He was a research associate at UCLA in infectious diseases and molecular biology. He then earned his medical degree in Canada, at Memorial University of Newfoundland. He completed his internal medicine residency at the University of British Columbia and his fellowship in medical oncology at the Medical University of South Carolina.

Verne Varona has become an internationally renowned keynote speaker with a captivating style that uses humor, insight, and practical science to improve and enrich the lives of many. He studied traditional Chinese medicine and nutrition at the East West Foundation of Boston, Massachusetts. With a physician associate, Verne cocreated The ODDS Program (Off Dangerous Drugs Safely), a dietary program designed to reverse pharmaceutical drug dependency. He is the author of *Nature's Cancer-Fighting Foods*. Varona's second book, *Macrobiotics for Dummies*, part of the internationally popular *For Dummies* series, is a comprehensive work that embraces a flexible, multicultural health perspective on body, mind, and spirit.

Timothy Wilson, MD is a board-certified urologist who specializes in minimally invasive, laparoscopic, and robotic-assisted urologic oncology. He is one of the top six surgeons in the world, in terms of the number of operations performed using robotic-assisted laparoscopic techniques. Dr. Wilson is a member of the American Urological Association and the Society of Urologic Oncology. Throughout his tenure, which spans nearly 30 years, he has published numerous peer-reviewed articles and book chapters in the areas of urologic oncology, urinary reconstruction, and robotic surgery. In 1995, *Los Angeles Magazine* deemed him one of 25 "Doctors Who Are Making a Difference," and in 1998, he was voted Professor of the Year by urology residents in training at the University of Southern California School of Medicine.

Henry Yampolsky, MD is a board-certified radiation oncologist practicing at The Center for Radiation Therapy of Beverly Hills. He completed his radiation oncology specialty training at the University of Southern

California/Norris Cancer Center and LAC+USC Medical Center. While at USC, Dr. Yampolsky acquired broad clinical expertise in the treatment of a wide range of cancers, as well as extensive experience with intensity-modulated radiation therapy (IMRT), stereotactic radiotherapy, and gynecologic brachytherapy.

Michael Zelefsky, MD is chief of Memorial Sloan Kettering's Brachytherapy Service. He was instrumental in pioneering the use of IMRT and IGRT for prostate cancer. Dr. Zelefsky is editor-in-chief of *Brachytherapy,* chairman of the National Patterns of Care Study for Genitourinary Cancers, and past president of the American Brachytherapy Society. He has received several awards, including the Boyer Award for Excellence in Clinical Research, the Outstanding Teaching Award in the Department of Radiation Oncology at Memorial Sloan Kettering, the 2009 Henschke Medal, and the 2009 Emanuel Van Descheuren Award for Excellence in Translational Research.

Zachary Zumsteg, MD completed his residency at Memorial Sloan Kettering Cancer Center and is presently a faculty member in the Department of Radiation Oncology at Cedars-Sinai Samuel Oschin Comprehensive Cancer Institute. In addition to his clinical practice, he is actively engaged in research spanning epidemiology, health services, clinical trials, and translational applications. Through this work, Dr. Zumsteg has developed a novel risk-stratification system for patients with intermediate risk prostate cancer that is widely used by oncologists in clinical practice and cited in National Comprehensive Cancer Network Guidelines. He is the author of numerous peer-reviewed publications, with articles appearing in journals such as *Lancet Oncology, Journal of Clinical Oncology, JAMA Oncology, European Urology, Clinical Cancer Research, Cancer,* and the *International Journal of Radiation Oncology, Biology, Physics.*

APPENDIX V

GLOSSARY

Ablation—Removal or destruction of a harmful growth, or any diseased part of the body, for medical reasons. It usually means getting rid of something altogether, rather than just reducing or mitigating a cancer or other diseased area. Cryoablation is ablating via freezing.

Abscobal Effect—Radiation-induced immune stimulation, whereby the immune system's killer T-cells can be enhanced via focused, high-dose radiation aimed at a single metastasis. As the cancer cells die, they release molecules into the bloodstream. These molecules can be detected by the T-cells, which can then use them to detect and attack other healthy cancer cells throughout the body (which contain the same kinds of molecules).

Active Surveillance—Also known as observation, active surveillance is the process of monitoring the cancer without any immediate medical intervention. Used mostly with *Low-Risk (Sky)* prostate cancer.

Adjuvant–Cancer treatment given right after the primary treatment, to increase the chances that cancer won't return. Sometimes called "adjunct" therapy or treatment, it enhances the effectiveness of the initial treatment. For example, after radical prostatectomy, a patient might be given adjuvant testosterone inhibiting drugs, even though there is no visible sign that any cancer remains.

Androgen Deprivation Therapy—"Androgen" refers to a male sex hormone, such as testosterone. See Testosterone Inactivating Pharmaceuticals.

Angiogenesis—The process of forming new blood vessels. As related to cancer, tumors need angiogenesis to occur in order to form new blood vessels that feed and provide oxygen to a tumor so the tumor can grow and spread, or metastasize. Thus, some cancer medications are designed as angiogenesis inhibitors. (In treating other conditions, such as heart disease, bone fractures, and even baldness, however, angiogenesis is encouraged, as more blood vessels are needed to provide extra nutrients and oxygen to appropriate tissue.)

Anterior—Situated toward the front of the body; opposite of posterior. The anterior prostate is typically undersampled during diagnostic biopsies.

Apex—Normally means the top of something; however, in prostate gland terminology, the apex is located at the lower portion of the gland. The prostatic apex is often undersampled by random biopsy. The *base* of the prostate is located at the top of the gland.

Assay—Medical term for a test to see what a substance is made of or what foreign substances it contains; a test that evaluates the purity or impurity of a substance or the activity of one part of a substance. An assay compares a sample and a control. One *genetic* assay tests for approximately 70 of the most common mutations seen in various cancers, including prostate cancer.

Bind—To form a weak, reversible chemical bond. Sometimes the binding of drugs to a receptor prevents another agent from attaching: "Both Casodex and Nilutamide bind the androgen receptor, blocking the activity of testosterone, thus inhibiting cancer cell growth."

Biopsy—Cancer is diagnosed by a biopsy, in which samples of prostate gland tissue are extracted and examined. Most common today is the 12-core *random* biopsy (a biopsy in which the samples are retrieved from random parts of the prostate gland). Because doctors do this type of random biopsy any time PSA is slightly elevated, over a million men are biopsied every year. This outmoded approach is no longer needed. *Targeted* biopsies are now made possible by new technology that allows the doctor to retrieve samples from the area in which cancer is almost certainly present, thus producing a more accurate (and oftentimes, for the patient, a less invasive) result.

Blood Tests—Blood tests diagnose and monitor disease. They may also detect treatment-related side effects or organ malfunction due to progressive cancer. Blood tests are an alphabet soup of initials! The most commonly performed blood tests are the CBC (Complete Blood Count), the BMP (Basic Metabolic Panel), and the Hepatic Panel. Several other blood tests are used to monitor prostate cancer, the most familiar being the PSA test. Appendix III explains blood tests in detail.

Bone Matrix—The part of the bone that makes it rigid. The matrix comprises about 30 percent of the bone, and is made of collagen, calcium, and a gel-like substance that cements it all together. Some cancer medications target bone matrix, hardening it in order to limit the access of cancer cells to substances found in the bone matrix that encourage cancer growth.

Bone Scan—Uses radioactive material to scan for cancer in the bones. Lymph nodes and bones are the most common sites of metastatic spread. However, bone scans can also indicate arthritis or other benign lesions that might be mistaken for cancer. When ambiguity persists after a bone scan, an MRI of the bone can give greater detail and help differentiate cancer-related abnormalities from benign ones.

Brachytherapy—See Radioactive Seed Implantation.

BRCA—A genetic mutation that can indicate a predisposition to various cancers, including breast, ovarian and prostate cancer.

Capsule—The outer boundary of the prostate gland. Extra-capsular means outside the prostate gland. This term is used when talking about the spread of cancer beyond the prostate gland. Typically, the term "extra-capsular" is reserved for cancer just outside the capsule. The term "metastases" is used for cancer in more distant areas of the body, such as the lymph nodes or bone.

Cancer—Disease characterized by abnormal, uncontrolled cell growth (which creates a tumor) and the ability of these cancerous cells to move away from the initial site and spread to other parts of the body (metastasize). Cancer cells are not as good at repairing themselves from radiation damage, so radiation is often used to damage and fight them. Cancer results from specific misbehaving genes; the genes that promote cell growth, for example, become locked in the "on" position due to a mutation in the gene.

Chemotherapy—Often shortened to "chemo" in speech. A type of systemic, whole-body treatment in which chemicals are injected into the bloodstream and circulate throughout the body to fight cancer cells.

Climacturia—Involuntary urination at the moment of orgasm. Although the exact mechanism of climacturia has not been well studied, men who have climacturia usually have urinary incontinence as well.

Clinical Stage—Not to be confused with pathologic stage. After determining the results of the digital rectal examination, the doctor records his findings—the size and extent of a prostate nodule, if a nodule is present—with a systematic lettering system that is described in Chapter 1. Also see Stage and Five Stages of Blue.

Clinical Trials—These are experimental trials of new drugs to treat cancer or other disease. Only certain patients will be eligible for clinical trials, and not all eligible patients will ultimately decide to participate. There are three types ("phases") of clinical trials, with pros and cons for participating in each.

Color Doppler Ultrasound (CDU)—An alternative type of high-resolution imaging used for the diagnosis and staging of prostate cancer. This is only available in a few centers around the US.

Combination Therapy—When a local treatment is combined with a systemic therapy, or if multiple systemic treatments are used at the same time, it is called combination therapy.

Cryoablation—See Ablation and Cryosurgery.

Cryosurgery—Also called Cryoablation, or Cryo for short. Usually a focal treatment in which the tumor is frozen to eradicate cancer. Sometimes cyroablation of the whole prostate is done, though this is less popular, as erectile dysfunction invariably occurs.

Computed Tomography (CT) Scan—Uses Xray technology to create a 3D anatomical image by rotating the Xray beam around the patient's body. It is used to detect tumors, measure them, and locate them. It can also be used to monitor the effectiveness of cancer treatment.

CyberKnife—A robotic radiosurgery system that was the original platform used to deliver SBRT. It is still the most commonly used form of SBRT. The "knife" in CyberKnife is actually radiation; it does not involve cutting. See Stereotactic Beam Radiation Therapy (SBRT).

Digital Rectal Examination (DRE)—In DRE, the doctor examines the patient's prostate gland by placing his finger inside the patient's rectum and feeling the prostate with his or her finger (digit) to check for prostate irregularities. Tumor size is the estimated size of an abnormality (termed a "nodule") that is felt by the doctor's finger. This is a useful first step in diagnosing and staging prostate cancer, but it provides information that is less precise than what can be obtained from a scan or a biopsy.

DRE—See Digital Rectal Examination.

EBRT—See External Beam Radiation Therapy.

Erectile Dysfunction (ED)—A risk of variable degree associated with every type of prostate cancer treatment, though not an inevitability in all treatments. ED varies in accordance with the type of treatment selected and physician skill.

External Beam Radiation Therapy (EBRT)—Radiation treatment in which radioactive beams target the whole prostate gland (and sometimes the adjacent lymph node area) in order to eradicate the cancer.

Extra-Capsular Extension (ECE)—See Capsule.

Five Stages of Blue—is a comprehensive system for allocating men with prostate cancer into separate categories, each of which can be further divided into three subtypes. Optimal treatment for prostate cancer varies widely depending on the Stage of Blue and the subtype. See Appendixes I and II for a summary of the Stages of Blue.

Focal Cryosurgery—See Cryosurgery.

Focal Treatments—A type of local treatment that treats only a subsection of the prostate gland, namely, the area where the cancer is located. This avoids complete removal of the entire prostate gland, thus sparing much of the surrounding normal tissue from unnecessary damage. Local and focal options, when administered by accomplished experts, eliminate the cancer in the gland with a reasonably high degree of consistency and are usually associated with a lower incidence of sexual, urinary, and rectal side effects compared with traditional radiation and surgery.

Foley Catheter (or simply "catheter")—A flexible tube inserted into the bladder through which urine can escape past a blockage in the prostate.

Gene—Genes control a person's inherited physical characteristics such as sex, eye color, height, etc. They are the reason your baby has your eyes, your wife's chin, and your great-grandfather's red hair. Because genes also control cell reproduction and growth, they play an important role in the field of oncology. Some genetic mutations (changes or corruption of the gene) cause cancer, which is uncontrolled cell growth. Genes that control cellular growth, for example, can get locked in the "on" position through a mutation. There are 25,000 to 35,000 genes *in each cell* in the human body! It's no wonder that a gene is mutated every so often; it's more of a wonder that the body reproduces so many genes so faithfully over and over again. Bad genes (mutated ones) can often be identified by genetic testing. This technology is an important new focus in oncology and is being studied intensively, so anything you read now may have already been improved upon by the time this book makes its way into your hands.

Gleason Score (Grade)—A number or grade assigned to cancer cells by a pathologist who examines biopsy samples under a microscope. The Gleason grade indicates how normal or abnormal the cells look on a 1-to-5 scale. Because prostate cancers in a single patient often have different grades, the grades are added together to come up with a score.

High-Dose-Rate Brachytherapy (HDR)—Also known as Temporary Seeds. See Radioactive Seed Implantation.

HIFU—High Intensity Focused Ultrasound—Equipment that transmits a destructive dose of focal treatment across the rectum into the prostate. It is used more commonly for *focal* therapy than for *whole-gland* ablation.

Hormonal Therapy—A type of systemic, whole-body treatment in which a hormone, usually testosterone, is manipulated in order to fight cancer cells. See also Testosterone Inactivating Pharmaceuticals (TIP).

Hormone-resistant Cancer—A type of cancer that can grow and thrive despite ongoing treatment with hormonal therapy. Hormone-resistant cancer needs to be fought aggressively as soon as it is detected, because it can grow exponentially.

IGRT—Image-guided radiation therapy. Most types of beam radiation—IMRT, SBRT, and proton therapy—use advanced targeting methods, sometimes requiring the implantation of a fiducial marker into the prostate gland, making it easier to accurately target the prostate gland.

Immunotherapy—A type of systemic, whole-body therapy that harnesses your body's immune system (T-cells) to fight cancer. One example is Provenge. The immune system can also be stimulated by radiation. (See Abscobal Effect.) At present, the field of immune therapy is advancing more quickly than any other area of cancer therapy.

IMPT—A recent advance in Proton Therapy, IMPT stands for *Intensity Modulated* Proton Technology.

IMRT—see Intensity Modulated Radiotherapy.

Incontinence—Loss of bladder control.

Intensity Modulated Radiotherapy (IMRT)—A type of External Beam Radiation Therapy (EBRT).

Intermittent Therapy—The intermittent use of TIP, especially for men with *Indigo*, but also used for *Royal*. A typical intermittent protocol consists of TIP administered for six to nine months followed by a treatment "holiday." After TIP is stopped, testosterone levels recover back to normal, thus relieving the patient of most of the negative side effects from low testosterone. However, since the PSA will also begin to rise when TIP is stopped, a second cycle of TIP is started when the PSA rises back to its original PSA baseline, or up into the 3-to-6 range, whichever is lower.

LDR—Low-dose-rate, a type of brachytherapy, also known as *permanent* seeds. See Radioactive Seed Implantation.

Lesion—A change in tissue caused by disease, like cancer, or a wound or injury.

Leukapheresis—A procedure that filters out a portion of the patient's white blood cells from the bloodstream in a process similar to dialysis.

Local Treatments—Treatments that focus on removing or eradicating cancerous tissue in the prostate gland. Examples are surgery (radical prostatectomy), radioactive seed implantation, varieties of external beam radiation therapy (IMRT, proton therapy, CyberKnife), and cryosurgery. Focal Treatment is another type of local treatment. Local and focal options, when administered by accomplished experts, eliminate the cancer in the gland with a reasonably high degree of consistency.

Lymph Nodes—Part of the body's immune system, the lymph nodes are small glands in various parts of the body, all linked by vessels that carry fluids and nutrients, and that get rid of waste material. You may have noticed that, when you have a bad sore throat, sometimes your lymph nodes are swollen. That's because they are filled with white blood cells to fight a bacterial or viral infection. Lymph nodes can also be "infected" with cancer, and cancer has the potential to spread through the lymph system.

Lymphocytes—A type of WBC that fights viruses and cancers. There are various subtypes of lymphocytes, such as the natural killer T-cells, which attack cancer directly; the dendritic cells, which detect and direct immune activity; and the regulatory cells, which guard against immune over activity, the so called "TRegs."

Median—If you were paying attention in math class, you may have learned that median is not the same as average. Instead, it is the *middle* number in a list of numbers ranked in order. For example, if you have the numbers 2, 3, 5, 8, 10, 27, 28, 41, 42, the *median* number is 10. However, if you know how to take the *average* of a group of numbers, you will recall that all the numbers are totaled, and the total is divided by the tally of the individual numbers, in this case 9. So, the *average* of these same numbers is *18,* which is different from the median. Median is used more often than average in medical statistics, because if the extreme numbers (in this case 41 and 42) were averaged into the equation, they would skew the results and possibly make them less representative of the majority of the numbers in the group.

Metastatic Prostate Cancer—Cancer that has spread beyond the prostate to a lymph node or bone, for example. Extra-Capsular prostate cancer is not considered metastatic, even though it is outside the gland. In its initial stages, metastatic disease is *microscopic*, and thus undetectable. After a period of time, once the metastases (sometimes called "mets" in medical lingo) increase in size, they become large enough to be detected on a scan. Men with either microscopic or visible metastases require *systemic* treatment that circulates through the blood and treats cancer throughout the whole body. See also Oligometastases.

MP-MRI—See Multiparametric MRI.

MRI—**Magnetic Resonance Imaging,** a type of body scan in which a strong magnetic field interacts with radio waves to create a highly detailed image. Because of the magnetic field, patients with metal implants will need to make sure the MRI technician knows about the implant, and special precautions might be necessary. Since MRIs don't use Xrays they are often considered to be safer. (See also 3-Tesla Multiparametric MRI, Multiparametric MRI.)

Multiparametric MRI (MP-MRI)—A highly specialized type of MRI that provides accurate images of the gland that can determine the absence or presence of prostate cancer, and sometimes determine if the cancer is spreading through the capsule or invading outside the gland into the seminal vesicles. Accurate results require optimal equipment, well-trained technicians, and experienced radiologists.

Mutation—See Gene.

Nadir—The lowest point. The PSA nadir is when the PSA arrives at its lowest point and thereafter stops dropping. A nadir of less than 0.1 is an important indication that TIP can be used as an effective long-term therapy. It is also an important measure for determining the effectiveness of other therapies.

Observation—See Active Surveillance.

Occult—Has nothing to do with the supernatural! Used in medical terminology, occult means "hidden," something that can't be detected easily. For example, "Men with *larger quantities of Gleason*

6 are known to be at higher risk of harboring occult, higher-grade cancer that may have been missed on the random biopsy."

Oligometastatic Disease—Early-stage metastatic cancer with relatively few metastases, usually less than five. Some cases of oligometastatic cancer are curable, but it is difficult to determine in advance which cases are curable. Treatment can consist of radiation therapy or surgery, sometimes combined with hormone therapy.

Oncologist—A doctor who is a cancer specialist. A prostate oncologist specializes in prostate cancer.

Pathologist—A specialized physician with many years of training in the study and diagnosis of specimens removed by surgery, needle biopsy, or other tests. The pathologist prepares the pathology report, which is sent to your doctor.

Pathology—Pathology is the study of disease, especially focusing on the causes of disease or changes in the body caused by disease.

Pathology Report—Explains the implications and the microscopic appearance of tissues removed from the body by either a needle biopsy or by surgery. The pathology report helps your doctor understand the extent of the disease in the prostate as well as the disease's aggressiveness.

Pathologic Stage—Uses a lettering and numbering system that looks quite similar to the system used for Clinical Stage that is described in Chapter 1. Despite these similarities, pathologic stage has nothing to do with how the prostate feels on DRE. Pathologic stage is determined by the pathologist in the pathology report.

PET (Positron Emission Tomography) Scan—Positrons are positively charged radioactive particles. In a PET scan, positrons are mixed in a solution that is injected into the patient's vein, and then a body scan is done to see in which tissues the positrons settle. The PET scan can be used to diagnose and locate cancer and metastases, including tiny lymph node metastases. This enables your doctor to decide whether or not treatment can be localized, or if more aggressive treatment is needed.

Prophylactic—In medical talk, this usually does not mean the birth control device. It refers to doing something to prevent something worse from happening. For example, you might hear someone recommend prophylactic radiation. This means that, although cancer isn't visible now, it is probably present in microscopic amounts. Thus, your doctor will recommend prophylactic treatment using radiation to knock out the cancer before it has a chance to grow larger.

Prostate Cancer—Coming in hundreds of varieties, it can be slow- or fast-growing, responsive or unresponsive to treatment, metastasizing early or not metastasizing at all. It is not a singular disease. There are *Low-*, *Intermediate-*, and *High-Risk* varieties, and each needs to be considered and treated in a unique manner. The right treatment means choosing the correct *intensity* of treatment, an intensity that matches the seriousness of each individual's cancer. Treatment, therefore, should be sufficient to control the cancer without overdoing it.

Prostate Gland—An exclusively male organ that helps create semen. Because of its location in the body, near the urethra, it can impede urine flow if it becomes enlarged, a condition called Benign Prostatic Hyperplasia (BPH). People often confuse the word prostate with another word, "prostrate," which means lying flat on the ground.

Prostate Specific Antigen—See PSA.

Prostatectomy—Surgical removal of the prostate gland. See Robot Assisted Radical Prostatectomy (RARP).

Proton Therapy—A local treatment that is a type of External Beam Radiation Therapy (EBRT).

Provenge—FDA-approved immunotherapy for prostate cancer, useful even in relatively advanced disease, and with an even greater benefit in men who begin treatment at an earlier stage. It is not as toxic as many treatments, so side effects tend to be mild, and treatment is less time-consuming than some other treatments. Provenge utilizes a patient's white blood cells, which are removed from his body through a procedure called leukapheresis. These white cells are then "trained" to recognize and attack prostate cancer.

PSA—Prostate Specific Antigen. A substance that is present in elevated quantities in men with prostate cancer and in some men with enlarged prostates. The blood test that detects and measures this antigen is called a PSA test. High or rising PSA levels are a potential early sign of prostate cancer. PSA plays a variety of different roles. The most familiar is screening for prostate cancer at an early stage. However, PSA has other uses. One example is how PSA helps to define the severity of the cancer (its Stage of Blue). PSA is also a sensitive indicator of cancer relapse after surgery or radiation. Lastly, rises or declines in PSA after hormone therapy or chemotherapy provide an important indication of whether a specific treatment is working. (See Nadir).

Radiation Therapy (Also called radiotherapy)—Any one of several treatments using radiation to eradicate cancer by damaging the DNA of cancer cells, causing them to stop reproducing. When we use the term "radiation," we are describing either *external* radiation, which is itself a broad term used to describe several different ways of delivering radiation beams to the prostate, or *internal* radiation—brachytherapy—in which radioactive pellets or seeds are surgically implanted into the prostate.

Radical Prostatectomy—The surgical removal of the entire prostate gland. See Robot Assisted Radical Prostatectomy (RARP).

Radioactive Seed Implantation (Brachytherapy)—A local treatment that uses internal radiotherapy in which the medical team strategically inserts small radioactive pieces of iridium, palladium, iodine, or cesium into the prostate gland in order to eradicate cancer. These pieces are called seeds, and they provide intense radiation in, and very close to, the cancer, but don't affect surrounding tissues; they usually stop producing radiation after a period of time. Brachytherapy comes in two varieties, *LDR* or *permanent* (low-dose rate, which delivers low-dose radiation over several months) and *HDR* or *temporary* (high-dose rate, which delivers a large dose over a few days).

Radiologist—A doctor who is specially trained to accurately interpret scans.

Relapsed Cancer—Also called "recurrent" cancer. This is when cancer that was previously thought to be in remission returns.

Remission—A *cured* cancer is a cancer in *permanent remission*. This is when all *signs and symptoms* of cancer are gone. Remission is no guarantee that all traces of the cancer are gone. There could still be cancer cells or microscopic metastases hidden in the body. This is why doctors continue monitoring with scans, PSA testing, etc. for a number of years after all treatment is completed (Chapter 46). *Partial remission* means that treatment has resulted in an improvement as a result of cancer treatment, but that 100 percent cancer eradication, otherwise known as a *complete* remission, has not occurred.

Robot Assisted Radical Prostatectomy (RARP)—Robotic surgery for prostate cancer was approved by the FDA in 2001. (You will often hear this called the *da Vinci* system surgery, which is the brand name of the equipment used for RARP.) Compared with open surgery, blood loss is less, hospitalization time is shorter, and men tend to bounce back more quickly after the operation, compared with nonrobotic surgery. Evidence is lacking that sexual or urinary function is less impaired with RARP.

Robotic Surgery—In this type of surgery, the surgeon controls robotic arms that cut with precision and make very small incisions, resulting in less pain and bleeding, quicker recovery time, and potentially less damage to surrounding nerves and tissue. Used in radical prostatectomy. See Robot Assisted Radical Prostatectomy (RARP).

Salvage Surgery—Salvage surgery is a surgical treatment for relapsed prostate cancer. Salvage surgery is performed after a patient has already pursued another treatment method (such as radiation) and suffered a recurrence of the disease.

SBRT—See Stereotactic Body Radiotherapy.

Seed Therapy—See Radioactive Seed Implantation

Sequential Therapy—Treatment by one drug at a time, which has traditionally been the most common way prostate cancer therapy is administered. Nowadays more doctors are opting for combination therapy, partly because recent treatments are less prone to cause extreme side effects, and research is showing that the earlier use of sequential therapy can be more beneficial.

Stage—Uses a system of rules for assigning men to a specific location in a sequence of options. The Stages of Blue system assigns men to five different categories. The Stages of Blue system incorporates components of other staging systems such as the D'Amico risk categories of Low, Intermediate and High-Risk for newly diagnosed men. The D'Amico system incorporates the staging findings of digital rectal exam, which is called the *clinical* stage. The Stages of Blue system also uses *pathologic* stage, which is information derived from the pathology report such as the percentage of biopsy cores positive for cancer.

Stages of Blue—is a comprehensive staging system for prostate cancer. See Five Stages of Blue

Standard of Care—A term meaning the diagnostic and treatment steps most commonly used in the medical community for treating a medical condition in a particular patient. For example, one might say that active surveillance is *becoming* the standard of care in *Low-Risk* prostate cancer patients. Different medical groups publish their own standard of care guidelines. Also, standard of care is used as a legal term in cases of medical malpractice. It is interesting to note that the standard of care may not represent the best care, because it takes time before the whole medical community adopts new technology. The "way it has always been done" (i.e. the standard of care), may not be the most optimal care in this modern era of rapidly improving technology.

Stereotactic Body Radiation Therapy (SBRT)—A local treatment that is a type of External Beam Radiation Therapy (EBRT). "Stereotactic" means the precise positioning in space, using 3D coordinates to locate and maintain the exact location of the tumor so that the radiation beams can be sent directly to the diseased area, avoiding nearby healthy tissue.

Stricture—Constriction or narrowing of a hollow tube or organ, such as the urethra or an artery, caused by scarring, inflammation, or external pressure.

Systemic Treatments—Medical treatments that circulate through the blood and treat cancer throughout the whole body (including the prostate). Men with either microscopic or visible metastases require *systemic* treatment. Examples are hormonal therapies, chemotherapy, immunotherapy, and, most recently, a new type of circulating radiation therapy called Xofigo.

Subtype—Each of the Five Stages of Blue can be divided into three subtypes: *Low, Basic* and *High* with information obtained from the patient's history, physical examination, scan results and pathology report. See Appendix I and II for the specifics.

T-Cells—A subtype of white blood cells. They are called T because some of them mature in the thymus. They attack substances that do not belong in the body (foreign antigens).

T Stage—A system of describing the size of a nodule on the prostate felt by the examining doctor's finger during the DRE. Also known as *clinical* stage.

Testosterone—The male sex hormone that stimulates the development of a man's reproductive organs, including the prostate. It also affects secondary sex characteristics, such as the growth of facial and other body hair, a deep voice, and muscle strength. (Women also produce testosterone, but much less.) Prostate cancer is exquisitely sensitive to the blockade of testosterone, and prostate cancer cells only grow and proliferate when testosterone is present; they shrivel and die when testosterone is absent. See Testosterone Inactivating Pharmaceuticals (TIP).

Testosterone Inactivating Pharmaceuticals (TIP)—A variety of different medications that block testosterone. TIP can be used alone or in combination with other therapies. TIP does cause numerous side effects, especially sexual, but these generally go away when TIP is ended.

TIP—See Testosterone Inactivating Pharmaceuticals.

Tumor—An abnormal growth of tissue in which the cells are multiplying in an uncontrolled way and, without treatment, eventually overtake normal tissue. Tumor size (not to be confused with prostate gland size) is an important predictive factor for every type of cancer, including prostate cancer. Bigger tumors are more dangerous than smaller ones.

Urologist—The most common type of doctor who typically manages prostate cancer. Urologists initially diagnose prostate cancer because of a high PSA, an abnormal digital rectal examination (DRE) or with a random biopsy.

White Blood Cells (WBC)—A component of the human immune system. Subtypes of WBCs are the neutrophils, which are the first line of defense for bacteria; and the lymphocytes, which fight viruses and cancer.

Xofigo—A new type of systemic treatment in which radiation is circulated throughout the body and concentrates near bone metastases to target the cancer.

INDEX